Healthy Bones

Healthy You!

www.healthyboneshealthyyou.com

Healthy Bones

Healthy You!

Lara Pizzorno, MDiv, MA, LMT

Author of the best-selling book
*Your Bones: How YOU Can Prevent Osteoporosis
& Have Strong Bones for Life—Naturally*

Dr. Joseph Pizzorno, N.D.

Author or co-author of over a dozen books, including
The Toxin Solution and *The Encyclopedia of Natural Medicine*

The material provided in this book is for informational purposes only and is not intended as a substitute for advice from your physician or other healthcare professional or any information contained on or in any product label or packaging. Facts and information are believed to be accurate at the time of publication.

Developments in medical research may impact the health, fitness, and nutritional advice that appears here. No assurance can be given that the advice contained here will always include the most recent findings or developments with respect to the particular material. You agree to hold the book's authors, the publisher and its employees, and all others involved in the writing, production, marketing, and distribution of this book harmless from all liability for damage claims due to injuries to you or third parties, including attorney fees and costs, incurred by you, arising out of any information or products discussed.

Published by: AlgaeCal Inc
#200 - 1286 Homer Street
Vancouver, BC V6B 2Y5
CANADA

ISBN (Softcover): 978-1-7777925-0-3   ISBN (Ebook): 978-1-7777925-1-0

Printed in the United States of America

Contents

Preface

I was only in my mid-40s when The Universe sent me a clear message: *Figure out what's causing your bone loss or die.*

You may have discovered your diminishing bone density after a fall or fracture—literally by accident. My realization was less dramatic. I was at a medical conference checking out the convention hall. One booth featured a new portable device to evaluate ankle bone density in doctors' offices. Back then, awareness of the osteoporosis tsunami was just beginning. DEXA (dual-energy X-ray absorptiometry) scans were expensive and not as commonly ordered. This piece of equipment could help doctors identify at-risk patients for far less money. While I was *way too young* to be concerned, I agreed to be scanned. The results sent my life irrevocably in a new direction—I was already severely osteopenic.

I knew osteoporosis *ran* in my family. My grandmother, aunt, and mother had all died after suffering hip fractures. My grandmother died within weeks. My aunt and mother endured a more protracted, painful journey, first in the hospital, then bedridden at home.

I Thought I was Doing the Right Things to Avoid this Family Curse

I'd always been an exercise junkie. I grew up in Florida, started swimming before I started kindergarten. Mucked out stalls and rode in junior hunter competitions until high school when I joined the swim team. Somehow got on the JV cheerleading squad. (I was energetic but so inept, so all I added was comic relief.) I kept swimming in college, a mile of laps most nights.

Then I moved to the Pacific Northwest and discovered hiking, jogging, and cycling—a necessity because I didn't have a car. I climbed Mount Rainier, twice. In sum, I considered myself *buff* and dramatically different from my grandmother's and mother's generation when a hard workout meant a challenging game of bridge.

My other saving grace was my diet. I became a vegetarian in high school.

Ate tons of vegetables, eggs, beans, tofu, yogurt, and cheese. Probably overdid it on the whole grains, especially wheat (which I no longer eat). But at least I avoided junk food and processed foods.

Despite my exercise and healthy diet, I was already osteopenic years before menopause when bone loss typically accelerates. I knew I had to figure out why—or break my hip. Or worse.

Seeking a Natural Approach to Treat My Osteopenia

I believe The Universe doesn't deliver a challenge without providing the tools to solve it. And I had the best resource anyone could hope for. My husband was Dr. Joseph Pizzorno, the founding president of Bastyr University, a pioneer in *science-based natural medicine*. Joe had not only coined that phrase, he also created the curriculum to popularize world-wide a naturopathic approach to maintaining health.

Joe's mantra is: *Diagnose first, then treat*. Diagnosis involves determining what's causing a dysfunctional outcome. And by treat, Joe doesn't mean *prescribing a drug that will suppress some symptoms and cause others*. Instead, he corrects the factors driving disease which naturally leads to restored health.

Joe's approach to restoring my vanishing bones did not include conventional osteoporosis treatments. Instead, we focused on figuring out the underlying causes, an effort that was greatly helped by Joe's prominence in the field. Some of our friends were physician-researchers on the cutting edge of genetic testing. One new test evaluated genetic risks for osteoporosis. They ran it on me, and I saw the light—more precisely my need for more sunlight.

Vitamin D: The First Ray of Sunshine in My Recovery

My genetic inheritance includes poorly formed vitamin D receptors, which greatly increase my needs for vitamin D to help me absorb calcium. I had managed to build bone growing up in Florida before the age of sunscreen. Lots of sun exposure let me produce lots of vitamin D when the sun's ultraviolet rays kissed my skin. But living in Seattle, where umbrellas are in use from September through July, had made me vitamin D deficient—for more than 20 years by the time we figured this out.

I started taking 10,000 IU of vitamin D3 daily—considered an outrageous amount at the time—to bring my levels to normal. Our doctor friends joked that this much vitamin D would turn me into a calcified version of Lot's wife, the Biblical figure who turned into a pillar of salt.

On the contrary, once I got an amount of vitamin D that even my cells could not ignore, I started absorbing enough calcium that my bones began to rebuild. Since then, I've discovered so much more about all the nutrients our bones need to stay healthy, a team of nutrients you'll learn all about in this book that includes far more than just calcium and vitamin D.

And I've learned about other genetic susceptibilities that increase our risk for osteoporosis. All of them can be corrected by simply providing the related nutrients in optimal amounts, which is really fortunate for me because I have every single susceptibility! It's no wonder osteoporosis ran in my family.

Moving to a Multi-Nutrient Version of Calcium Made the Difference

In 2011, I published my first edition of *Your Bones: How You Can Prevent Osteoporosis & Have Strong Bones for Life—Naturally*. While still slightly osteopenic, I was slowly gaining bone every year and knew I had found a safe, effective approach. My mother had died before what I had learned could help her, a source of great sadness for me but also inspiration. I have dedicated my life to share this lifeline with all the women (and men) fighting osteoporosis.

A few months after *Your Bones* was published, my daily morning review of the breaking research on bone health revealed something intriguing. Dean Neuls, the owner of AlgaeCal, was conducting research on a unique red algae called *Lithothamnion superpositum*, the richest plant source of calcium on the planet, as a possible bone-health supplement. The initial research conducted on bone cells produced such spectacular results that a 6-month study had just been completed in humans that compared two versions of an AlgaeCal supplement.

Both versions produced dramatic benefits and the one resulting in higher bone-density gains is now available as AlgaeCal Plus. That formulation includes not just all the minerals naturally present in *Lithothamnion superpositum* (calcium, magnesium, and more than a dozen other trace minerals that play key roles in bone-building) but also vitamin D3 and vitamin K2 (in its most potent form of MK-7), extra magnesium, boron, and vitamin C. In my years of research, this comprised all of the nutrients I had discovered were most critical for bone health.

The AlgaeCal protocol combined this supplement with a partner product (Strontium Boost) that provided a safe, natural form of the mineral strontium. At the time, strontium was making big news in research circles. Impressed by what I read, I reached out to Dean directly for more information and began using AlgaeCal Plus in July 2011.

My next DEXA scan, just 10 months later, showed amazing results. The bone mass density (BMD) in my hip/femur had improved by 2.4%, and my spine improved 5%. As women typically experience *bone losses* of 1% to 2% every year after age 50, these results were extraordinary. I was still slightly osteopenic, but in 10 months, I'd improved more than I had in the past 3 years. I was finally rapidly rebuilding my bones.

Unfortunately, I feared my progress would be derailed when, several months later, I suffered a serious car accident.

The Ultimate Test: Could My Bones Still Heal After Injury?

The driver gunned his engine to beat a yellow light. Everyone ahead of him had stopped. He couldn't. The resulting collision threw my tiny Smart car under the SUV in front of me. I felt like I was inside a trash compactor. The rear and front ends of my car tried to become one. My neck, chest, and hips were badly bruised. I was slammed into something so forcefully that I broke a tooth.

My back hurt, and the pain kept getting worse. The cause remained a mystery for almost two years, when I was referred to an orthopedic surgeon. He ordered an MRI and discovered a fluid-filled cyst had developed that was pressing on nerves between 2 of my lumbar vertebrae. Surgery was immediately scheduled, and I finally began to recover.

My ability to exercise—and many aspects of my active life—had been derailed for 3 years as I went from physical therapist to chiropractor to massage therapist, all to no avail. I lived on ibuprofen, which barely dulled the pain. Plus, I knew this drug, like all non-steroidal, anti-inflammatory medications, was damaging my gut and my liver.

A month after my surgery, my next DEXA was past due and I was nervous. For the past 3 years, I'd been in a state of constant pain and inflammation that kept my cortisol levels unhappily elevated. And chronically elevated cortisol and inflammation promote bone loss. I did gentle Pilates mat work as often as possible. I kept eating well and taking my AlgaeCal Plus and Strontium Boost. *Would that be enough?*

From Osteopenia in My 40s to Strong, Healthy Bones at 66

I cried when I saw my DEXA scan report. Then I called Dean Neuls to personally thank him for creating AlgaeCal.

My Z-score, a measure comparing me to other women my age, was +0.6, better than the healthy/normal score of 0. More amazing, my T-Score, which compared me to young, healthy women, was -0.2, well within the –1.0 to +1.0 considered *normal*. All this, despite a devastating car accident that prevented me from properly caring for my bones!

After decades of researching bone science and learning how to correct for my body's lousy genetics, I finally had fully healthy bones with *no signs of osteopenia!* And I gotta tell you, if I can do it, SO CAN YOU!

Your Bone-Health Challenges are a Mystery We Can Solve Together

People ask me the one or two things they can do to prevent osteoporosis. Unfortunately, no magic bullet or one-size-fits-all approach can address everyone's individual needs, but there are definitely some basics.

A healthy, whole-food diet and exercise are essential. So is minimizing your exposure to environmental toxins. And choosing the right supplements to ensure you're getting all the key nutrients your bones require.

We explore all of these throughout *Healthy Bones Healthy You!*

Outside these general recommendations, each of us is unique and may have individual challenges to address. My most important Achilles heel was my lousy vitamin D receptors. Yours may stem from something completely different, like other nutrient deficiencies, digestive difficulties, sensitivity to gluten, a sedentary lifestyle, or toxic levels of lead, mercury, or cadmium accumulated over your lifetime.

As I continue to learn more each year, I recognize that my vitamin D problem was one of many factors causing my bone loss. I have other genetic anomalies that increase my need for certain nutrients. For example, I don't activate several of the B vitamins very well, including B6. If I don't take a supplement providing B6 in its already active form of pyridoxal-5-phosphate (P5P), I do a lousy job of absorbing magnesium. For years, I suffered from indigestion that made me miserable and lessened my ability to absorb nutrients. That was due to infection with a very common bacterium, *Helicobacter pylori*. When that was identified and treated—thankfully ending my constant gas, bloating, and belching—my improved digestion enhanced the health of my bones.

Figuring out what is putting you at risk for osteoporosis—what necessary things you're not getting and what harmful things you're exposed to—is like playing a mystery board game. We've written *Healthy Bones Healthy You!* to serve as a road map to your own game of *Bone-Health Clue*, so you can find what's most relevant for your unique physiology. Winning will take a bit of work, but you have several advantages going for you:

- You don't need to spend 30 years researching bone health. I've done this and can help point you in the right direction. In addition, recent research provides a trove of knowledge into the bone-building process—far more than I had when starting my journey.

- You can't marry Joe, but you can get his cutting-edge guidance on healing. As my co-author, he provides his insights and the latest guidance on how to avoid toxins, fortify your body's defenses, and promote optimal health to support your bones.

- You don't need science-geek friends with access to a DNA lab. Affordable tests now allow you to easily check genetics, your blood levels of vitamin D, and the other key measures that affect bone health. Joe and I will help you identify which tests may be best suited for your situation and how to interpret your results.

I'm now 72 and have gorgeous bones—far stronger and healthier than they were 30 years ago. I live fully, enjoying an active, energetic life without limits. And I'll be the first woman in my family in all the generations I know to not die due to osteoporosis. This is what I want for you, and I know you can have it!

Just think: I am truly the poster woman for osteoporosis with every genetic susceptibility and other major risk factor I've learned about. So if I can beat this, I know you can, too! Regardless of your age, family history, or health challenges, you have the power to restore the health of your bones.

And you'll discover that following the guidance in *Healthy Bones Healthy You!* delivers results beyond just your bones to improve your overall health and quality of life. You *can* remain strong and vibrant throughout your golden years. Actually, gold isn't good enough. Let's go for platinum. Joe and I are here to support you every step of the way!

— Lara Pizzorno

Introduction

Here's a fact you may not hear elsewhere: **Healthy, vibrant bones are your birthright!**

Don't expect to see that on news reports touting the epic levels of osteoporosis. Or from the conventional medicine world that accepts chronic disease as a *natural* part of aging. Instead, you're told frail, crumbling bones are something you'll just have to accept, especially if osteoporosis *runs* in your family. Balderdash!

Bone loss is not a mysterious process nor an inescapable one we can do nothing about. Our bodies come programmed to create healthy bones throughout our lives. An elaborate process to continually remove old bone and replace it with strong new bone renews around 10% of your skeleton every year. Provide the necessary ingredients to build new bone and protection from things that disrupt this process, and you get a brand new skeleton every 10 years!

Get the Knowledge to Take Control of Your Bone Health

You picked up this book for a reason. Perhaps you've recently been diagnosed with osteoporosis or its precursor, osteopenia. Maybe you've suffered a fracture and don't have great confidence in the options you've been offered (or their potential side effects). Or you could simply want a natural way to build healthy bones, so you can continue to work in your garden, keep up with your kids/grandkids, bike or hike on woodsy trails, and do whatever other activities bring a smile to your face.

You're in the right place. Researchers now understand what causes osteoporosis, and we know how to stop it. No one needs to experience this frightening, life-robbing disease. We don't say that out of blind optimism. Our confidence springs from more than 30 years of studying bone health and reading countless medical journal articles, coupled with Lara's personal experience beating this disease and that of many others following our recommendations.

In 2013, I (Lara) published the second edition of *Your Bones: How You Can Prevent Osteoporosis & Have Strong Bones for Life—Naturally.* I've since been overwhelmed by the positive reception at medical conferences and from physicians who applied this guidance to help their patients.

Most gratifying is my experience moderating an online community of more than 17,000 people, many facing a diagnosis of osteoporosis or osteopenia. I've listened to their concerns, shared my research, and corresponded extensively with the amazing women and men in this group. By following my protocol, hundreds of them have reported back on the restored ability of their bones to rebuild. Many even sent me the DEXA scan reports showing their bone density improvement! Throughout this book, we include *Cases from the Community* to document some of their inspiring journeys. By following the recommendations in this book, we have no doubt you will have similar success!

New Developments Illustrate What Your Body Needs for Healthy Bones

While *Your Bones* was the culmination of decades of bone research, science continues to illuminate the complex processes that maintain our bones, the myriad factors that disrupt this process, and natural ways to counteract their effects.

An enormous amount of research sheds new light on the role of specific nutrients (beyond calcium, vitamin D, and even vitamin K) in the bone remodeling process. I've also learned more about genetic variations that affect our individual ability to absorb or activate those nutrients as well as chronic diseases that provide unique challenges for bone growth. Those elements could be the key to helping you determine *your* optimal level of nutrient intake to fuel healthy bones.

Plus, we now understand how exposure to the tsunami of chemical toxins in our modern lives—plastics, food additives, pesticides, and heavy metals—creates the perfect recipe for bone loss, along with chronic diseases that further promote bone loss. That's why I co-wrote *Healthy Bones Healthy You!* with my husband Dr. Joe Pizzorno, author of *The Toxin Solution*, a guide to cleansing our bodies from the poisons in our water, air, food, and everyday products.

As a leader in naturopathic medicine, who helped launch the field of *science-based natural medicine*, Joe is uniquely qualified to advise on avoiding and mitigating toxins to restore the natural ability of our bodies to heal.

How this Book is Different than Others on Bone Health

Don't take the material in *Healthy Bones Healthy You!* as simply our opinions. We examined thousands of clinical studies to create this book and included only respected, peer-reviewed research that is credible, relevant, and statistically valid. Where possible we've cited the reference number (PMID) in PubMed, the premier source for biomedical literature. Through this database, you can access abstracts of these papers or locate them in their entirety. That allows *Healthy Bones Healthy You!* to serve as a practical how-to health guide for individuals as well as a reference for medical professionals who wish to investigate topics in more detail.

In many cases, we provide intricate details of study design that would be ignored elsewhere. However, these elements often give critical context and determine the validity of what's been studied. Our goal is to equip you to confidently share these findings with your doctor, so you can advocate powerfully for your health interests and make choices that boost your overall level of wellness.

Ultimately, we want you to join a steadily growing group of people who have recaptured the health of their bones—a feat that would have been considered impossible not so long ago. No matter your situation, health, or genetics, we're confident that the positive, proactive strategies outlined in *Healthy Bones Healthy You!* will work for you because we've seen it happen—over and over!

Here's the Amazing Part! (Though Not Unexpected)

Though the approaches suggested in this book are designed around building healthy bones, expect to experience benefits that go well beyond. The things your bones require—an array of key nutrients, reduced exposure to harmful chemicals, and weight-bearing exercise—match the needs of all of your organs to remain healthy and vibrant.

Follow the recommendations contained here and your overall health is likely to improve. For example, reducing chronic inflammation naturally leads to a reduction in those aches and pains you've become accustomed to. Ensuring you get the full complement of B vitamins will not only benefit your bones; you'll see your energy level rise (without the need for caffeine and sugar-packed drinks you find in those fluorescent cans). And weight-bearing exercises, such as barre3, Pilates, or yoga, that stimulate your bone-building sensors, will also improve your flexibility, balance, and mood.

When you have *Healthy Bones*, you will find that you have a *Healthy You!* We're honored that you've chosen to take this important journey with us and want to hear about your progress. Please keep in touch! Connect with us at www.HealthyBonesHealthyYou.com.

— Lara and Joe Pizzorno

How to Get the Most Out of
Healthy Bones **Healthy You!**

Consider this book an *advanced* guide designed for those with a personal interest in their own bone health as well as for clinicians to serve their patients. We identify what's fueling the firestorm of osteoporosis and low bone density and show you how to extinguish the burning in your bones. The predominant factors involve lifestyle, our modern one being exceptionally suited to putting a wrench in the machinery of our bone-building process.

Here's how the book is organized:

- **Part One: What's Causing Your Bone Loss?** reveals why osteoporosis has become so prevalent. We explore why our typical diet fuels bone loss, toxic metals and chemicals that disrupt the process, and the resulting chronic diseases that further disrupt bone remodeling. The good news is that most of these causes can be avoided or mitigated, and we show you how.

- **Part Two: Nutrients Your Bones Need to Rebuild** reports the latest research on what minerals and vitamins you need, well beyond just calcium and vitamin D. Learn what you can get from your diet, when supplements are needed, and how to make adjustments based on your lifestyle and genetics.

- **Part Three: Tools to Support Healthy Bones** ties together the earlier sections by providing resources on diet, exercise, and lab testing.

  » Find out the basic principles of a bone-building diet, so you can create recipes (or adapt your favorites) to provide the nutrients missing from the average diet and support bone health.

  » Discover our favorite weight-bearing exercises—barre3, Pilates, and yoga—all of which can be modified for any age or fitness level.

  » Use the diagnostic scans and lab tests listed to provide insight on your vitamin status; hormone levels; digestive, parathyroid, kidney, liver, and thyroid function; and other factors specific to your needs for strong, healthy bones.

Strategies to Best Use this Book

Read this book from cover to cover. We've structured each section to build on the information in the previous ones. And each chapter illustrates different aspects of how the cells affecting your bones interact with enzymes, nutrients, and other substances. Reading the whole book will leave you with a deep understanding of how to support the bone remodeling process.

Realize that topics that don't seem to apply may be more relevant than you think. For example, people who don't work in a factory may feel at little risk for heavy metal exposure. However, you'll discover in Part One that we're all at risk of such exposures, from cadmium in conventionally grown foods, mercury in ocean fish and dental fillings, and lead our bones accumulated decades ago from leaded gasoline and paint.

Similarly, you'll learn important health strategies in the disease chapter even if you don't have a particular disease (or don't know it, as many diseases go undiagnosed). For example, even if you don't have chronic kidney disease (CKD), you may be suffering from reduced kidney function like many as we age (needlessly so—we show how to keep your kidneys healthy).

Use the bulleted note sections and headings as a quick guide: In Parts One and Two, we begin each topic area with Bone Essentials, a summary of key chapter takeaways. We end each section with Bone-Healthy Action Items, the most important things you can do to support your bone health. In addition, we include many subheadings and bolded summaries to start paragraphs, so you can effectively scan chapters and quickly take away key points.

Look for icons that highlight content: Throughout the book, we've used icons to flag particular topics or mark expanded discussion on a point. These icons include:

Genetic anomalies, which can affect how well we absorb or utilize nutrients, occur much more often than people realize. Look for the DNA strand to note when we discuss such factors that could be contributing to your bone loss (though fair warning these can get a bit technical).

For those who love diving into the details (like Joe and me), this microscope alerts you where we're taking a closer look at a topic.

Take inspiration from these stories from an online community of people just like you. Each one highlights one person's bone-health journey. While the research we share provides the roadmap to better bones, nothing beats seeing real people overcome their bone-health challenges.

Share this material with your doctor. This book is your guide to providing the support your bones need to become healthy and strong. And to empower you to share this knowledge confidently with your healthcare professional, so you can work as partners on your treatment.

Naturopaths and doctors who have done the additional work to become certified in functional medicine are often most open to looking at nutrients and toxins in relation to disease. However, every day, more conventionally trained physicians recognize the need for a natural and holistic approach to osteoporosis, particularly when they see the research. By educating your doctor on these developments, you can improve your own care and that of others.

Take action even if you start small. This book contains everything you need to know to safely, naturally improve the strength of your bones. However, just *knowing* this information doesn't help unless you put it into action. Don't feel you need to do everything all at once or you may get overwhelmed. Instead, read the book and focus on the areas that seem to best fit your situation, and make changes that will have the most impact.

We *know* you can reclaim your bones' health, and we promise you will be so glad you made the effort!

PART ONE

What's Causing Your Bone Loss?

Many factors in our modern lifestyle can disrupt the healthy balance between bone resorption and formation. In medical literature, they're called *secondary causes of osteoporosis*. Some ramp up the cell signals that trigger overactivation of *osteoclasts*—our cells that clear out old bone. Others hamper the production of our *osteoblasts*, preventing their ability to produce new bone. These disruptions wreak havoc on the bone remodeling process and the quality (strength) and quantity (density) of our bones.

What causes this? The standard American diet, food additives, environmental toxins, and quite a few chronic diseases. The list of bone-wreckers appears daunting, but there's a silver lining. These factors are largely within our control. We'll share strategies to greatly lessen the harmful impact of every single one of them—naturally and safely. Implementing changes takes some effort and investment, but you'll quickly see a huge payoff, not just in the strength of your bones, but your general health.

CHAPTER 1

The Standard American Diet Eats Your Bones

Aptly abbreviated as SAD, the *Standard American Diet* is the perfect recipe for osteoporosis. The SAD's abundance of sugars, refined carbohydrates, sodium, inflammatory oils, gluten, and chemical additives, all too frequently swallowed with a dose of alcohol, combine to destroy the health of our bones. Research revealing how each ingredient in the SAD promotes bone loss has been around for many years. It has just been ignored. The scientific data, however, is substantive and incontestable.

The SAD causes inflammation and promotes an acidic pH in the body. In an attempt to restore our cells' optimal alkaline state, calcium is withdrawn from our bones. To make matters worse, the SAD lacks sufficient calcium and other key nutrients our bodies need to build healthy bones. We'll dive more into those specific nutrients in Part Two.

In this section, you'll discover which foods (or *food products*) are most damaging, which provide the most nutritional benefit, and how to make smart choices that protect your bones.

Dietary and Metabolic Acidosis:
Our Diet Promotes an Ideal State for Bone Loss

BONE ESSENTIALS

- The SAD is imbalanced. Too few vegetables and too little calcium are consumed to healthfully balance protein from meat, dairy products, eggs, and fish. This causes a drop in the body's pH from optimal (slightly alkaline) to acidic.
- As we age, our kidneys' ability to remove excess acid declines.
- Bone loss occurs because a pH below 7.5 (an acidic pH) triggers osteoclast activity and inhibits osteoblasts' ability to lay down new bone.
- Consuming more vegetables, which promote an alkaline pH, helps maintain balance.
- When high protein intake (1.2 grams/kg of body weight per day) is accompanied by adequate calcium intake (1,200 mg daily), a high protein diet does not increase fracture risk, and, in fact, *lowers* the risk of hip fracture.

Calcium Deficit Sets the Stage for Bone Loss

The standard American diet provides insufficient calcium and causes inflammation. One of the most insidious ways the SAD causes inflammation is by promoting an acidic pH in the body. (This is not about the pH of the food, but rather the results of how it is metabolized in the body.) In an attempt to restore our optimal alkaline state, calcium is drawn from our bones. The foods we eat are literally eating our bones.

Exacerbating its negative effects, the SAD lacks the foods (e.g., leafy greens and other vegetables, whole grains, legumes, nuts, and seeds) that contain the vitamins and minerals bones *require* to rebuild. Americans fall short of virtually all the key bone-building nutrients, including calcium. The typical diet in the United States today delivers only 600 to 700 mg of calcium per day, way below the recommended 1,200 mg per day.[1]

Calcium Recommended Dietary Allowance		
Age	Woman (mg/day)	Men (mg/day)
19 to 50	1,000	1,000
51 to 70	1,200	1,000
Over 70	1,200	1,200

Source: Institute of Medicine Dietary Reference Intakes for Calcium and Vitamin D, Nov. 2010
www.nap.edu/resource/13050/Vitamin-D-and-Calcium-2010-Report-Brief.pdf

Our bodies seek to remain slightly alkaline. Similar to maintaining a healthy temperature, our bodies work to keep our cells, body fluids, and organs at a slightly alkaline level (7.35 on the pH scale). (The only exception is in the stomach, which secretes gastric acid to help digest food.)

This process, called *acid-base homeostasis*, is critical for virtually all normal cellular functions. Disruptions can cause an acid overload in the body, leading to a pH below 7.35 and a condition called acidosis. A diet high in acid-forming foods and low in alkaline-forming foods promotes such an imbalance.

SAD causes chronic elevation of acid levels. Foods contribute a net acid or base effect due to the balance between their acid-forming and alkaline (base-forming) constituents.

• *Acid-forming constituents* (e.g., sulfuric acid) are released when dietary proteins rich in the sulfur-containing amino acids, methionine, and cysteine are broken down. These typically are from animals (meat, eggs, and dairy products).

• *Alkaline (base-forming) constituents* (e.g., bicarbonate and citrate) are produced from our bodies' metabolism of plants. (While some plants, such as soybeans, contain methionine and/or cysteine, they don't have the same acidizing effect as animals due to smaller concentrations, along with their rich potassium levels.)[2]

Our modern diet generates higher overall acid load, expressed as our *net endogenous acid production* (NEAP), than our biological ancestors. The average American diet produces a NEAP of *positive* 48 mEq/d, according to the US Third National Health and Nutrition Examination Survey (NHANES III). Contrast that with our hominid ancestors, whose diet produced a far lower overall NEAP. In a recent study estimating the acid load of 159 hypothetical pre-agricultural diets, 87%

were found to be alkaline-producing with an average NEAP of *negative* 88 mEq/d.[3] The 60% shift (hominid diet NEAP of -88 mEq/d to SAD diet of +48 mEq/d) shows the major increase in acid our bodies are now forced to neutralize.

Acidosis leaches calcium from our bones. Our kidneys are our primary means of eliminating excessive acid. As we age, their effectiveness decreases, and our bodies seek to maintain acid-base homeostasis by withdrawing calcium from our bones.

Even minor disruptions of our necessary slightly alkaline pH can cause calcium to be leached from our bones. When our diet causes chronic acidity, as does the SAD, the continual calcium loss translates as we age to a loss of bone. Highly acidic diets have been shown to cause bone loss in postmenopausal women, even when their intake of calcium is adequate.[4]

Acidosis ramps up osteoclasts and inhibits osteoblasts. Chronic low-grade acidosis was thought to passively reduce bone mass, simply as a result of exposure to acidic bodily fluids. However, we now know that an acidic pH affects both osteoclast and osteoblast activity, directly impacting bone loss.

Osteoclasts are almost inactive at a pH above 7.4, but pH reductions of as little as 1/10th of a pH are sufficient to cause a doubling in the areas where osteoclasts are at work.

A number of *in vitro* (test tube) studies have shown that even small changes in pH both increase osteoclasts' resorptive activity and inhibit osteoblasts' ability to mineralize bone.

Numerous studies have shown that acid-promoting diets cause increased excretion of both calcium and *bone matrix protein* (BMP), a urine marker used to estimate the rate of bone loss. Restoring a slightly alkaline 7.35 pH by eating more vegetables or taking bicarbonate or citrate supplements decreases the amount of calcium and BMP excreted.[5]

Prevent Acidosis-based Bone Loss with Adequate Protein

Your bones need protein, possibly more than you're currently getting. The right type and amount can go a long way to protect your bones from acidosis. Research shows that older adults need at least 1.2g/kg body weight (BW)—50% more than the Recommended Dietary Allowance (RDA) of 0.8 g/kg BW.[6] Undernourished or frail elders need even more, as much as 1.5 g/kg BW.[7] Getting enough protein may lower your risk of hip fracture by as much as 16%.[8]

If you eat animal protein, make sure you get enough calcium. While we need protein, a diet high in *animal* protein can almost triple your risk for hip fracture. *How can you prevent this?* Simply by getting enough calcium:

- Calcium loss in urine increases with high-protein diets: 1 mg of calcium is lost for every 10 grams of protein consumed. But the increased incidence of fractures seen in the research typically occurs in individuals who are consuming little dairy protein. It's not the dairy foods, specifically, but the high concentration of calcium in dairy foods that offsets their protein-induced loss.[9]

- Several studies have indicated that "protein and calcium act synergistically on bone—*if* both are present in adequate quantities in the diet." Only when calcium intake is low, does calcium loss caused by animal protein become a problem.[10] [11]

- A study following middle-aged individuals found that the risk of hip fracture in the group consuming the highest amount of animal protein (compared to those eating the least protein) was 2.8x higher when they consumed less than 800 mg/day of calcium. However, the higher animal protein eaters had an 85% reduced risk of hip fracture (compared to those eating the least protein) when consuming at least 800 mg/day of calcium.[12]

- Data collected on 2006 postmenopausal women in the 1999-2002 NHANES (National Health and Nutrition Examination Survey) found those consuming too little protein (less than 46 grams per day) had a far higher risk of fracture—even if they were getting 1,200 mg of calcium daily. In contrast, women consuming 70 grams of protein daily along with at least 1,200 mg of calcium had a 31% lower risk of fracture.[13]

The message is clear. Getting enough protein is essential for bone health, and balancing that protein with sufficient calcium is equally so. That's especially true for meat sources of protein.

BONE-HEALTHY ACTION ITEMS

- Eat plenty of vegetables to maintain a slightly alkaline pH.
- Get enough protein (1.2 g/k BW) *and* adequate calcium (1,200 mg daily).
- Dairy foods' high calcium content offsets the tendency of animal protein to promote bone loss.

Sodium:
Excess Salt in Processed Foods
Leaches Calcium from Our Bones

BONE ESSENTIALS

- Americans age 2 years and older average a whopping 3,436 mg of sodium daily—well above the RDA of 2,300 (about 1 teaspoon per day) for adults.
- In postmenopausal women, excessive salt causes the loss in urine of both calcium and hydroxyproline, a major component of collagen which makes up 90% of the protein matrix in bone.
- Excessive salt intake causes the average postmenopausal woman to lose 1 mmol every day from her total bone mass. This totals 14 grams per year. Since our bodies contain 1,200 g of calcium, at this rate, we've lost half our bone mass in 40 years. Obviously, bones start to break much, much sooner.

We're all told to take it easy on the salt. You've undoubtedly heard how sodium consumption can raise blood pressure and that high blood pressure is a major risk factor for heart disease and stroke.

You may not know that sodium threatens your bones as well. Sodium causes calcium to be lost in your urine, in turn, stimulating bone resorption. Sodium and calcium compete for reabsorption in the kidneys. For every 2,290 mg of sodium excreted in urine, 40 mg of calcium is also lost.[14]

And the SAD diet delivers a lot of salt. Adults 19 and older are recommended a daily allowance of no more than 2,300 mg of sodium—the amount in just 1 teaspoon of salt.[15] Even if you lay off the saltshaker, you're likely to get more sodium than that from hidden sources. The average daily sodium intake for Americans age 2 and older, mainly from processed and restaurant foods, is a whopping 3,436 mg.[16]

Did you catch that? Salt consumption far above the safe upper limit begins in the U.S. at age 2! And we wonder why we are experiencing an osteoporosis epidemic.

Salt hurls a double-whammy at postmenopausal women. Compared to premenopausal women (or men), postmenopausal women lose more calcium relative to sodium in urine. In addition, postmenopausal women lose a similar amount of *hydroxyproline*, a major component of collagen. Since 90% of the protein matrix in bone is composed of collagen, the daily loss of hydroxyproline caused by the SAD's excessive sodium content really boosts bone loss. The good news is that restricting salt intake lowers not only the amount of sodium our kidneys must excrete in urine, but also the amounts of both calcium and hydroxyproline we lose.[17]

Postmenopausal women lack the sodium safeguards of young women and men. Young women and all men have an increased ability to absorb calcium, which makes up for sodium-caused losses. In those with normal parathyroid gland function, the kidneys will be sent a message to increase their conversion of vitamin D into *1,25-D*, the hormonal form in which vitamin D increases our intestines' ability to absorb calcium. This protective *absorb-more-calcium* response doesn't kick in for postmenopausal women. Why remains unclear, though the results are seen in the increased calcium and hydroxyproline excreted in postmenopausal women—those with and without osteoporosis—but not in premenopausal women.[18]

Reading your food labels carefully to ensure you're not getting too much salt is especially good advice for women as we get older. Better yet, just avoid processed foods, which add salt to make up for their lack of true flavor. Fresh, organically grown food doesn't need an overdose of salt to taste good. For even more flavor, add bone-boosting spices.

BONE-HEALTHY ACTION ITEMS

- Keep your sodium intake below 2,300 mg or 1 teaspoon of salt per day.
- Postmenopausal women must be especially careful to watch their sodium intake to avoid losing calcium.
- Beware of hidden salt in processed foods and when dining out.
- Get creative. Season your food with a variety of natural spices, many of which, unlike salt, have bone health benefits.

Refined Sugars:
Not so Sweet for Your Bones

BONE ESSENTIALS

- The average American consumes 125 grams of sucrose (nearly 10 tablespoons) and 50 grams of high fructose corn syrup (HFCS) every day in processed foods.
- Our high intake of refined sugar raises blood insulin levels which contributes to bone loss.
- Providing male subjects 100 grams of sugar increased the amount of calcium the men lost in their urine by about 30% and increased the amount of magnesium (another essential mineral in bone) lost in their urine by about 40%.
- Consumption of refined carbohydrates, which your body sees as another form of sugar, greatly increases the amount of calcium excreted in urine.
- HFCS alone causes high triglycerides, insulin resistance, increased total and visceral fat (belly fat), which promote cardiovascular disease, fatty liver, and sarcopenia. All of these cause bone loss.

Paleolithic humans ate very differently. For them, a high-carb snack was a piece of very ripe fruit, and the most concentrated sugar they encountered was a very occasional bit of honey. Our genetic profile matches our ancient ancestors by 99.9%. Yet, the average American gets 70% of total calories from food products that didn't even exist 150 years ago, much less millions of years.

Our bodies are unprepared to process the tsunami of sugars in the modern diet. Just as with salt, processed foods are packed with refined sugar, delivering more than 6 ounces per day to the average American. That's 137 pounds of sugar per year and is a *very conservative* estimate which doesn't even include sugar-laden carbonated beverages.

The average American consumes 125 grams (4.4 ounces or nearly 12 tablespoons) of sucrose (table sugar, produced from sugar cane and sugar beets) and 50 grams of high fructose corn syrup (HFCS) *every single day* in processed foods. These *Big Farma* foods of commerce (but not of health!) also attack your bones with other refined simple sugars (e.g., dextrose). This refined sugar overload causes your body to lose calcium and promotes diseases that cause further bone loss.

High insulin contributes to bone loss. When foods containing high sugar are consumed, the pancreas reacts by secreting more insulin. The SAD, which is loaded with processed foods high in refined sugars, causes large amounts of insulin to be secreted into the bloodstream at virtually every meal and snack. Studies show several different ways this weakens our bones:

- High blood levels of insulin (hyperinsulinemia) are a key contributing factor to osteoporosis (not to mention metabolic syndrome, type 2 diabetes, and cardiovascular disease—ok, we just did). Chronically elevated insulin inhibits your kidney's ability to reabsorb calcium leading to more calcium loss in the urine, increasing bone loss over time.[19]

- Substituting sugar for unrefined starch in the diet of lab rats caused bone mineral density to drop in the femur and tibia, and lessened tibia bending strength. The bones of the sugar-fed rats became weaker and more brittle. Unrefined starch is good for healthy bones! Find it in root vegetables like carrots and yams, baked potatoes, and in whole grains, like old-fashioned rolled oats, brown rice, millet, and quinoa.

What does this mean for your bones? Eat more root vegetables and skip the processed *food-like* stuff. Those hidden spoonfuls of sugar send your calcium down the toilet and increase your risk for hip fracture.[20]

How the glucose in HFCS decimates your bones. While sucrose is still used in plenty of processed foods, the cheaper high fructose corn syrup predominates in processed foods and beverages. HFCS is composed of both fructose and glucose in approximately equal parts. The glucose HFCS adds to our diet is bad news for your bones.

- In studies using human cells, high-dose glucose consumption inhibited osteoblast proliferation, leading to bone loss.
- In human studies, 100 grams of glucose per day increased the amount of calcium men lost in their urine by about 30%. Participants also lost about 40% more magnesium, another essential mineral in bone.[21]

In this last study, participants were not given candy, cake, cookies, or other foods we consider desserts. They ingested only 100 grams of glucose, an amount of sugar present in a can of soda, a typical serving of fruit juice, or virtually any processed food made from refined flour, corn or potatoes.

Your body treats the carbohydrates in refined grains as just another form of sugar. Even *natural* granola cereals and energy bars are loaded with sugars and refined carbohydrates in at least 100-gram amounts. Even in young, healthy adults, an increase in the amount of refined carbohydrates consumed causes a significant increase in the amount of calcium lost in urine.

Researchers varied the amount of refined carbohydrates in an otherwise standardized diet in 18 healthy young subjects. While the amount of calcium in urine varies throughout the day, higher refined carbohydrates caused a significant increase in the number of single urines with a calcium concentration above 360 mg.[22] This is a lot of calcium to lose! To put it in perspective, the normal amount of calcium that should be found in *an entire day's* (24-hour) urine collection is about 600 mg.[23]

HFCS promotes diseases that cause further bone loss. The health effects of sugar are hardly limited to your bones. As it has gained prominence in our diet, HFCS has been shown to promote a host of ailments, which in turn contribute to bone loss. Some of those include:

- Increased triglycerides, which promotes cardiovascular disease, which promotes bone loss.[24]

- Insulin resistance, which promotes type 2 diabetes, which promotes bone loss.[25]

- Increased total fat, particularly visceral (belly) fat, activates osteoclasts and promotes bone loss.[26]

- Fat deposits in the liver and in muscle, which cause both fatty liver disease and sarcopenia. Fatty liver disease impairs your liver's ability to convert vitamin D3 into 25(OH)D, the form in which vitamin D circulates in your bloodstream. Sarcopenia, when fat infiltrates skeletal muscle, also promotes osteoporosis.[27] [28] [29]

The sugar and salt in processed foods contribute to a variety of chronic diseases. Later, we'll explore how those conditions further degrade bone health and steps you can take to counteract their effects. (See Chronic Diseases, Chapter 4.)

BONE-HEALTHY ACTION ITEMS

- Avoid sodas and limit or dilute juices, which contain sugar whose absorption is not slowed by fiber.

- Beware of foods that contain high fructose corn syrup or are high in glucose or other sugars.

- Avoid or limit refined breads, crackers, bagels, potato or corn chips, pretzels, white rice and extruded cereals like corn flakes and toasted oat rings. While these foods don't taste sweet, the body reacts to them like sugar.

- Add unrefined starches to your diet. Find them in beans; root vegetables, like carrots, yams, and potatoes; whole fruits like apples, peaches, and plums; and whole grains, like old-fashioned rolled oats, brown rice, millet, and quinoa.

Imbalanced Fats:
Inflammatory Fatty Acids
Cause Skinny Bones

BONE ESSENTIALS

- A healthy diet contains 25% to 35% of calories from healthy fats, which enable us to absorb fat-soluble vitamins, including vitamins A, D, and K.
- The right fats, monounsaturated fats, polyunsaturated fats, and essential fatty acids, in the right balance, protect and build bone.
- The wrong fats, saturated and trans fats, make you fat and your bones skinny.
- Omega-3s (e.g., EPA and DHA) are essential for healthy bones. These fats increase osteoblast production and activity.
- Omega-6s also promote bone health when not consumed in excessive amounts.
- You want to consume enough omega-3s to produce a ratio of no more than 4:1 omega-6: omega-3, though the SAD dishes up a highly imbalanced ratio of 20:1.

Fats get an unfair rap, often seen as the dietary bad guy. The truth is your bones—and your entire body—need healthy fats. Along with providing calories for immediate use and storing energy, fat is required to:

- Absorb and transport the fat-soluble vitamins, including those critical to our bones. Vitamin D allows us to actively absorb calcium, vitamin K1 has significant protective effects on bone, and vitamin K2 activates the proteins that pull calcium into bone (*osteocalcin*) and keep it out of our arteries, breasts, brain, and kidneys (*matrix Gla protein*).
- Help produce bone-maintaining hormones, including thyroid hormones, parathyroid hormone, estrogen, progesterone, and testosterone
- Cushion and protect our organs (in healthy amounts) and keep skin healthy and unwrinkled

The problems arise when we get too much fat and/or the wrong kinds.

The wrong fats make you fat and your bones skinny. The right fats protect and build bone. Take a look at the latest statistics on obesity. In January 2021, the American Obesity Association projected that in 2025, 50% of Americans will be obese. By 2030 that number jumps to 60%. Pretty obvious we are getting too much of the wrong kinds of fat![30]

How much fat do we need? A healthy diet contains approximately 20% to 35% (we recommend the lower end of this range) of calories from fat (around 40 to 70 grams per day for women and 45 to 77 grams for men), depending upon age and activity level. To find out how many grams of fat you need daily, check out this handy calculator: (www.healthcalculators.org/calculators/fat.asp).

Too much fat will increase your risk of osteoporosis, as well as obesity, heart disease, cancer, and diabetes. Even the proper amount can harm your bones if your intake of omega-6 fatty acids is out of proportion to that of omega-3 fatty acids.

By now, you won't be surprised to learn that the SAD delivers too much fat in the form of omega-6s and not enough omega-3s. Here's a primer on the types of dietary fats and how some simple changes can prevent imbalances that destroy your bones.

While saturated fats typically promote bone loss, fat from organically-raised animals can protect bones. Saturated fats, which are solid at room temperature, can be found in meats, dairy products, and processed baked goods. Excessive consumption of saturated fat gets a lot of press for increasing the risk of heart disease. However, the real story is more complex. Some saturated fats can actually support your body and bones if they contain a bone-protecting fatty acid called *conjugated linolenic acid* (CLA). Whether they do depends on how the animals are fed and raised.

Meat and dairy products from organically raised animals—grass-fed beef, free-range chicken, and pasture-raised dairy cows—produce saturated fat with significant amounts of CLA. Over the last twenty years, research has shown that CLA improves bone mass; reduces body fat; lowers the risk of cardiovascular diseases and cancer; and modulates immune and inflammatory responses.[31]

In contrast, conventionally raised livestock live on a diet split between 50% hay and silage and 50% genetically modified corn or other grains.

This animal version of the SAD similarly promotes inflammation because the saturated fats these animals produce are high in omega-6s and contain little to no CLA. Meat and dairy products from grass-fed animals contain 300% to 500% more CLA than products from cattle fed a conventional diet.[32] [33] [34]

The CLA found in organically raised animal products calms the chronic low-grade inflammation that is now so common and protects your bones. The bottom line for your healthy bones: if you enjoy meat and dairy foods, choose organic to get the bone-protecting benefits of CLA found in grass-fed cattle and free-range poultry.

Processing Foods Destroys the Benefits of Unsaturated Fats

Unsaturated fats, found in vegetables, plants, nuts, and seafood, are grouped into two main types: *monounsaturated fats* and *polyunsaturated fats.* Both types remain liquid at room temperature, though monounsaturated fats start to solidify at refrigerator temperatures.

Both types of these fats offer necessary nutrients and can be healthy. However, as with saturated fat, their overall positive or negative effect largely depends on their processing. Unfortunately, many processed foods contain polyunsaturated fats that are partially or fully hydrogenated to increase product shelf life or create a more spreadable form (such as margarine). The resulting unhealthy saturated fats are called *trans fats.* The good news is that all the publicity around the bad effects of trans fats has resulted in their levels being lower in foods than 20 years ago. The bad news is that they still lurk in many foods.

Trans fats promote inflammation, osteoclast activation, and bone loss. Rarely found in nature—and then in just tiny amounts—trans fats have generated healthy profits for the food processing industry but are destructive for us. You can find them hiding out in all kinds of processed foods, including chips, cookies, cakes, pies, pastries, donuts, fried foods, artificial creamers and whipped cream, and French fries.

Avoid trans fats like the plague. These *franken-fats* increase your risk for cardiovascular disease and heart attack (raising potentially harmful LDL cholesterol while also lowering protective HDL cholesterol) and decrease insulin sensitivity (promoting type 2 diabetes and obesity). From a bone health perspective, they're also a disaster:

- Trans fats are loaded with pro-inflammatory omega-6 fats that activate your osteoclasts.
- Hydrogenation changes the vitamin K1 found in polyunsaturated fats into dihydrophylloquinone, a form that is no longer anti-inflammatory and can no longer be converted by your body into a short-lived version of vitamin K2 called MK-4. We need K2 to activate osteocalcin and matrix Gla protein, to direct calcium into our bones and keep it out of our arteries.[35]

No wonder the Dietary Guidelines for Americans and the Institute of Medicine have recommended keeping trans fat intake as low as possible, ideally none. Yet, trans fat can still be hiding in your food, as amounts of 0.49 grams or less per serving can be rounded down to 0 grams on the Nutrition Facts label, even though realistic serving sizes may be much greater.[36]

While saturated and unsaturated fats have both healthy and unhealthy attributes, trans fat is a clear no-no when it comes to health. Avoid it by staying away from processed foods likely to contain hydrogenated oils.

Monounsaturated fats like olive oil promote bone health. *Monounsaturated fats*, which include olive oil, avocado oil, canola oil, and peanut oil, offer some bone-protective effects. Research has associated a reduced risk of fracture in elders with a higher ratio of monounsaturated fat in their diet. In addition, several studies point to olive oil as a boon for bones:

- Olive oil as the primary source of added fat has been positively associated with bone density.[37]
- Two polyphenols in olive oil, oleuropein, and hydroxytyrosol, inhibit osteoclasts and promote the proliferation of osteoblasts. In a study of rats, whose ovaries were removed to simulate human menopause, these polyphenols were able to totally prevent bone loss.

Olive oil is also rich in vitamin E, a powerful antioxidant which helps lessen osteoclast activation.[38] Considering all of this, use olive oil as your go-to to dress salads. Don't use olive oil to cook at high temperatures, but do rely on it to add flavor to cooked grains, beans, or roasted vegetables. Whisk some into soups or use it to add richness to sauces and dips. Choose organic, *extra virgin* olive oil over refined versions to get far more vitamin E and bone-protective polyphenols. Store your oil in an opaque container or at least out of direct light and in a cool place to protect the potency of its bone-protective compounds. [39]

The SAD's polyunsaturated fats deliver an unhealthy balance of omega-6 and omega-3 fatty acids. *Polyunsaturated fats* contain the essential fatty acids omega-6 and omega-3. Our bodies can't synthesize these fats, which is why they're called *essential* fatty acids. Both are critical for healthy immune and nervous systems, plus healthy bones. However, the SAD, with its reliance on refined safflower, soybean, and corn oils, delivers excessive omega-6s and provides few omega-3s. Here's how the imbalance negates the positive effect of these oils:

- We rely on the omega-6 fatty acid *arachidonic acid* (AA) to produce *prostaglandins,* including PGE2, a hormone-like compound that controls inflammation and aids healing. However, PGE2 *produced in excess* promotes excessive, *chronic inflammation*, which overly activates osteoclasts. Excess omega-6 fats also inhibit the production and activity of osteoblasts.[40]

- In contrast, omega-3 fats are metabolized into anti-inflammatory *prostaglandins* (PGE3) and protect our bones through a bunch of mechanisms, all of which *decrease* the production and activity of osteoclasts and *increase* osteoblast production and activity.[41] [42]

- A more nefarious effect of excess omega-6s is to cause precursors of osteoblasts (mesenchymal stem cells) to turn into fat cells instead. Talk about adding insult to injury![43]

The good news is that omega-6s can *promote* bone formation when consumed in lesser amounts and in healthy balance with the omega-3s. Since omega-6 oils are everywhere in the processed food supply, you should plan your diet to include foods rich in omega-3s.

- Plant sources of omega-3s, called *alpha-linolenic acid* (ALA), include nuts and seeds, and their oils. Chia seeds, walnuts, and flaxseed oil, in particular, are good sources of ALA.

- Cold-water fish, like Alaskan salmon or sardines, are an excellent source of the longer chain—and most bone-protective—omega-3s, *docosahexaenoic acid* (DHA), and *eicosapentaenoic acid* (EPA).

However, beware of farmed fish, which are the aquatic equivalent of cattle in feedlots. The fishmeal, vegetable proteins, vegetable oils, and binding agents used to make their feed pellets contain way more omega-6s than omega-3s. To top it off, farmed fish often have high levels of polychlorinated biphenyls (PCBs), man-made toxic chemicals our bodies find very difficult to excrete, so they accumulate in fat.

What balance of omega oils is best for bone health? Experts disagree on the optimal balance of omega-6: omega-3, with recommendations ranging from a ratio of 1:1 to at most 4:1. However, the SAD's ratio of at least 15:1 (and more likely 20:1) is clearly skewed towards inflammatory omega-6. In unpublished research, as part of a corporate wellness program, Dr. Pizzorno measured the omega-6: omega-3 ratio in several thousand Canadians and the typical ratio found was 20:1.

- Many studies have now shown that omega-3s lower osteoclast activity and thus reduce bone resorption.[44] [45] [46] [47] [48]

- The Framingham Osteoporosis Study evaluated 623 individuals whose average age was 75 years and found that *both* omega-6 and omega-3s fatty acids (DHA and EPA) protect hip bone health—*provided* intake of EPA and DHA is high enough to produce a ratio of no more than 4:1 omega-6: omega-3.

The takeaway is that we need healthy fats! Monounsaturated fats and even some saturated animal fat from pastured animals can be a healthy part of our diets, though we should favor polyunsaturated fats with higher omega-3 fatty acids. The key comes down to choosing meat and dairy products from pastured animals fed natural diets, fish that are wild-caught, organically grown nuts and seeds, and cold-pressed vegetable oils that have not been subjected to hydrogenation (to avoid trans fats).

BONE-HEALTHY ACTION ITEMS

- If you enjoy meat and dairy foods, choose organic to get the anti-inflammatory, bone-protective benefits of conjugated linolenic acid (CLA) found only in grass-fed cattle and free-range poultry.

- Increase your use of monounsaturated fats, especially organic, extra virgin olive oil.

- Avoid processed and other SAD foods where inflammatory trans fats lurk: cookies, cakes, and other baked goods; French fries and other fried foods; non-dairy creamers; and anything containing hydrogenated oils. Some brands of frozen pizza and microwave popcorn contain 5 grams and 7 grams per serving, respectively.

- Introduce more omega-3 fatty acids by eating nuts and seeds, such as chia seeds, walnuts, and flaxseed.
- Eat cold-water fish, like Alaskan salmon or sardines, to get the longer chain—and most bone-protective—omega-3s, DHA and EPA. Choose only wild fish, as farm-raised fish are more likely to contain toxic PCBs and are a less healthy ratio of omega-6s: omega-3s.
- Aim for fat to make up a maximum of 25% to 35% of calories, primarily from healthy fats. To customize based on age, weight, and height, use this online Fat Intake Calculator: www.healthcalculators.org/calculators/fat.asp

Wheat and Gluten:
Less Staff of Life and More a Club Bludgeoning Your Bones

BONE ESSENTIALS

- Gluten, the major protein in wheat, disrupts gut function in about 80% of us (not just those with celiac disease), causing chronic inflammation.
- Eating wheat causes most people's intestines to release a compound called zonulin, which opens the *tight junctions* between the cells that make up the walls of your digestive tract.
- By increasing intestinal permeability, zonulin also opens our intestinal *doors* to whatever is in the gut, including pathogens and toxins.
- Gluten protein contains at least 50 toxic epitopes (strings of amino acids) that provoke inflammation and a hyperactive pro-inflammatory immune system in susceptible individuals.
- Wheat has been significantly altered over the last 50 years, changes that make it appear far more dangerous to your immune system.

Way back in 460 BC, Hippocrates, the father of western medicine, asserted, "All disease begins in the gut." In 2010, Dr. Alessio Fasano put this medical insight into modern terms saying, "The gut is not like Las Vegas. What happens in the gut does not stay in the gut."[49] Naturopathic doctors have been advising their patients for over a century that health begins with a properly functioning gut.

Fasano was alluding to the fact that gluten, the major protein in wheat, disrupts gut function, not just in those with celiac disease, but in approximately 80% of us who are eating wheat several times a day. This causes chronic inflammation that promotes numerous diseases, including osteoporosis.

Fasano discovered this while seeking a vaccine for cholera, a disease that still kills 5 million children every year in the developing world. Fasano's team discovered that the tight junctions in our intestinal cell walls—believed to be a static barrier wall—act more like doors the body opens as a defensive mechanism. The key that opens these doors is a protein our bodies produce called *zonulin*, for which only three agents have been discovered that trigger its release:

- Vibrio cholerae (specifically, its toxin)[50]
- pathogenic intestinal bacteria
- a polypeptide in gluten called gliadin, which contains an indigestible peptide fraction called alpha-gliadin (α-gliadin).

The body's dramatic release of zonulin to open the intestinal wall to flush out cholera and other pathogens is potentially life-saving. Yet, this same mechanism comes into play whenever we eat gluten-containing grains. While the effect is less dramatic, the loss in control of intestinal permeability promotes a wide range of inflammation-related diseases, including osteoporosis because chronic inflammation causes excessive osteoclast activation.

How gluten (α-gliadin) promotes bone loss—and not just for those with celiac disease. For those with celiac disease, any exposure keeps their intestinal doors open unless gluten is eliminated and permanently avoided. About 20% of the population doesn't produce zonulin. These individuals can consume some wheat and other gluten-containing foods without the risk of developing celiac disease (unless they are part of a minority of people who produce antibodies to wheat proteins), but they will still be under attack by the many other inflammatory peptides found in gluten.

For the majority of us (about 80%), zonulin's effects are quickly reversible, with our intestinal doors closing about 3 hours after exposure. However, those following the SAD often consume gluten at every meal and snack, creating a *leaky gut* whose chronically open doors unleash bone-destroying inflammation.

This leaky gut greatly increases the load of undigested food components, toxic bacterial molecules, and inflammatory microorganisms sent to our body's next line of defense, the liver. While a healthy liver converts invaders into compounds that can be excreted in urine or bile for removal, the ability of an overwhelmed or unhealthy liver (such as one loaded with fat) to handle the job is compromised. That increases the amount of inflammatory debris circulating throughout the body, which, in itself, is detrimental to bones.

Plus, the liver is responsible for the first step of vitamin D's metabolism into the form in which it helps us absorb calcium. A sick, overtaxed liver can't perform any of its jobs very well. (See NAFLD, Chapter 4.)

Unfortunately, the inflammatory effects of gluten don't stop there. Our bodies lack the enzymes to completely digest gluten, so we break it into polypeptides (i.e., gliadin) and peptide components. Similar to how α-gliadin triggers zonulin release, gliadin contains other peptide sequences with toxic actions.

A DNA map of α-gliadin reveals a number of detrimental activities on human cells:

- **inducing apoptosis** (cell suicide)
- **creating superantigens**, which create an oversized immune response. They, in essence, activate Godzilla to neutralize Bambi.
- **attracting neutrophils** (our immune system's inflammatory first responders) to the intestine, again causing an unneeded immune response.

Should you avoid gluten to protect your bones? Everyone has their own individual sensitivity to gluten, which can change over time. Some attribute our society's dramatic increase in gluten sensitivity, which is now thought to affect 13% of the general population, to changes in wheat production over the last 50 years:[51]

Different strains of wheat have been combined through *hybridization*, altering gluten's protein sequence by as much as 5% to create *new and improved* versions.[52] [53]

Deamidation, a common food-industry practice, renders gluten water-soluble by using acids or enzymes. This improvement in the ability to process wheat has been shown to create substances our digestive tract doesn't recognize, generating an immune response in susceptible people.[54] [55] [56]

If you've been diagnosed with osteopenia or osteoporosis, gluten may be a contributing factor. Run tests for celiac disease and wheat allergy. Even if both are negative, consider trying a gluten-free diet to evaluate gluten sensitivity. Notice whether you experience relief from the symptoms (see box below), which should become apparent within a matter of weeks, provided you don't have celiac disease. If you discover that gluten is contributing to your bone loss, avoid it!

Symptoms of Gluten Sensitivity:

- Osteopenia, osteoporosis
- Dermatitis (eczema or skin rash)
- Bone, joint or muscle pain (e.g., rheumatoid arthritis)
- IBS-like symptoms (abdominal pain, bloating, bowel habit abnormalities - either diarrhea or constipation)

- Weight loss
- Leg or arm numbness
- Muscle cramps
- Anemia
- Foggy mind, headache, fatigue
- Depression

Source: Non-Celiac Gluten sensitivity...[57] , Divergence of gut permeability...[58] Spectrum of gluten-related disorders...[59]

BONE-HEALTHY ACTION ITEMS

- If you have osteopenia, osteoporosis, or any symptoms of gluten sensitivity, ask your doctor to order the tests needed to check for celiac disease and wheat allergy.
- Even if both are negative, consider trying a gluten-free diet for at least one month to evaluate gluten sensitivity.
- For a list of common food items that contain gluten, check out www.celiac.org/gluten-free-living/what-is-gluten/sources-of-gluten

Excessive Alcohol:
A Little Helps, Too Much Harms Bone

BONE ESSENTIALS

- Light alcohol consumption (for women, one 4-ounce glass of wine or a 12-ounce glass of beer; for men, two drinks per day) has been found to improve BMD, particularly in postmenopausal women and men over age 50.
- Alcohol, regardless of the type consumed, causes blood levels of several markers of bone resorption (osteocalcin, CTx and NTx) to drop and estrogen levels to rise.
- Beer's beneficial effects on bone are thought to be due to its silicon as well as ethanol content.
- Wine's bone benefits are likely linked in part to its phytochemical content, especially the resveratrol in red wine, which both inhibits the formation of osteoclasts and boosts that of osteoblasts.
- Too much alcohol, however, decreases the production of osteoblasts, increases that of fat cells, causes liver damage, lowers estrogen levels, increases free radical production/inflammation, and destroys osteocytes, the bone cells that regulate bone remodeling and new bone formation.

Poet Ogden Nash quipped that *candy is dandy, but liquor is quicker.* He could have been referring to bones, not prospective beaus. Just as refined sugars cause bone loss, alcohol consumed in excess can have significant detrimental effects. Moderate use of alcohol, however, has positive effects: reducing bone resorption and promoting bone formation.

Various studies show benefits from light alcohol consumption, considered 14 grams/d ethanol for women or 28 grams/d for men. That equates roughly to about one 4-ounce glass of wine or 12-ounce bottle of beer for women, or two similarly sized drinks for men.

- Light alcohol consumption has been shown to *improve* bone mineral density and bone mass, especially for postmenopausal women and men over age 50.
- Fourteen grams of alcohol has been associated with increased

lumbar spine bone mineral density (BMD) and whole-body BMD in postmenopausal women.

- Beer offers similar beneficial results for pre- and postmenopausal women drinking 4 beers per week and in men consuming one beer or other alcoholic beverage per day. [60]

Note that the alcohol content of a standard drink can vary dramatically. While beer is assumed to contain 5% alcohol by volume (ABV), it can contain from 3% to over 12% ABV depending on style and brewer.[61] Wine ranges vary wildly from 5.5% to over 20% ABV, with bolder and richer wines tending to have more alcohol.[62] Hard liquor ABV can also vary, so a good rule of thumb is sticking to one mixed drink, cocktail, or shot (1.5 ounces of spirits). For more precise measurements, check the ABV marked on the bottles.

How a wee bit of alcohol helps our bones:

- A *small* amount of alcohol, regardless of type, causes blood levels of several markers of bone remodeling (osteocalcin, CTx, and NTx) to drop.[63]
- Estrogen level has been observed to increase in women drinking no more than 10 grams/d of alcohol as well as men with light alcohol consumption. Men convert testosterone into estradiol in small but crucial amounts for their bone health, which could partly explain the increased BMD observed in light drinkers.
- Beer contains silicon, which has beneficial effects on collagen formation and bone. (See Silicon, Chapter 6.) A glass of beer contains 7 mg of the bone-building mineral, while a glass of wine (4-ounces) provides 1 mg. (Your bones and your waistline might fare better with spinach, which contains around 5 mg of silicon per half cup for just 20 calories.)
- Wine's bone benefits are linked in part to its phytochemical content, especially the resveratrol present in red wine. Resveratrol inhibits the activation of *RANKL*, whose actions ultimately produce bone-removing osteoclasts. In addition, resveratrol significantly enhances bone formation by increasing the production of Cbfa-1/RunX2, a transcription factor that causes bone marrow cells (specifically, mesenchymal stem cells) to become bone-building osteoblasts rather than *adipocytes* (fat cells).[64] Lead inhibits Cbfa-1/RunX2, another reason it destroys bone. (See Heavy Metals, page 75)

How too much alcohol destroys bone. Drinking more than a serving of alcohol per day (one drink for women, two drinks for men) decreases bone formation through a variety of mechanisms:[65]

- Excessive alcohol results in mesenchymal stem cells becoming adipocytes (fat cells) rather than osteoblasts. Too much alcohol suppresses insulin-like growth factor (IGF-1), which causes osteoblasts to proliferate and inhibits lipid (fat) accumulation in bone marrow.

- Reduced IGF-1 activity also lessens the bone-building actions of *parathyroid hormone* (PTH), which increases production of 1,25-D, the active, hormonal form of vitamin D, when blood levels of calcium drop too low. By interfering with PTH production, excessive alcohol consumption decreases blood levels of calcium, triggering its removal from bone.

- Alcohol damages the liver, which is the primary place where vitamin D3 is converted to 25(OH)D, the form in which vitamin D circulates in the bloodstream.

- Excess alcohol lowers blood levels of estrogen (specifically, estradiol) in women. Estradiol has many anti-inflammatory actions, including inhibiting the production of RANKL, which causes osteoclast production and activity to increase. (As seen previously, moderate alcohol consumption is associated with an increase in estrogen levels.)

- Alcohol increases the production of free radicals (reactive oxygen species, ROS) in osteoblasts. This damages these bone-building cells causing them to age and die more rapidly. ROS also increases RANKL, increasing osteoclast activity.

- Alcohol destroys *osteocytes*, the most abundant cell in bone tissue. Osteocytes are osteoblasts that have become embedded in the bone they laid down and continue to orchestrate new bone formation. Healthy osteocytes prevent osteoclast activation. Too much alcohol causes osteocytes to commit apoptosis (cell suicide). Dying osteocytes send signals that recruit osteoclasts, so an increase in osteocyte death increases bone loss.

- Alcohol suppresses the bone-building *Wnt signaling pathway* and increases the activity of its antagonist, DKK1. Wnts are proteins that direct cell signaling. In the most studied pathway through which Wnt signaling occurs, the Wnt/β-catenin pathway, β-catenin moves into the nucleus of bone cells and tells them whether they should proliferate and build new bone or die. Emerging research shows the Wnt/β-catenin pathway also regulates how osteocytes respond to weight-bearing exercise by orchestrating the production of new bone. In animal studies, when too much alcohol is consumed, all the major bone-building components of the Wnt signaling pathway are suppressed, and *adipogenesis* (fat cell production) is enhanced.

- Alcohol increases production of *acetaldehyde*, the main metabolite of ethanol, which directly inhibits osteoblast proliferation and activity.

BONE-HEALTHY ACTION ITEMS

- Drink beer, wine, or spirits *in moderation.* Beer and wine are definitely healthier choices for bones.

- One drink per day for women or two for men helps improve bone mineral density and bone mass, particularly in postmenopausal women and men over 50.

- Avoid drinking more alcohol than this. A very occasional extra glass of wine or beer won't hurt, but if you often overindulge, you'll produce fewer osteoblasts and more fat cells, and kill off your osteocytes, the bone cells that regulate new bone formation. Plus, you'll damage your liver, lower your estrogen levels, and increase inflammation, a recipe for wrinkles, fat gain, and bone loss.

CASES FROM THE COMMUNITY

The Community is a sponsored group of more than 17,000 men and women supporting each other to build stronger bones naturally.
(www.algaecal.com/community)

Emily's Story

Emily's first concerning DEXA scan was in 2004, showing low bone density. She then underwent four months of chemotherapy treatments for breast cancer which plunged her into early menopause at only age 47, increasing her risk of osteoporosis and fractures. Seven years later, her ovaries were removed to lower her risk of cancer recurrence. This only made things worse for her bones, and sure enough, her subsequent DEXA scans showed her bone density continuing to go downhill. Emily thought declining bone density was just her fate.

When her spine T-score got to -3.0, her doctor told her how serious this was. Emily was committed to finding a natural solution. She got a copy of *Your Bones* (Lara's book) and, based on the research covered, began taking AlgaeCal Plus and Strontium Boost in January 2019. She also took extra omega-3 using a plant based supplement since she was following a vegan diet. She worked to minimize gluten in her diet, get enough protein (70 grams), and maintain healthy blood levels of vitamin D (70.3 ng/ml). She also walked daily, started running, and took yoga classes several times per week.

In April 2021, Emily wrote to Lara and *The Community*: "OK here you go! I no longer have osteoporosis!!" The T-score in her spine had moved from -3.0 (osteoporosis) to -2.2 (osteopenia) in the 2 years and 3 months she had been on the plan. She also showed improvement in her left hip, and her femoral neck numbers had stabilized. "I am incredibly grateful for you and for all the women in this group who support and encourage each other," says Emily. "I can now ride my bike without the fear a minor fall will fracture my bones."

Lara's Take: Treatments for other conditions can make improving bone health more challenging. However, Emily shows that dietary changes (such as eating an organic plant-based diet and limiting gluten and processed foods), regular weight bearing exercise, and getting the proper amount of nutrients and protein can lead to significant gains.

See details on supplements for calcium on page 135, strontium citrate on page 273, and omega-3 oil on page 208. Learn more about bioidentical hormone replacement therapy (BHRT) on page 265 and determining vitamin D levels on page 176. Statements regarding the products above have not been evaluated by the Food and Drug Administration. These products are not intended to diagnose, treat, cure, or prevent any disease.

CHAPTER 2

Toxins Hiding in Your Food Destroy Your Bones

You've seen how the standard American diet both lacks the necessary nutrients for bone health and delivers foods that actively derail it. Sadly, you're facing another threat to your healthy bones that's even more insidious. The production, packaging, preservation, and storage of food bombards us with hundreds of known toxins.

Plastics release chemicals that cause inflammation and disrupt hormones. Conventional farming introduces pesticides that damage our kidneys, liver, and thyroid glands, while promoting further inflammation. Phosphate additives overload our bodies with phosphorus, disrupting our endocrine system's regulation of calcium. Fluoride in toothpaste and our water supply damages bone quality and depletes key minerals healthy bones need.

All of these toxins damage our ability to create strong, healthy bones. Unlike the ingredients in foods, these chemicals are not disclosed on nutrition labels. This chapter shows you where your risk lies and how to make safe choices that protect your bones.

Pesticide Residues:
Contribute to Chronic Diseases
Affecting Bone Health

BONE ESSENTIALS

- Dietary exposure to pesticide residues, even very low doses of pesticide mixtures, is now well known to damage human health.
- Organochlorine pesticides (OCPs) have a very long *half-life* in the body. They accumulate in body fat and have toxic effects on a wide variety of bodily systems, particularly the kidneys.
- At levels supposedly *safe* for us, organochlorine pesticides promote bone loss by causing chronic low-grade inflammation and impairing lipid (cholesterol) and protein metabolism, and liver, kidney, and thyroid function.
- Exposure to organochlorine pesticides greatly lowers our production and recycling of glutathione, the most important antioxidant our bodies produce to protect us.

Organically grown fruits and vegetables contain a wealth of vitamins, minerals, and phytonutrients vital for bone health. Yet, consumers eating the SAD get far fewer nutrients and are also exposed to a mixture of pesticides in what should be health-promoting foods. Even dietary exposure to very low doses of pesticide mixtures is now recognized as harmful to human health (and ultimately our bones).

Acceptable **daily intakes (ADIs) produce toxic actions when combined.** The U.S. Environmental Protection Agency (EPA) sets *safe* ADI levels of individual pesticides by evaluating them *one at a time*. That's not how they're encountered in the real world. Animal studies have constructed models to examine pesticides both singly and when combined (as occurs in our conventionally grown food). The results are not pretty!

Four widely-used *organophosphate pesticides* **(OPPs) produced toxic results** in rats dosed with residues in their drinking water at supposedly safe levels of each. The combined pesticides produced several effects with nasty implications for bone health, including:[66]

- **Liver and renal dysfunction**, which interferes with our removal of toxins from the body and vitamin D's conversion into its active form, as well as the kidneys' reabsorption of calcium and magnesium, increasing their loss in urine.

- **Disruption of lipid and amino acid metabolism**, initiating more inflammation and encouraging cardiovascular disease.
- **Thyroid gland dysfunction**, which disrupts bone remodeling, leading to bone loss.

Organochlorine pesticides (OCP), another class of pesticide, were found to disrupt bone-marrow cell signaling in the offspring of pregnant and breastfeeding mice. Such damage affects oxygen throughout our bodies, lessens our production of lymphocytes (immune cells), and can lead to anemia. This study evaluated *endosulfan*, a widely used OCP now being phased out, which is well-known to be a pro-oxidant, meaning it generates free radicals that attack our cells.[67]

Endosulfan creates chronic inflammation by activating signaling pathways (NF-kappa B and JNK) that trigger the production of other pro-inflammatory mediators (i.e., TNFa and IL-6), which then restimulate the original inflammatory compounds. This vicious cycle perpetuates the subclinical chronic inflammation that drives metabolic syndrome, with its resulting disease consequences, including type-2 diabetes, cardiovascular disease, and osteoporosis.

Damaged bone marrow cells, seen in the research animals' offspring, further inflammation through anemia, a condition where blood cells are unable to carry sufficient oxygen (hypoxia). The resulting damage to immune cells (lymphocytes) lowers our ability to clear pathogens, toxins, and cellular debris. Research shows that lymphocyte numbers decrease in proportion to the level of exposure to many common toxins in the environment.

OCPs impair our kidneys' ability to filter out toxins, which makes them less able to excrete toxins to protect the rest of our body. Researchers studied 270 chronic kidney disease (CKD) patients and found much higher levels of pesticides (OCPs) compared to a healthy control group, especially those whose genetic inheritance rendered them less able to detoxify these harmful compounds.

For individuals who had issues with the production and recycling of *glutathione*, a protective antioxidant, CKD risk was increased by 80%.[68]

Unfortunately, inheriting slow versions of the enzymes involved in utilizing glutathione for detoxification is all too common, affecting between 20% and 50% of us.[69] (See Chapter 7, The B Vitamins, page 329)

Along with CKD, exposure to persistent OCPs is associated with diabetes and cardiovascular disease. Pesticides, especially OCPs, accumulate in body fat, and some have a long biological half-life (time they remain in the body). All of these degenerative conditions are characterized by low-grade, chronic inflammation, and each is *strongly* associated with an increased risk of osteoporosis.[70 71 72 73 74 75 76 77 78]

Environmental toxins, particularly OCPs and OPPs, are ubiquitous around the world because they have been widely used in agriculture, and—this will upset you—in *public health programs*. Your taxes have contributed to the poisoning of our food, air, and water.

We now know that pesticides, at levels we continue to be told are *safe*, cause chronic inflammation, disrupt the function of our organs (liver, kidneys, and thyroid), and threaten the health of our bones. Eat organically grown food and avoid pesticides like the plague they are! Your bones (and the rest of your body) will thank you.

BONE-HEALTHY ACTION ITEMS

- Choose organic produce whenever possible.
- Shop at farm stands and at farmer's markets, where you can ask farmers about their pesticide use.
- Grow your own fruits, vegetables, and herbs in a garden or greenhouse. Be sure to use organic methods.
- To identify the most and least contaminated fruits and vegetables, check out the Dirty Dozen™ and Clean Fifteen™ lists released each year by the Environmental Working Group, a non-profit group that compiles the lists based on public government data (www.ewg.org/foodnews/dirty-dozen.php).

Phosphate Additives:
Deliver Toxic Phosphorus Levels in Processed Food

BONE ESSENTIALS

- Phosphorus in food additives is rapidly and almost completely absorbed, unlike phosphorus in real food.
- Healthy regulation of calcium requires that calcium and phosphate be in balance, optimally an equal (1:1) balance.
- Due to phosphate additives in processed foods, the calcium to phosphorus ratio in the typical U.S. diet is about 0.6:1, way below recommended guidelines.
- When phosphorus intake is too high, two hormones are secreted: parathyroid hormone (PTH) and fibroblast growth factor-23 (FGF-23), both of which, if chronically elevated, cause bone loss.
- PTH increases osteoclast activity. FGF-23 prevents the production of 1,25-D, the form in which vitamin D helps us absorb calcium.

Phosphorus is an essential nutrient—it occurs in most foods as a natural component. However, phosphorus is also approved as an additive and is now used in countless processed foods. Our increasing consumption of processed foods in the U.S. over the past decades has caused phosphorus consumption to rise to a level that not only far exceeds our requirement for phosphorus, but is destroying our bones.

CKD patients show the risk of our high phosphorus intake. In patients with chronic kidney disease (CKD), high blood levels of phosphate are strongly associated with cardiovascular and *all-cause mortality* (death for any reason). Since their kidney function is impaired, CKD patients are unable to clear excess phosphorus, so they must greatly limit their intake of processed foods. Seems logical to avoid the phosphates before kidney failure!

Recently, the high load of phosphates Americans eat has been associated with cardiovascular disease and all-cause mortality in *everyone in the general population*. In effect, CKD patients have been our *canaries in the phosphate toxicity coal mines* for an issue that now affects us all.[79]

How much phosphorus is the SAD inflicting on us? No one knows the full extent to which we are being phosphate poisoned by the SAD. Current databases, including those based on the updated USDA Nutrient Content Databases, underestimate the phosphorus content of processed foods by at least 25% to 30%.

How did our phosphorus intake become so high? Over recent decades, phosphorus has been added to many foods as a processing agent with a variety of functions. Today, look in the average person's refrigerator or pantry, and you'll find the majority of processed foods contain one or multiple ingredients that contain phosphorus. People consume phosphate additives at breakfast, lunch, dinner, and snack time. While the amount in each item may be low, the total phosphorus load each day really adds up.[80] (See box, Where Phosphates Hide in Foods.)

Making matters worse, manufacturers aren't required to specify how much they've added since phosphorus is on the Generally Recognized as Safe (GRAS) list. With over 40 phosphorous compounds on the GRAS list, calculating how much we're consuming in the form of food additives is impossible. While at modest dosages they are considered *safe*, with so many sources, the total far exceeds the safe level.

Even with an accurate assessment of our dietary phosphorus intake, we'd still have only a poor guess as to how much phosphate is floating around in our bloodstream. The phosphorus in food additives is rapidly and almost completely absorbed, unlike phosphorus in real food, which is bound to protein and other food molecules that slow the speed and amount of absorption. In addition, the phosphorus in plant protein sources, such as soybeans or whole grains, is mostly present as phytate and is far less easily absorbed.

How high dietary phosphorus intake causes bone loss and cardiovascular disease. Though there are several mechanisms, here's one that has received a lot of attention: the disruption of our endocrine system's regulation of calcium. The fact is: calcium and phosphate have to be in balance, optimally a 1:1 balance. When the calcium-to-phosphorus dietary intake ratio is less than 1:1 (almost always because dietary phosphorus intake is too high), parathyroid hormone secretion can increase to potentially bone destructive *levels*.

Where Phosphates Hide in Foods

Foods High in Phosphates

- Milk and dairy
- Mixed dishes (grain-based)
- Breads, rolls, and tortillas
- Quick breads, bread products, and sweet bakery products
- Poultry
- Pizza
- Vegetables
- Meats
- Mixed dishes (meat, poultry, and seafood)
- Cured meats and poultry
- Plant-based protein foods
- Cereals
- Eggs
- Seafood
- Savory snacks, crackers, and snack/meal bars
- Other desserts
- Candy (chocolate)
- Beverages (sugar-sweetened, diet, and alcoholic)
- Juice (100%)
- Fruits
- Soups
- Condiments and sauces

Ingredient Names that Indicate Phosphate Additives

- Calcium acid phosphate
- Calcium phosphate
- Dicalcium phosphate
- Disodium hydrogen pyrophosphate
- Disodium phosphate
- Lecithin
- Modified corn starch
- Modified food starch
- Mono-calcium phosphate
- Mono-potassium phosphate
- Mono-sodium phosphate
- Phosphoric acid
- Potassium tripolyphosphate
- Sodium acid pyrophosphate
- Sodium aluminum phosphate
- Sodium hexa-meta-phosphate
- Sodium hexa-mono-phosphate
- Sodium phosphate
- Sodium tripoly/sodium hexa-meta-phosphate blends
- Sodium tripolyphosphate
- Tetrapotassium pyrophosphate
- Tetrasodium pyrophosphate
- Tricalcium phosphate
- Trisodium phosphate

Source: Accessing the Health Impact of Phosphorous...Advanced Nutrition... [81]

In both animal models and human clinical studies, a high phosphorus diet has been shown to trigger the secretion of two hormones that, if excessively elevated, cause bone loss:

- Parathyroid hormone (PTH): Although it increases activation of vitamin D, PTH increases osteoclast activity, thus causing bone resorption when chronically elevated.

- Fibroblast growth factor-23 (FGF-23) inhibits the synthesis in the kidneys of the hormonal form of vitamin D (1,25-dihydroxyvitamin D3), the only form in which vitamin D helps us absorb calcium. FGF-23 is secreted by osteocytes, the type of bone cell that controls the rate of remodeling.

The combined effects of elevated PTH and FGF-23—increased bone breakdown and greatly impaired ability to absorb calcium—deliver a double bone-breaking punch. In addition, the PTH and FGF-23 combo causes significant harmful cardiovascular effects, such as arterial calcification, endothelial dysfunction, and left ventricular hypertrophy (thickening of the muscle in the left ventricle of the heart in response, a marker of heart disease).

PTH is persistently elevated in response to weeks of consuming processed foods high in phosphate additives (which is what anyone eating the SAD is doing all the time) and is significantly higher in young women whose habitual diets have calcium-to-phosphorus ratios of less than 0.6:1.

A number of animal studies have shown that high dietary phosphorus relative to calcium causes secondary hyperparathyroidism, bone resorption, lower peak bone mass, and fragile bones in young and old animals. Studies in healthy adult humans have shown that, even in these healthy subjects, oral phosphate loading increases levels of markers of bone disease and cardiovascular disease.[82]

Meat products are a concentrated source of highly bioavailable phosphorus. While meat naturally contains phosphorus, *meat products* contain phosphorus additives as well. For example, the majority of fresh frozen chicken products contribute *an average* of an additional 84 mg of phosphorus in a 3-ounce (100 grams) serving. (*And who eats just 3 ounces of chicken?* That's an amount 25% smaller than a deck of cards.)

Similar analyses of other meat and poultry *products* found a range of 6.1 to 21.5 mg of phosphorus in *each gram* of protein (1 ounce = 28 grams). *Enhanced* meat products are those that have been injected with a solution of water and other ingredients (e.g., salt, phosphates, antioxidants, and flavorings). These have a 28.4% higher phosphorus-to-protein ratio than natural meat products, though their phosphorus content had not previously been in the nutrient database.[83]

No wonder estimates of phosphorus intake from processed foods are at least 30% too low. National surveys show that at least one-half of the U.S. population consumes phosphorus above the 400 mg/d Estimated Average Requirement (EAR). In fact, the phosphorus intake of many individuals is quite likely to be greater than the upper safe intake level of 4,000 mg/d (except for rapidly growing adolescents).

That's a scary thought when you consider that research shows a direct and significant relationship between higher dietary phosphorus intake (greater than 1,400 mg/d) and all-cause mortality in healthy people participating in NHANES III, even after adjusting for other lifestyle and demographic factors.[84]

Drink a cola each day; your bones will rapidly go away! Colas are not only especially rich in phosphoric acid, they're loaded with refined sugars and contain no redeeming calcium, magnesium, or other bone-essential minerals. A perfect recipe for bone loss!

And phosphoric acid has an absorption efficiency approaching 100%. In English, that means nearly *all* of the phosphate goes rapidly from your digestive tract into your bloodstream and thence, everywhere in your body. This phosphate additive is used in products ranging from commercial salad dressings to dairy products. And you'll find it in all carbonated cola beverages, including diet.

- Researchers speculate that, due to the extremely rapid and efficient absorption of phosphorus from phosphoric acid in cola beverages, drinking colas would lead to even greater harmful effects on bone than the same amount of phosphorus from less well-absorbed food sources.

- Other research in postmenopausal women has shown that femoral neck bone mineral density (thigh bone BMD, a marker of bone fragility and risk of hip fracture) decreased more and more as the number of cola servings consumed per week increased.

- Earlier studies, dating back to 1999, had found an association between cola consumption, low blood levels of calcium, and increased PTH levels and bone resorption in adult women.[85]

Researchers decided to look at what would happen to bone in healthy young men if a protein and calcium-rich drink (milk) was replaced with cola. For 10 days, eleven healthy young men drank 2.5 liters of cola each day, then they took a 10-day break, followed by another ten days during which they drank 2.5 liters of semi-skimmed milk every day. They ate the same basic diet throughout. During the cola period, they consumed 470 mg of calcium and 1,690 mg of phosphorus each day. During the milk period, their calcium intake was 3,500 mg and phosphorus was 3,640 mg daily. Within just 10 days of drinking cola, blood levels of phosphate, PTH, and markers of bone breakdown (serum CTx and NTx] rose dramatically.[86] [87] [88]

Remember, dietary guidelines recommend that calcium and phosphorus should be consumed in a 1:1 molar intake ratio or even a 1.5:1 ratio of calcium-to-phosphorus. In reality, the calcium: phosphorus ratio in the typical U.S. diet is nowhere near these recommended guidelines. For at least 25% of the U.S. population, the calcium: phosphorus ratio is less than 0.6. In animal studies, mass intake ratios of less than 0.5 promote bone loss—and here's the kicker—bone loss occurs even when calcium intake is adequate.[89]

The phosphate additives that are now added to virtually every processed SAD food cause bone loss. By avoiding those items, especially meat products and colas, you can go a long way towards protecting your bones.

BONE-HEALTHY ACTION ITEMS

- Avoid colas (including diet) and other products with highly absorbable phosphoric acid.
- Avoid *enhanced meat products,* so you don't get phosphorus additives on top of the phosphorus naturally occurring in meat. Eat only fresh (ideally free-range or grass-fed) meat.
- Check out the *Where Phosphates Hide in Foods* table to identify what processed foods contain phosphates and the names these additives could be disguised as on ingredients labels.

Plasticizers:
Food Packaging Destroys Your Bones

BONE ESSENTIALS

- Plastic is everywhere. Our food, drinking water, and bodies now contain plastic. In the U.S., 94% of tap water samples were contaminated with plasticizers in 2019.
- Plasticizers (such as BPA and phthalates) are chemicals that migrate out of their host plastics. Once inside our bodies, they cause inflammation that promotes bone loss.

- Plasticizers disrupt the normal production and signaling of our thyroid, parathyroid, adrenal, and sex hormones.
- Women with higher urine levels of phthalates have lower hip and femur BMD and are at higher risk of osteoporosis.
- BPA directly suppresses osteoblast and osteoclast development, inhibiting bone renewal, and also inhibits the secretion of calcitonin, a hormone that counterbalances PT hormone's effect of removing calcium from bone when blood levels are low.
- BPA even increases your risk of being overweight.

Your body is being invaded by plastic, and that's really bad news for your bones.

Plastic is everywhere—including your food and drinking water. In 2019, *microplastics* were detected in 83% of tap water samples from around the world. The highest concentrations were seen in the U.S., where 94% of tap water samples were contaminated.

Research presented at a gastroenterology conference in Vienna informed us that microplastic, tiny bits of plastic from decomposing plastic bottles, containers, plastic wrap, and plastic grocery bags—which have been showing up in our oceans, fish, and tap water—are now residing inside us! The real concern is not the shards of plastic in our digestive tract themselves, but rather that the chemicals they contain leach out during gut passage, get absorbed, and accumulate in human tissues.

Plasticizers, **the chemicals in plastic, cause inflammation and bone loss** by disrupting the functioning of our endocrine system, the glands that secrete all our hormones. Plasticizers disrupt the normal production and signaling of our thyroid, parathyroid, adrenal, and sex hormones. And don't forget vitamin D, whose active form (1,25-D) is a hormone with numerous endocrine effects.[90 91 92 93]

Normally, the interplay among all our hormones is carefully orchestrated—until plasticizers nuke it. Obviously, throwing a wrench into the workings of our endocrine system can make lots of things go awry—including our ability to rebuild and maintain healthy bones. Plasticizers are not your bones' friends.

The Dangers of Phthalates and BPA: Common Food Packaging Materials

We focus here on two very commonly used plasticizers—*phthalates* and *bisphenol A* (BPA), both of which you are definitely exposed to. We'll share research-backed ways you can protect yourself against these bone-busting compounds.

Phthalates are incorporated into plastic to increase its flexibility, transparency, and durability. They're found in plastic bottles, all kinds of containers, food wraps and packaging, medical device tubing, water fountains, soda dispensers, and the equipment used to add liquids in the production of processed foods. And most distressing to Lara, the plastic tubing in espresso machines!

They're also present in places you might not expect, such as food additives, controlled release medicine, children's toys, cosmetics, and perfume. About a third of nail polishes, glosses, enamels, and hardeners contain phthalates, as well as many shampoos, sunscreens, skin lotions, and insect repellents. By design, phthalates are not strongly bound to the plastic to which they are added, so phthalates are highly susceptible to leaching. Plasticizers migrate out of their host plastics, and once in our bodies, disrupt normal endocrine function and affect our bones.

While phthalates make plastic soft, BPA makes plastic hard. BPA-based plastic is clear and tough and is made into a variety of common consumer goods, such as plastic water bottles. Epoxy resins containing BPA are used to line water pipes, as coatings on the inside of many food and beverage cans, and in making the thermal paper used in sales receipts. And, like phthalates, BPA is bad news for your bones:

- In cell studies, BPA directly suppresses both osteoclast and osteoblast cell development and shuts down bone alkaline phosphatase (B-ALP), an enzyme used by osteoblasts in new bone formation.[94]

- BPA also inhibits Wnt signaling, which is a key part of the process through which new osteoblasts develop, and then causes any osteoblasts that still manage to grow up to commit suicide.[95][96]

- Both phthalates and BPA decrease circulating levels of vitamin D (25[OH]D) in adults, increasing the risk of deficiency by about 20%.[97]

BPA also harms bone by inhibiting *calcitonin* secretion. Calcitonin is a hormone secreted by the thyroid gland that lowers blood levels of calcium. In other words, it opposes the effects of parathyroid hormone (PTH), which causes the release of calcium from our bones to increase levels in the bloodstream when needed. When PTH has done its job, and blood levels of calcium have been restored to normal, calcitonin is supposed to be secreted to stop further calcium removal from our bones. BPA prevents that from happening.

BPA can even make you fat! A study found a correlation between BPA plasma levels and waist circumference, which indicates belly fat (a.k.a., visceral adipose tissue)—the worst, most inflammatory kind of fat.

What can you do to protect yourself? Fortunately, plenty! Overall, food packaging is *the* major source of exposure to phthalates and BPA. Happily, a study published in *Environmental Health Perspectives* has now provided proof that simply eating a diet composed primarily of fresh, not plastic-packaged foods, significantly reduces the level of these chemicals in our bodies in just three days.

During the 3-day fresh food diet in this study, participants ate organic meals with no canned food and minimal plastic packaging and stored their food in glass and stainless-steel containers. Their average urine levels of phthalates dropped by more than 50%, and levels of BPA dropped by more than 60%.[98] [99] [100]

By avoiding food packaging, plastic water bottles, and other plastic or plastic-lined containers, you can go a long way towards reducing these chemicals in your body. A tool that can help is Detox Me, a free smartphone app from the Silent Spring Institute (www.silentspring.org/detox-me-app-tips-healthier-living), which walks you through simple, research-based tips to reduce your exposure to plasticizers and other harmful chemicals.

BONE-HEALTHY ACTION ITEMS

- Eat fresh or frozen food! BPA and phthalates migrate from the linings of cans and plastic packaging into food and drinks.
- Cook and eat more meals at home, preferably with fresh, organic ingredients. Studies have shown that people who eat

more meals prepared outside the home have higher levels of BPA. If you absolutely loathe cooking or truly don't have time, buy organic prepared foods from your grocery store delicatessen. Transfer food from plastic to glass containers as soon as you get home.

- Store your food and beverages in glass, ceramic or stainless steel. Plastic containers leach chemicals into food and drinks, especially if they are fatty (meat, fish, cheese, full-fat dairy products, dips, and oils) or acidic (vinegar, salad dressings, juices, and many condiments).

- Never microwave anything in plastic! *Microwave safe* means the container won't melt—not that cooking in it is safe for your health. Warmer temperatures increase the rate at which chemicals leach into your food and drinks. Use only heat-resistant glass or ceramic containers to cook or reheat your food.

- Brew your morning java the old-fashioned way. Automatic coffee makers may have BPA and phthalates in their plastic containers and tubing. Call the manufacturer to find out. If your coffee maker flavors every cup with plasticizers, use a glass French press and start your day without a dose of phthalates and BPA.

Fluoride:
in Toothpaste and Tap Water Damages Your Bones

BONE ESSENTIALS

- Fluoride contains the toxic chemical element fluorine. As the strongest oxidizer currently known, fluorine easily rebuffs the liver's attempts to prepare it for excretion and passes into the bloodstream, from which it is rapidly distributed to all tissues, including our bones.

- High levels of fluorine overwhelm bone cells' ability to protect themselves with glutathione, then shuts down osteoblasts, increases osteoclast production and activity, and triggers the secretion of PT hormone, whose chronic elevation causes bone loss.

- Although fluoride activates both osteoblasts and osteoclasts, so fluoride may increase bone mass, the newly formed bone lacks normal structure and strength.
- Fluorine exposure also reduces levels of copper, zinc, manganese, and other required trace minerals involved in building bone.

Fluoride, a common element in the earth's crust, is naturally present everywhere— in the soil, rocks, plants, and water all over the earth. Many industrial processes use or release fluorides, including coal burning, oil refining, aluminum production, and the production of phosphate fertilizers. (Yet another reason to eat organically grown foods!)

Our primary sources of exposure to fluorides are our food and water, and fluoride-containing dental products, such as toothpaste. Despite its association with preventing tooth decay, fluoride may hurt your health, including your teeth as well as your bones. The fluoridation of public drinking water, in an effort to prevent tooth decay, has resulted in a significant increase in dental fluorosis—a disturbance in the production of dental enamel when teeth are developing (between the ages of 3 months and 8 years). This causes tiny white streaks or specks in the tooth enamel, and in more severe cases, pitting and brown discolorations. As of 2005, 23% of people in the U.S. age 6 to 39 had mild or worse dental fluorosis.[101] High-systemic (whole-body) fluoride exposures can cause skeletal fluorosis, a condition in which bones become hard and brittle, ligaments calcify, and bone pain and loss result.

How does fluoride weaken bone? Fluoride activates both osteoblasts and osteoclasts. At very low and localized concentrations in dental implants, fluoride encourages osteoblast production and new bone formation. At higher concentrations, fluoride blocks new bone formation.

While fluoride may increase bone mass, the newly formed bone lacks normal structure and strength. Under a microscope, the crystallization pattern of bone from fluoride-treated animals and humans reveals itself to be abnormal. In *trabecular bone*, the spongy interior portion of our bones, fluoride increases bone volume and thickness but does not increase connectivity. This lack of trabecular connectivity reduces bone's ability to resist fracture despite the increase in bone mass.

Fluoride releases fluorine, which is toxic. Fluoride is a compound that contains the chemical element *fluorine,* a highly toxic, reactive, yellowish-green gas. Fluoride is found in higher concentrations in the southern United States and in all areas where the waters are soft, alkaline, and calcium-deficient. Fluoride compounds that occur naturally in drinking water are almost totally bioavailable—at about 90%! The fluorine they contain is virtually all absorbed from the gastrointestinal tract and enters our circulatory system.

At that point, fluorine reacts with stomach acid to form hydrogen fluoride. Hydrogen fluoride is absorbed from the gastrointestinal tract and sent into the portal vein, which delivers it to the liver. In the liver, harmful compounds are usually transformed into something we can send out of the body in urine or bile. Fluorine, however, is itself such a strong oxidizer—the strongest oxidizer currently known—that it easily rebuffs the liver's attempts to prepare it for excretion and passes into the bloodstream, from which it is rapidly distributed to all tissues, including our bones.[102] The primary way the body gets rid of fluorine is through the kidneys. Unfortunately, excessive dietary acidity impairs the kidneys' ability to excrete fluorine, so more ends up in tissues, such as teeth and bones.

Once inside bones, fluorine attacks through several mechanisms:

- Fluorine is so toxic that it overwhelms bone cells' ability to produce their most important antioxidant defender, glutathione. Once defenses have been eliminated, fluorine is free to shut down osteoblasts and cause inflammation that increases osteoclast production and activity.[103] [104]

- Fluorine accumulates in bone, binding to and shutting down alkaline phosphatase, an enzyme that, in bone, is involved in the production of osteoblasts. Fluorine exposure also reduces levels of copper, zinc, manganese, and other trace minerals that enzymes involved in building bone require for their activity. The end result: osteoblast production and bone-building stops.[105]

- Our bones are largely composed of calcium compounds, up to 50% of which are hydroxyapatite. Fluorine converts hydroxyapatite to fluorapatite. This changes bones' crystalline structure, delays further mineralization with calcium, and greatly reduces bone quality and resilience.[106]

- Hydrogen fluoride reacts with calcium to form an insoluble salt, CaF_2. This salt then must be eliminated by the body, and as it goes, takes out calcium from the bone matrix.[107]

- Fluoride induces the secretion of parathyroid hormone, which triggers the production of osteoclasts. Increased fluoride intake has been repeatedly shown to cause hyperparathyroidism, which causes bone loss. (See Hyperparathyroidism, Chapter 4.)

Protect your teeth without fluoride. The Institute of Medicine's 1997 guidelines on fluoride say 3 mg/d and 4 mg/d for adult women and men, respectively, are adequate to prevent tooth decay with upper limits at 10 mg/d for anyone older than 8 years. However, even that lowest amount of fluoride may be unnecessary for dental health.

Consider choosing a toothpaste or mouthwash with xylitol, a natural sugar our bodies produce in tiny amounts and is also found in very tiny amounts in berries and vegetables. Xylitol not only prevents plaque formation and cavities but has also been shown to reverse developing cavities and restore healthy tooth enamel—safely.[108] Studies demonstrate that 4 to 12 grams of xylitol per day is effective, and this is most easily delivered in xylitol-containing chewing gums, which keep the xylitol they contain in contact with teeth longer.

Be aware of foods and beverages with high fluoride content. See table below and access the USDA's list of the fluoride content in more than 400 foods (data.nal.usda.gov – bit.ly/3ew71Xd).

Tea contains fluoride, the amount depending on variety and origin. The Camellia sinensis plant is the source of tea leaves for white, green, black and oolong teas. (And matcha, which is very finely ground up tea leaves). As the Camellia sinensis plant grows, its roots efficiently absorb fluoride from the soil, depositing most of it in the leaves, which are used to produce tea. Green, black, and oolong tea, which are made from older, more mature leaves, contain up to 20 times more fluoride than white tea, made from younger tea leaves and buds.

According to the World Health Organization, the soil in Japan is naturally lower in fluoride than that in China, so Japanese green tea contains less fluoride than Chinese green tea. WHO also notes several areas of the world where high naturally occurring fluoride concentrations affect tea crops and drinking water: India, Sri Lanka, parts of Africa and the Middle East.

Bottom line: Unless you are drinking more than 2 to 3 cups of tea each day, don't worry about its fluoride content. Tea is loaded with anti-inflammatory phenols with bone protective effects. To minimize your fluoride intake, drink white tea or get the best quality Japanese green tea and matcha you can find.[109]

Fluoride Content of Common Foods and Beverages	
Water	**mg/100 grams (3 oz)**
Municipal water, tap (mid-west)	99
Municipal water, tap (south)	93
Municipal water, tap (northeast)	74
Well water, tap (mid-west)	53
Municipal water, tap (west)	51
Well water, tap (west)	24
Well water, tap (south)	10
Well water, tap (northeast)	9
Other Beverages	**mg/100 grams (3 oz)**
Tea, instant (prepared with tap water)*	335
Tea, brewed (microwave)*	322
Tea, brewed (decaffeinated)*	269
Grape juice white	204
Wine (white)	202
Carbonated water, fruit flavored	105
Wine (red)	105
Fruit juice drink (apple)	104
Grape/apple juice blend (Juicy Juice)	102
Coffee	91
Foods	**mg/100 grams (3 oz)**
Raisins	234
Crab, canned	210
Shrimp, canned	201
Shrimp, fried	166
Fish sticks, baked	134
French fries (McDonald's)	115
Oatmeal, cooked	72

Source: data.nal.usda.gov/ – Shortcut link: bit.ly/USDA-Fluoride

BONE-HEALTHY ACTION ITEMS

- Include calcium-rich foods in your diet to reduce fluoride's bioavailability.[110]
- Avoid fluoride-containing toothpaste. Check the ingredient list for sodium fluoride (NaF), stannous fluoride (SnF_2), olaflur (an organic salt of fluoride), or sodium monofluorophosphate (Na_2PO_3F).
- Use toothpaste, mouthwash, or gum containing xylitol to promote dental health.
- Avoid or limit foods containing high fluoride content, such as tea, whose leaves contain more fluoride than any other plant. Drink tea grown in Japan where the soils contain less fluoride and don't consume more than 3 cups of tea daily.

CHAPTER 3

Heavy Metals Poison Your Bones

Remember back in the `70s when heavy metal meant Led Zeppelin? Unfortunately, today when we hear *heavy metal*, we're talking about environmental poisons, not music. Lead accumulates in our bones over decades. Cadmium in our soil and chemically grown food prevents bone mineralization. Mercury harms the kidneys. All of them destroy our bones. Let's look at the latest research on each of these bone poisons.

Gasoline:
Now Unleaded but Bone-Breaking Lead Remains in Bones

BONE ESSENTIALS

- Current exposure to lead continues from old pipes and paint in our homes, batteries, ammunition, and other industrial uses.
- If you're 50 or older, the lead in the gasoline you encountered during your teenage years got stored away in your growing bones. For women, that lead comes out as you reach menopause/peri-menopause.
- Lead decreases osteoblast formation, increases osteoclast activity, causes kidney disease, prevents your kidneys from activating vitamin D, and promotes high blood pressure.
- Having low blood levels of lead only tells you about recent exposure, not how much is lurking in your bones.

Beginning in the 1970s, the EPA began banning lead in gasoline, paint, and for other uses. Lead levels in the population have dropped significantly since then, and we've been reassured that lead is no longer a problem. Unfortunately, that's not true!

- Accumulated lead remains in the bones of virtually all of us over age 50, as we were exposed during our youth when growing bones are most vulnerable. Children absorb 40% of a dose of lead, compared to 10% in adults, and retain 30% of lead absorbed compared to 1% in adults.[111]
- A paper published in March 2019 in *Reviews on Environmental Health* notes: "…in the United States exposure sources include paint, the industrial legacy of lead exposure and batteries. In high-income countries, the legacy of lead exposure keeps populations continuously exposed."[112]

More than 90% of the lead in our bodies resides in our bones, which are constantly being remodeled. In the process of bone resorption, that quarantined lead is released into our blood right along with calcium. As we enter menopause (or andropause – men are not immune!), our rate of bone loss increases, releasing more of the sequestered lead from our bones.[113] Clear associations have now been found between increased bone levels of lead and osteoporosis, kidney disease, cataracts, high blood pressure, heart disease, and death rate.[114]

Continued lead exposure puts everyone at risk. Lead continues to contaminate many U.S. homes. In 2006, an estimated 22% of U.S. homes—23.2 million—still contained lead-based paint. Paint deteriorates, flakes, and becomes lead-laden dust in the air, on the floors, in bedspreads and pillows—you get the idea. Copper water pipes used lead-containing solder prior to 1987. Worse, houses built before the 1930s may have lead pipes. If the water supply is at all acidic or corrosive, lead leaches into the water as happened in Flint, Michigan, resulting in thousands of poisoned children. Remember, children are particularly sensitive to lead's effects. Current research has led to strong recommendations to further lower the presently allowed blood lead level to minimize chronic cumulative lead toxicity.[115] [116]

How Lead Promotes Bone Loss – Let Us Count the Ways

Lead decreases the formation of our bone-building osteoblasts, while keeping bone-removing osteoclast production and activity rolling right along. To finish this death blow to our bones, lead short-circuits our ability to absorb calcium by harming our kidneys, preventing them from activating vitamin D into 1,25-D, the form in which it helps us absorb calcium. [117] [118] [119]

Hormone-Affecting Levels of Uric Acid: The retention of uric acid, another damaging effect of lead on the kidneys, disrupts hormone production in premenopausal women by preventing progesterone production during the menstrual cycle. This significantly inhibits the production of our bone-building cells, the osteoblasts. (This also results in infertility in women and reduces sperm count in men. Couples trying unsuccessfully to conceive may wish to consider testing for heavy metal toxicity.)[120]

High Blood Pressure: Higher lead levels, as measured in the tibia (shinbone), are a significant predictor of hypertension (high blood pressure), with above-average levels in study participants increasing their chance of having high blood pressure by 24%. High blood pressure indicates and causes chronic inflammation in our blood vessels and chronic inflammation activates osteoclasts.

Kidney disease: Like other heavy metals (e.g., mercury and cadmium), lead has a bunch of toxic effects, resulting in kidney tissue becoming fibrotic, scarred, and atrophied. Since the kidneys are the primary place where vitamin D is converted into the form in which it works for us, malfunctioning kidneys undercut our ability to absorb calcium.

The Scientific Scoop on Lead's Nefarious Mechanisms of Bone-Destruction

Lead makes you fat and your bones skinny via its effects on several bone-cell signaling pathways:

Lead slams the production of a transcription factor in bone marrow cells called *Cbfa-1/RunX-2* (core-binding factor-1/runt-related transcription factor-2). *How do they come up with these names?* Fortunately, you don't have to remember this one or even the acronym. The important point is that the bone marrow cells in question (mesenchymal stem cells) are the precursors for both bone-building osteoblasts and fat-storing adipocytes (fat cells). Mesenchymal stem cells' choice to become osteoblasts instead of fat cells is dependent upon Cbfa-1/RunX-2. Lead shuts down Cbfa-1/RunX-2, so precursor bone marrow cells grow up to be fat cells, not osteoblasts.

Lead increases the production of *sclerostin* and *peroxisome proliferator-activated receptor-γ* (PPAR-γ), both of which prevent the formation of new bone.

- **Sclerostin** stops the bone-building process. Sclerostin is produced by osteocytes—which are what osteoblasts turn into after they begin laying down the matrix for new bone. Sclerostin's job is to shut down proteins involved in bone formation in areas where new bone formation has already been completed or where new bone formation is not needed.

It may sound like sclerostin is a very undesirable fellow but think about what would happen to you if bone formation got out of control and kept going rampantly on and on. You wouldn't be able to think about this for very long because the bones in your skull would grow until no room remained for your brain. You'd die before that though as the nerves in your spinal column would be squished to smithereens by expanding vertebral bones.

Normally, sclerostin is produced and activated just enough to gently prevent excessive or unneeded bone formation. When lead is around, however, sclerostin production escalates to the point that it slams the brakes on all bone formation.

- **PPAR-γ** is a cellular receptor that gets turned on by the insulin-sensitizing drugs, the glitazones (rosiglitazone and pioglitazone) and is the reason these drugs cause bone loss. *Why?* Because PPAR-γ's activation in mesenchymal stem cells (those precursor cells for both osteoblasts and fat cells we just talked about) causes these precursor cells to become fat cells, not osteoblasts. Lead ramps up PPAR-γ activation.

The combination of these factors—Cbfa-1/RunX-2, sclerostin, and PPARγ— is called the Wnt/β-catenin pathway. When Cbfa-1/RunX-2 is not inhibited, and sclerostin and PPAR-γ are, this pathway builds bone. Your bones are like a beautifully orchestrated symphony in which each instrument has certain notes to play. Lead destroys this harmony, distorting the normal balance among the bone-remodeling actions of the Wnt/β-catenin pathway.

Blood levels of lead only show recent exposure, not levels in bone. Testing your *blood* level of lead shows only recent environmental exposure, such as from old piping or exposure to lead dust from ammunition. (During a daily firearm training course at an indoor range, blood-lead levels were found to have doubled in participants after 6 weeks.)

You need to test *bone* lead level to evaluate the amount your bones have accumulated over a lifetime's exposure, particularly if you are elderly (65 years or older – which sounds younger and younger to us as we are now 72 (Lara) and 73 (Joe). If you are doing the right things—healthy diet, supplementing with proper nutrients, and doing weight-bearing exercise—but still losing bone, consider testing if lead or other toxic metals could be why. (See Lab Tests, Chapter 10.)

BONE-HEALTHY ACTION ITEMS

- Check your house for the presence of lead in old paint and pipes.
- If over 65 and losing bone despite healthy eating and exercise, consider having your *bone lead levels* tested for cumulative lead exposure.

Cadmium:
Destroys Bones in Amounts Well Below OSHA Safe Levels

BONE ESSENTIALS

- Recent studies confirm urine cadmium levels of 0.50 mcg/g creatinine—far lower than the 3 mcg/g OSHA considers safe—damage the kidneys and promote bone loss, fragility, and fractures.
- The use of high-phosphate fertilizers, which contain cadmium in amounts up to 300 mg/kg, on conventionally grown foods is the primary source of cadmium-related osteoporosis in U.S. women 50 or older.
- Twenty-one percent of osteoporosis prevalence among women 50 years or older may be attributable to cadmium.
- Cadmium causes bone loss by disrupting the kidney's production of 1,25-D, the active hormonal form of vitamin D, increasing calcium loss in urine, interfering with osteoblasts' bone-building actions, and increasing the formation and bone-resorbing activities of osteoclasts.

In 1968, mining operations introduced cadmium into the water supply in Toyama Prefecture, Japan. People eating the local rice, which was grown with the poisoned water, developed *itai-itai* (it hurts, it hurts), a disease that caused kidney stones, kidney failure, bone pain (osteomalacia), and osteoporosis.

Cadmium accumulates for decades in the kidneys and bone. Those afflicted with *itai-itai* disease had more than 10 times the urinary cadmium level of 3 mcg/g creatinine the U.S. Occupational Safety and Health Administration (OSHA) deems safe.[121] [122]

Yet, recent studies indicate that urinary excretion of cadmium greater than 0.50 mcg/g creatinine damages the kidneys and promotes bone loss, fragility, and fractures.[123] Like lead, there is no *safe* level.

- In 1999, a study in Belgium of populations living in the vicinity of zinc smelters found that urinary cadmium excretion of just 1 mcg/g creatinine—just one third of OSHA *safe* level—was associated with a 73% increased risk of bone fractures in women and a 60% increased risk of height loss in men.

- In China, osteoporosis prevalence in women 50 or older who lived near a smelter, increased from 34% in the control group (less exposure) to 51.9% in heavily polluted areas.

- Early kidney damage, osteoporosis, and a 300% increased risk of fractures were found in the 1,000 people living in Southern Sweden near a nickel-cadmium battery plant. Urinary cadmium levels of 3.48 mcg/g creatinine—just over the OSHA safe level—were found to cause osteoporosis.

- Another Swedish study assessed the cadmium urine levels of 2,688 women along with a DEXA scan of their bone mineral density (BMD). Those with cadmium levels of 0.75 or greater mcg/g creatinine had a much greater chance of osteoporosis—245% at the femoral neck and 197% at the lumbar spine—than those with less than 0.50 mcg/g creatinine.

In the last study, results were even more dramatic for women who didn't smoke, increasing osteoporosis risk of those with higher cadmium levels to 347% at the femoral neck and 326% at the lumbar spine. Cadmium in cigarette smoke, inhaled into the lungs, is more effectively absorbed than food sent through the digestive tract. However, this study pokes holes in the belief that, if we don't smoke, our bones are not at risk of osteoporosis from cadmium toxicity.

Dietary cadmium exposure, shown to damage bones, is increasing. When researchers drew data from two National Health and Nutrition Examination Surveys (NHANES III) involving 4,258 women age 50 or older, their findings on cadmium and risk for osteoporosis were shocking.

- Women with urinary cadmium levels between 0.50 and 1.00 mcg/g creatinine (compared to those under 0.50 mcg/g) had a 43% greater risk for hip-BMD-defined osteoporosis.

- Of U.S. women 50 or older, 73% are estimated to have cadmium body burdens above 0.50 mcg/gram creatinine—a level repeatedly found significant for increased risk for osteoporosis and other diseases.[124]

This data and other recent studies suggest that 21% of osteoporosis prevalence among women 50 years or older may be attributable to cadmium. Another interesting finding from NHANES III was that smokers didn't show a statistically increased risk. Instead, the SAD is our primary source of cadmium.[125] [126]

Small levels of cadmium may be found in all foods, as the metal exists at low levels in the earth's crust. However, high-phosphate fertilizers used on conventionally grown crops can contain cadmium in amounts up to 300 mg/kg, causing high cadmium content in agricultural soils. (Another reason to eat organically grown produce!)[127] [128]

An FDA study points to dietary cadmium exposure increasing 26% from 1990 through 2003, up to 11.06 mcg per person per day. This translates to 21% of the *safe* intake of cadmium after just a week.[129]

The most recently conducted studies clearly show it is *dietary cadmium*, not *smoking*, that is the primary source of cadmium-related osteoporosis risk in the U.S. female population 50 years or older. While comparable research has not yet been done on aging men, we predict it will reveal a serious osteoporosis risk from dietary cadmium.

How Cadmium Destroys Our Bones

Cadmium prevents bone mineralization thus directly causing osteoporosis by:

- Inhibiting calcium's incorporation into bone cells.

- Inhibiting alkaline phosphatase, an enzyme involved in new bone formation produced by osteoblasts.

- Diminishing osteoblasts' ability to mineralize bone and produce collagen. Cadmium also lowers bone's collagen content by stimulating osteoclasts, which break down the collagen matrix in bone.

- Activating gene expression of toxic response pathways in bone cells, which further stimulate osteoclasts' bone resorption.

Cadmium harms the kidneys, which indirectly leads to bone damage, by:

- Disrupting parathyroid hormone's signaling to kidney cells to convert 25(OH)D, the form in which vitamin D circulates in the bloodstream, into 1,25-D, the form in which vitamin D increases our intestinal absorption of calcium. (See Vitamin D, page 164.)
- Cadmium also directly inhibits the kidney enzymes that convert 25(OH)D into 1,25-(OH)2D3.
- Cadmium damages the kidney's filtering and reabsorption apparatus (specifically, the renal tubules), causing even more calcium to be lost in the urine. High urine levels of calcium, a condition called hypercalciuria, are considered a possible marker of cadmium exposure.

Other sources of cadmium exposure: Clearly, those who aren't near a smelter or mining operation are still at risk for cadmium poisoning, largely through conventionally grown food.[130] However, coal burning releases cadmium into the air, where it deposits on agricultural lands, in the water supply, on our streets, our backyards, our windows—basically everywhere. Our homes can become exposure sources, as we track cadmium in on our shoes, pull it in with window fans, or find ourselves near someone who is smoking. Cadmium is also used in rechargeable nickel-cadmium batteries, in some paint pigments (notably, cadmium red), and even in some cosmetics.[131]

BONE-HEALTHY ACTION ITEMS

- Eat organic vegetables, fruits, grains, eggs, and meats. Plants grown with high-phosphate fertilizers will accumulate more cadmium as will farm animals fed such foods.
- Don't smoke and avoid those who do.
- Avoid eating oysters, scallops, and shellfish from areas with high cadmium levels, such as coastal areas along New England and the Great Lakes.
- Prevent cadmium contamination of your home by using HEPA air filters and cleaning your windowsills, screens, and fans regularly. Avoid wearing shoes in your home. Leave them in a shoe rack in your garage or next to your front door.

- Don't touch unprotected or damaged nickel-cadmium (Ni-Cd) rechargeable batteries.
- Consume zinc-rich foods as this important trace mineral competes with cadmium.
- Be wary of children's jewelry imported from China; an analysis by the Consumer Product Safety Commission found 12% contained at least 10% cadmium (with one item containing 91% cadmium).[132]
- Get tested to determine your body burden of cadmium, ideally lower than 0.50 mcg/g creatinine. (See Lab Tests, Chapter 10.)

Mercury:
Destroys Bone by Harming the Kidneys

BONE ESSENTIALS

- Mercury is everywhere in the environment, but our most common sources of exposure are dental amalgams and fish, with lesser amounts coming from air, water, some vaccinations, and cosmetics.
- Mercury accumulates in and damages the kidneys, interfering with their activation of vitamin D and increasing calcium loss in urine.
- Mercury is directly toxic to brain cells and has been associated with an increased risk of autism, cognitive decline, and Alzheimer's disease.
- Mercury poisoning plays a significant role in high blood pressure, cardiovascular disease, stroke, mitochondrial dysfunction, and oxidative stress—all of which increase chronic inflammation, promoting excessive osteoclast activation and bone loss.

Mercury and its compounds have been used for thousands of years, long before its toxic effects were known. The liquid metal's unique properties have made it useful for pigments, cosmetics, scientific equipment, and a number of industrial applications. Mercury may be lurking in your eye drops, mascara, or vaccinations (as thiomersal).[133] The burning of coal, disposal of municipal and hazardous waste, gold mining, and cement production also release mercury into the environment.

Inorganic mercury compounds, found in some vaccinations and cosmetics, are water-soluble with a bioavailability of 7% to 15% after ingestion, and accumulate mainly in the kidneys, causing damage.

However, our most common sources of mercury exposure are *silver* dental fillings (amalgams) and fish. Of the types of mercury, these are also the most readily absorbed.

- Elemental mercury, such as from dental amalgams, is lipid (fat)-soluble and can cross the blood-brain barrier. This is mainly inhaled, causing rapid absorption and distribution to all major organs, though primarily the brain and the kidneys.[134]

- Methylmercury, found in contaminated fish, accounts for the majority of human exposure. This mercury compound is absorbed from the gastrointestinal tract into the bloodstream and rapidly to target organs, primarily the kidneys.[135]

Mercury harms bones, starting with the kidneys. A few hours after exposure to methylmercury, approximately 50% of a dose of mercury has made its way to the kidneys where it's highly toxic. If the dosage is high enough, kidney cells swell, rupture, and die within as little as 12 hours. Even below the levels that kill kidney cells, methylmercury causes a series of bone-damaging results:

- As mercury continues to accumulate and the kidney's supply of defensive antioxidants decreases, the uncontrolled *oxidative stress* (free-radical overload) damages the kidney's delicate filtration system (glomeruli) which become fibrous.[136]

- A damaged kidney's ability to convert vitamin D into its active form is greatly impaired.

- By preventing vitamin D's activation, mercury causes hypocalcemia (low blood calcium), which triggers calcium's withdrawal from bone.

Emerging research is also showing that mercury poisoning plays a significant role in high blood pressure, cardiovascular disease, stroke, mitochondrial dysfunction, and oxidative stress.[137] [138] *What do these conditions have in common?* All promote chronic inflammation, which promotes excessive activation of osteoclasts, excessive bone loss, and osteoporosis.

How to lighten your body's load of bone-destroying mercury. If you have *silver* dental fillings, have them removed by an ecologically trained dentist who will know how to minimize the release of mercury (so it does not end up in your brain or your kidneys) during extraction.

Eat smaller species of wild-caught fish, such as salmon and sardines. The Natural Resources Defense Council lists which fish are lowest in mercury (www.nrdc.org/stories/smart-seafood-buying-guide).

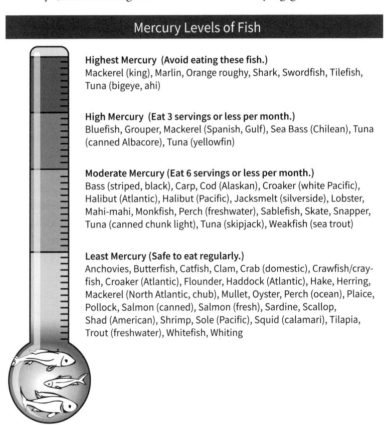

Mercury Levels of Fish

Highest Mercury (Avoid eating these fish.)
Mackerel (king), Marlin, Orange roughy, Shark, Swordfish, Tilefish, Tuna (bigeye, ahi)

High Mercury (Eat 3 servings or less per month.)
Bluefish, Grouper, Mackerel (Spanish, Gulf), Sea Bass (Chilean), Tuna (canned Albacore), Tuna (yellowfin)

Moderate Mercury (Eat 6 servings or less per month.)
Bass (striped, black), Carp, Cod (Alaskan), Croaker (white Pacific), Halibut (Atlantic), Halibut (Pacific), Jacksmelt (silverside), Lobster, Mahi-mahi, Monkfish, Perch (freshwater), Sablefish, Skate, Snapper, Tuna (canned chunk light), Tuna (skipjack), Weakfish (sea trout)

Least Mercury (Safe to eat regularly.)
Anchovies, Butterfish, Catfish, Clam, Crab (domestic), Crawfish/crayfish, Croaker (Atlantic), Flounder, Haddock (Atlantic), Hake, Herring, Mackerel (North Atlantic, chub), Mullet, Oyster, Perch (ocean), Plaice, Pollock, Salmon (canned), Salmon (fresh), Sardine, Scallop, Shad (American), Shrimp, Sole (Pacific), Squid (calamari), Tilapia, Trout (freshwater), Whitefish, Whiting

Source: Natural Resources Defense Council, www.nrdc.org/health/effects/mercury/guide.asp

Enhance your Body's Protective Defenses Against Mercury

Glutathione, a powerful antioxidant, is the body's best defense against mercury toxicity. Glutathione neutralizes mercury, transports it out of cells for elimination from the body, and helps reduce the oxidative stress caused by mercury. You can support glutathione production by:

- **Decreasing glutathione depletion**. Toxins and anything that increases oxidative stress rapidly use up glutathione. Decreasing alcohol intake and cleaning up the diet helps to maintain the body's natural glutathione levels.

- **Supplementing with glutathione**. Liposomal glutathione (which can survive the digestive process) is now available as a supplement.

- **Supplementing with alpha-lipoic acid**, which can help replenish the sulfur-containing antioxidants that mercury inactivates.[139]

- **Supplementing with oral N-acetylcysteine (NAC) and/or whey**. Both are very effective delivery forms of cysteine, whose availability is the rate-limiting factor in our body's production of glutathione.

In addition, you can support mercury's elimination from your body:

- **The medication *DMSA*** (2,3-dimercaptosuccinic acid) is a water-soluble, low-toxicity molecule developed in the 1950s as an alternative to more toxic chelating agents. While IV injection of DMSA has been associated with adverse events, oral use is much gentler and rarely causes problems when at lower levels. DMSA chelates all forms of mercury (and is even more effective for lead) and has the added benefit of increasing glutathione production. Oral DMSA must be prescribed and monitored by your physician.

- **Ensure optimal intake of dietary fiber.** A key reason toxic metals like lead, cadmium, and mercury accumulate in our bodies is the dramatic reduction in dietary fiber—a drop from our evolutionary level of 100 to 150 grams/day to today's 10 to 20 grams/day. When sufficient fiber is present, we excrete toxins via stools. When insufficient fiber is present, instead of moving out of the body in stool, toxins are reabsorbed from the small intestine and sent back to the liver.

BONE-HEALTHY ACTION ITEMS

- Choose seafood and fish with lower mercury levels and limit higher-mercury species.

- Don't get *silver* dental amalgams and consider having an ecologically trained dentist remove yours if mercury toxicity could be an issue.

- Increase your glutathione stores by consuming organic dairy foods rich in whey and supplementing with N-acetyl cysteine, alpha-lipoic acid, and liposomal glutathione.

- Increase the fiber in your diet to support the elimination of toxic metals.

- Consider running the lab tests that assess body burden of heavy metals, and if indicated, oral use of DMSA as a chelating agent.

CASES FROM THE COMMUNITY

The Community is a sponsored group of more than 17,000 men and women supporting each other to build stronger bones naturally.
(www.algaecal.com/community)

Tracie's Story

"Oh my! Miracles are real!" exclaimed Tracie's post to *The Community*. "I just had my second DEXA scan today, and the results made me cry!" *What was Tracie beaming about?* In just 14 months between scans, she experienced increases in bone mineral density across the board, including her spine (+9.6%), left hip (+10.2%), and right hip (+6.9%).

At only 59 years old, Tracie was diagnosed with advanced-stage osteoporosis. Then and there, she decided to make some serious lifestyle changes. She started on a Mediterranean diet* and replaced plastic cooking utensils, sunscreens, and other household items with non-toxic alternatives. At Lara's suggestion, she sought out a naturopathic doctor who put her on collagen and bio-identical hormones, which made a world of difference. (Tracie says her husband agrees!) She also began a once-per-week weight-resistance training designed for bone health.

But what Tracie credits as making the biggest difference was starting on AlgaeCal, a plant-based calcium that includes a host of nutrients bones need, including vitamin D. Given that Tracie lives in rainy Tacoma, Washington (just a half-hour drive from us, Lara and Joe), her skin likely produces little if any vitamin D.

Tracie says she is now focused on her wellness, so she can continue to stay active in her church and enjoy spending time with her grandkids.

Lara's Take: What amazing progress! But not surprising because Tracie decided to prioritize her health and sought improvements in several areas: creating a healthier diet, eliminating toxins, testing her hormones, starting an exercise program, and getting the supplemental nutrients she needs.

See details on supplements for calcium on page 135. Learn more about the Mediterranean diet on page 355 and bioidentical hormone replacement therapy (BHRT) on page 265. For information on vitamin D levels, see page 176. Statements regarding the products above have not been evaluated by the Food and Drug Administration. These products are not intended to diagnose, treat, cure, or prevent any disease.

CHAPTER 4

Chronic Degenerative Diseases that Promote Bone Loss

All the factors driving bone loss that we've discussed so far—the standard American diet, nutrient insufficiencies, and environmental toxins—also promote the chronic degenerative diseases that plague our society. The actions of these diseases further promote bone loss in a variety of ways. The illustration below connects the dots between our ultra-processed foods, chemical agriculture, chronic diseases, and osteoporosis.

Like osteoporosis, many of these diseases sneak up on us over time. Even if you don't have a particular disease, we urge you to review this chapter as you may unknowingly have a condition that contributes to your unexplained bone loss. We include strategies to address each of these that safeguards your bone and builds your health.

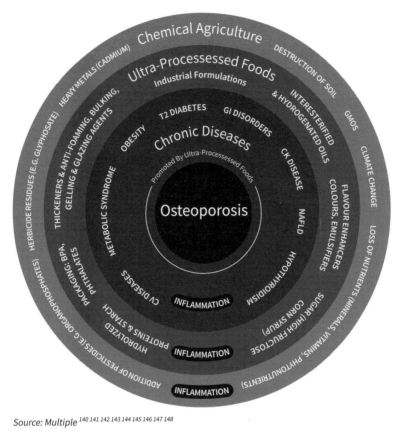

Source: Multiple [140][141][142][143][144][145][146][147][148]

Cardiovascular Diseases:
High Blood Pressure, Atherosclerosis

BONE ESSENTIALS

- Cardiovascular disease and osteoporosis share the same mechanisms and risk factors. The worse the DEXA score, the greater the risk of high blood pressure, heart attack, and stroke.
- High LDL cholesterol often leads to high blood pressure, a combination that promotes bone loss by:
  - » Reducing intestinal absorption of calcium and increasing its

elimination in urine, a combination that lowers blood levels of calcium, which is then withdrawn from bone to restore necessary blood levels.

» Damaging the kidneys, impairing their ability to reabsorb calcium and convert vitamin D into the form in which it helps us actively absorb calcium.

- Elevated LDL cholesterol promotes chronic inflammation, increasing the risk that osteoblast precursors in the lining of our blood vessels will become active and deposit calcium there.

» Osteoblast precursor cells in our blood vessels are activated by high blood sugar, high blood pressure, and oxidized (damaged) LDL cholesterol.

» Vitamin K2 activates matrix Gla protein, which prevents calcium from depositing in blood vessels.

» Exercise causes increased production of a protein produced by the liver called Fetuin-A, which also inhibits blood vessel calcification.

- If you must take a statin to lower cholesterol, check your dosage. Low doses may be protective, but higher doses triple the risk for osteoporosis in both women and men.

- If you must take a blood-pressure-lowering medication, thiazide diuretics are protective, but loop diuretics and calcium channel blockers harm bone.

It's now well accepted that cardiovascular disease and osteoporosis share many of the same mechanisms and risk factors. Each increases the likelihood that the other will be present. Bone loss and the development of calcium deposits within blood vessel walls occur in tandem. Osteoporosis is now considered a marker for increased risk of stroke and cardiovascular death—and vice versa.[149] [150] [151] [152] [153] [154] [155]

- Postmenopausal women with osteoporosis are at an increased risk for cardiovascular events that is proportional to the severity of their osteoporosis. The worse the DEXA score, the greater the risk of high blood pressure, heart attack, and stroke.[156]

- Even in postmenopausal women who have no other ailments or symptoms, a high coronary artery calcium score is associated with a greatly increased risk of having osteoporosis.[157]

What promotes cardiovascular disease? High LDL cholesterol and high blood pressure are the two key risk factors—and they are linked. High LDL cholesterol often leads to high blood pressure and increases the risk of other conditions including coronary heart disease, stroke, peripheral arterial disease and even type 2 diabetes.

When chronic inflammation oxidizes LDL cholesterol circulating in the bloodstream, plaque deposits can form in the walls of our arteries, causing them to harden and narrow, a condition called *atherosclerosis*. In response, the heart has to work much harder to pump blood through these stiff, narrowed blood vessels. As a result, blood pressure increases and remains high, and that further damages arteries and veins.

Even if your LDL cholesterol and blood pressure levels are just mildly elevated, when both risk factors are present, they interact to more quickly damage blood vessels throughout the body. One area especially vulnerable to damage is the tiny delicate blood vessels in our kidneys.[158] [159]

Why do high LDL cholesterol and/or high blood pressure promote bone loss?

Reduced nutrient delivery and waste removal. High blood pressure and atherosclerosis combine to lessen the flow of blood through your vasculature. That hinders the delivery of nutrients throughout your body—including to your bones—and the delivery of inflammatory wastes to your kidneys for excretion.[160]

Reduced intestinal absorption and increased urinary elimination of calcium, in those with high blood pressure, reduces the amount of calcium in the bloodstream. This triggers activation of the parathyroid glands, which then causes calcium to be withdrawn from bone to restore necessary blood levels.[161]

Damage to the kidneys from high blood pressure impairs their ability to reabsorb calcium and convert vitamin D into 1,25-D, the active hormonal form in which vitamin D helps us absorb calcium from our intestines.

Elevated LDL cholesterol also promotes chronic inflammation, increasing the risk of calcium deposition in blood vessels rather than bone. *Why does this happen?*

Osteoblast precursors—cells that are able to develop into calcium-depositing osteoblasts—are found not only inside our bones but also in the vascular smooth muscle within our blood vessels. When these cells are triggered into action in the vasculature, they deposit calcium in our blood vessels—which we obviously do not want.[162]

What activates these osteoblast precursor cells in our blood vessels?

- **Chronic inflammation**, delivered by *cytokines* like TNF-α and NF-κB, which rise in response to high blood-sugar levels, high blood pressure, and oxidized LDL cholesterol.

- **A lack of vitamin K2**, which activates matrix Gla protein to prevent calcium from depositing in blood vessels.

- **Low blood levels of fetuin-A**, a protein produced by the liver that inhibits blood vessel calcification.[163] Regular exercise increases production of fetuin-A. In elders, VO2max, a measure of aerobic fitness, positively correlates with fetuin-A levels. A higher VO2max (the more oxygen your body can use) equates to higher blood levels of fetuin-A and lower coronary artery calcification. *What's your VO2max?* You can find simple, quick tests to estimate it (www.shapesense.com/fitness-exercise/calculators/vo2max-calculator.shtml).

BONE-HEALTHY ACTION ITEMS

- Don't consume the standard American diet. It promotes high cholesterol, high blood pressure, and high blood sugar. (See SAD, Chapter 1.)

- Ensure your intake of vitamin K2 is optimal. (See Vitamin K, Chapter 5.)

- Get regular weight-bearing exercise! (See Exercises, Chapter 9.)

- If you must take a statin to lower cholesterol, check your dosage. Low doses (up to 10 mg/d) may be protective, but higher doses triple the risk for osteoporosis in both women and men.[164]

- If you must take a blood-pressure-lowering medication, ask your doctor if a thiazide diuretic can be prescribed. Thiazide diuretics have been shown to protect bone, while loop diuretics and calcium channel blockers harm bone.[165][166]

Chronic Kidney Disease (CKD)

BONE ESSENTIALS

- Chronic kidney disease is very common as we age and promotes bone loss by lessening our ability to absorb calcium and eliminate inflammation-producing toxins in urine.
- CKD is caused by excessive intake of phosphate additives and insufficient intake of calcium, vitamin D, K2, and magnesium.
- If you have CKD, the most commonly used markers used to check bone formation (P1NP, and CTx) won't be reliable for you because they are cleared by the kidney. Check your level of iPTH and bone-specific alkaline phosphatase (BSAP) instead.
- Loss of kidney function is not an inescapable part of aging and can be improved with the right actions.

Approximately 33% of U.S. adults age 60 or older have chronic kidney disease (CKD), and due in part to CKD's effects on bone, also have osteopenia or osteoporosis.[167] Fragility fractures are 2 to 14 times more common in CKD patients than in the general population.[168]

Why does CKD cause bone loss? CKD harms bone because it disrupts our ability to absorb calcium from our intestines and to reabsorb calcium and magnesium from our kidneys. By doing so, CKD causes secondary hyperparathyroidism and chronic inflammation. Put this all together, and it spells bone loss.[169]

The central trigger for this whole bone-breaking process is our consumption of too much phosphorus, primarily from the phosphate additives used in processed foods.[170][171] (See Phosphate Additives, Chapter 2.)

Lack of calcium, vitamin D, and vitamin K2 further promote CKD-related bone loss. Now, add to the SAD phosphate overload situation (pun intended) the fact that many of us are not consuming the nutrients critical for healthy bone remodeling:

- **Calcium**: Fewer than 10% of U.S. females age 13 years and older meet the recommended amount of dietary calcium from foods, and even with dietary supplements, few consume 1,200 mg of calcium daily. You cannot absorb calcium from your intestines that you have not consumed in the first place!

- **Vitamin D** must be present in adequate amounts to help you absorb calcium. Vitamin D levels in the majority of adults in the U.S. are below the far from optimal levels of 30 ng/mL even when accounting for dietary supplement use.[172] (See Vitamin D, Chapter 5.)
- **Vitamin K:** Recent papers also show that up to 90% of patients with CKD are vitamin K deficient and that poor vitamin K status is strongly associated with low bone mineral density and increased fracture risk in individuals with CKD.[173] (See Vitamin K, page 5.)

It's now also well established that vitamin K insufficiency promotes calcification in our blood vessels, including the tiny delicate blood vessels in the kidneys. Vitamin K2 supplementation has been shown to prevent further calcification, improve kidney blood vessel function, and improve eGFR in patients with CKD.[174] [175]

A Final Nail in The Kidney Disease Bone Health Coffin: Uremic Toxins

What are uremic toxins? Toxins produced from urea by unfriendly gut bacteria.

What's urea? Urea is a waste product of the liver's metabolism of protein and amino acids. Your liver breaks down the proteins and amino acids absorbed from your digestive system and in the process creates blood urea nitrogen (BUN). BUN is then released from your liver into your bloodstream, which takes it right to your kidneys for elimination in urine.

When your kidneys are not healthy, their ability to remove BUN is impaired, so more is left in your blood. Unfriendly gut flora, whose levels are markedly increased in individuals with CKD, can also contribute to high blood levels of BUN. Certain species convert an amino acid (tryptophan) into uremic toxins, including one (indoxyl sulfate) that has been shown to both damage osteoblasts and prevent osteoclasts from responding to PTH, causing a condition called *dynamic bone disease* typically seen in CKD patients.[176]

What promotes these unhappy changes in gut flora? The low-potassium, low-phosphorus diet recommended for patients with CKD, which is low in fiber and probiotic-rich dairy (e.g., yogurt). Yes, lowering phosphorus intake is necessary, but the way to do so is to stop consuming phosphate additives (i.e., processed foods)—not vegetables, fruit, and yogurt. The phosphorus in real food is far less effectively absorbed than the phosphate additives in processed food, and phosphate binders can be taken to further lower its absorption.

What else might help? Activated charcoal, which safely binds uremic toxins in the gut for elimination via stools. You can also supplement with beneficial gut bacteria (probiotics) and prebiotics (food for those probiotic organisms), the latter consumed via food or supplements.

If you have CKD, what blood tests can tell you how well your bone health protocol is working? You can check your level of *intact parathyroid hormone* (iPTH) and a bone formation marker called *bone-specific alkaline phosphatase* (BSAP).* The other most commonly used markers (P1NP, and CTx) won't be reliable for you because they are cleared by the kidney.

In studies of CKD patients, higher levels of PTH and BSAP were associated with lower cortical and trabecular bone density, and fracture risk was greater in patients with both low (<150 pg/mL) and high (>300 pg/mL) PTH levels, and with higher BSAP levels.[177]

How to Maintain Healthy Kidney Function at Any Age

The accepted dogma in conventional medicine is that kidney function *necessarily* worsens as we age, even if we do not develop CKD. The Baltimore Longitudinal Study of Aging, which followed 446 volunteers over 23 years, demonstrated this does not have to be the case. When excluding those with chronic diseases that affect kidney function, 36% of subjects had no decrease in kidney function. Some even showed a statistically significant *increase in function* as measured by creatinine clearance. [178]

The standard of care interpretation is that a slow decrease in eGFR is normal with aging and a low eGFR in an elderly person (anyone older than 65) is not something that can be addressed. *So, why bother looking at what can be done to improve kidney function?* Sorry, we're not buying

---

* Also known as bone alkaline phosphatase (bone-ALP, B-ALP or BAP). Since all of these terms commonly appear in research, we use them interchangeably in this book.

it! Particularly as we have seen kidney function improve in individuals who followed our recommendations:

Stay well hydrated. When the amount of fluid in the body drops too low, this activates the renin-angiotensin system, a hormone system involved in the body's control of blood pressure and fluid volume. *Angiotensinogen* is produced in the liver and sent to the kidneys, where it is ultimately converted to angiotensin I and further into angiotensin II as needed. Chronic elevation of angiotensin II is damaging to the tiny, delicate blood vessels in the kidneys.

As we age, because our sense of thirst often diminishes, we can more easily become dehydrated. Even mild dehydration triggers the production of angiotensin II, which, along with oxidative stress and chronic inflammation, is believed to be behind the age-associated decline of kidney function. Another function of water is to help the kidneys remove water-soluble toxins from the body via urine. Having enough water present helps dilute these toxins, lowering their concentration in the urine, so they are less likely to damage your kidneys on their way out.

Get plenty, but not too much protein. Older adults need about 30 to 45 grams of protein per meal (1.5 grams of protein per kilogram of body weight per day) to optimize maintenance of muscle. But you do *not* want to consume more protein than this. Overloading your system with protein is really hard on the kidneys and increases your risk of producing those uremic toxins.[179] [180]

If you're consuming more protein than 30 to 45 grams per meal, lessen your intake. And do it by decreasing your consumption of meats because their breakdown products, including urea, are hardest on the kidneys. Plus, if you eat meat, choose organic certified meat from pastured animals. Chemical and metal toxins that damage the kidneys concentrate in the flesh of conventionally raised animals, so avoiding their meat further decreases the load of toxins your kidneys must try to clear out.

Don't eat processed foods—they're loaded with sodium as well as phosphates! Researchers now think that lifelong consumption of salt at the current typical amount of 3.4 grams per day is a significant reason people's kidneys degenerate as they age. Too much salt seriously stresses the kidneys to work overtime to get rid of the excess. Decrease your consumption of salt to less than 1/2 gram—approximately 1/8 tsp—per day. If you eat processed foods, you will find this surprisingly difficult.

Phosphorus is an essential mineral for cell structure and function, but when consumed in excess—as when processed foods make up the bulk of the diet—it damages the kidneys.[181] In fact, one of the early signs of kidney failure is increasing phosphate levels in the blood. (See Phosphate Additives, Chapter 2.)

For plenty of quick, easy ideas that will help you reclaim your kitchen (and your health) from the processed food industry, we recommend a website called *The World's Healthiest Foods* (www.whfoods.org), which Joe's medical team, including Lara, created for the George Mateljan Foundation 20 years ago. Our only directive in creating this website was to provide top-quality, science-based nutritional advice. This totally free and ad-free website gets over 10 million unique visitors every month—and has for many years now.

Minimize your exposure to toxic metals:

- **Arsenic** is found everywhere in the earth's crust, accumulates naturally in aquifers and, if not filtered from the water supply, contaminates drinking water.[182] Rice and chicken are the commonly eaten foods most contaminated with arsenic.[183] [184] [185]

- **Cadmium** is a widespread environmental pollutant and kidney toxin. Chronic exposure to even low levels of cadmium can damage the kidneys and promote kidney stone formation. Cadmium both damages the kidneys' filtration system and shuts down their ability to convert vitamin D into its active hormonal form, which helps us absorb calcium. (See Cadmium, Chapter 3.)

- **Lead** causes free radical damage in the kidneys and reduces their production of the enzymes necessary to fight it, particularly glutathione, the body's most important, internally produced antioxidant.[186] Your best protection against lead is ensuring optimal intake of calcium. Both use the same absorption pathways, and calcium is preferentially absorbed over lead. (See Lead, Chapter 3.)

- **Mercury** accumulates in the kidneys, again depleting defensive antioxidants. The resulting free-radical overload damages the kidneys, which become fibrous and unable to effectively filter out toxins. In order to efficiently remove mercury from kidney cells, a chelating agent, such as DMSA, is required.[187] (See Mercury, Chapter 3.)

Ensure optimal intake of calcium, magnesium, vitamin D3, and vitamin K2. These nutrients support the health of your kidneys. Calcium restriction is no longer advised for the prevention of stone formation. In fact, diets with a calcium content ≥ 1 g/day (that are low protein, low sodium) have been associated with reduced kidney stone formation, even in stone-forming adults with high urine calcium output. Vitamin D3 is required for our active absorption of calcium.[188]

Vitamin K2 is the cofactor that activates the enzymes that ensure our healthful use of calcium: osteocalcin, which pulls calcium into our bones and matrix Gla protein, which prevents calcium from depositing in soft tissues—including our kidneys. Calcium and magnesium should be present in a 2:1 balance. Since you are consuming 1,200 mg of calcium daily, 600 mg of magnesium is required. (See Calcium and Magnesium, Chapter 5.)

One word of caution regarding the richest food sources of magnesium. Spinach is high on the list. Spinach is one of our favorite greens, but it's high in oxalates, so spinach is not a leafy green to overindulge in if your kidney function is compromised. Your best food choices for magnesium are pumpkin and sesame seeds, soy and black beans, Swiss chard, and beet greens.

If you like peanut butter, 2 tbsp. contain 49 mg of magnesium. Black beans are another great magnesium booster—just 1/2 cup contains 60 mg. Serve them with avocado (1 cup cubed contains 44 mg).

And, finally a prescription you'll love: don't forget chocolate! One ounce of dark chocolate containing at least 60% cacao will give you 50 mg of magnesium. Plus, dark chocolate (choose a low- or no-sugar version with at least 65% cacao) supports the kidneys not just with its magnesium, which improves blood flow, but also with active compounds, such as the catechins found in chocolate, which protect the kidneys from oxidative stress.

Support your kidneys by consuming citrate. Try to have two servings of *whole* citrus fruits (except grapefruit *if* you take any of the numerous medications that are detoxified by the Phase 1 liver enzyme CYP3A4) each day. Drinking lots of juice may be hard on your teeth, and juices also contain too high a dose of concentrated sugars—natural sugars but still sugar.[189]

Take a large bottle of sparkling mineral water (Lara's favorite is Pellegrino), drink about one third of it, and pour in enough lemon, lime, or orange juice (fresh squeezed, not the highly processed concentrate stuff) to fill the bottle again—then drink this throughout the day. Mineral waters are a surprisingly good source of calcium, and the added fluids and citrate will be very good for your kidneys. Citrus (lemons, oranges, and lime) and non-citrus fruits (melon) have been shown to be protective against the risk of stone formation. Be sure to choose mineral waters low in sulfur compounds as these make the mineral water acid forming. In contrast, mineral waters high in bicarbonate are alkaline forming.[190]

Increase your consumption of nitrate-rich vegetables, especially beets. Beets are brimming with naturally occurring nitrates, which convert to nitric oxide when you consume them. Nitric oxide dilates the blood vessels, leading to significantly increased blood flow. One study found that beetroot juice greatly improved the distance people with peripheral vascular disease can walk before they experience severe pain—evidence of its ability to improve circulation by dilating blood vessels.

Enjoying a delicious glass (8 oz) of beet juice spiced up with some freshly grated ginger (one cubic inch) twice a day will greatly improve microcirculation—the flow of blood through your kidneys' tiny blood vessels. Adding some freshly grated ginger to your beet juice will increase the activity of the kidneys' own antioxidant enzymes and improve kidney function—in part because ginger specifically protects the kidneys from cadmium, alcohol toxicity, and pesticides.

You can also drink ginger tea: just grate some fresh ginger to make tea, steep, and add a bit of honey. You can use ginger in salad dressings, and to add spice to soups, stir-fries, salads. Get creative! I often add both cinnamon and ginger to my homemade granola. Check out my super-easy recipe here (bit.ly/LaraGranola).[191]

BONE-HEALTHY ACTION ITEMS

- Decrease salt and phosphates—skip the processed food-like stuff and eat real organically grown foods you prepare at home.
- Drink plenty of clean water, 3 to 4 quarts daily.
- Ensure you're getting enough calcium, magnesium, vitamin D3, and K2.

- Get plenty of citrate by enjoying fresh whole citrus fruits or adding freshly squeezed juice to a large bottle of mineral water and drinking it throughout your day.
- Increase your consumption of nitrate-rich vegetables and ginger. Drink a couple of glasses of beet juice spiced with ginger daily. Or try ginger tea and add ginger to your home-cooked meals.

Chronic Gastrointestinal Conditions

When your digestive tract's ability to release and absorb nutrients is chronically short-circuited, that promotes bone loss. When your digestive tract is chronically inflamed, that also promotes bone loss.

A variety of gastrointestinal diseases, and the drugs used to manage them, produce both effects, increasing your risk for osteoporosis. Here's what you need to know about some of the most common bone-busting gastrointestinal conditions.

Gastroesophageal Reflux Disease (GERD)

BONE ESSENTIALS

- Gastroesophageal reflux disease (GERD) by itself does not cause bone loss. The proton pump inhibitors (PPIs) used to manage it do. The use of a PPI increases risk of developing osteoporosis and fractures.
- One dose of a PPI completely prevents stomach acid production for 24 hours. Stomach acid is required to digest food and to prepare minerals, including calcium, for absorption.
- If you are taking a PPI, you must work with your doctor to *slowly* get off the drug, so you do not experience the *rebound effect* of excessive stomach acid production.

Gastroesophageal reflux disease (GERD), by itself, does not cause bone loss. The proton pump inhibitors (PPIs) used to manage it do. The use of a PPI increases the risk of developing osteoporosis by 50% and is strongly associated with the risk of hip fracture:[192]

- A review of 24 observational studies, which included 319,568 hip fracture patients, found those using PPIs faced a greater risk of hip fracture: increases of 17% with a low dose, 28% with a medium dose, and 30% with a higher dose. Even short-term PPI therapy increased hip fracture risk by 20%, while long-term PPI therapy increased risk by 24%.[193]

- A meta-analysis revealed that proton pump inhibitors increase the risk of hip, spine, and any site fractures by 30%, 56%, and 16%, respectively.[194] [195]

Why do PPIs promote osteoporosis? Pop just one little PPI pill and your ability to produce stomach acid completely shuts down for a full 24 hours. Your stomach acid is needed to release calcium from its stabilizing partner, such as carbonate. That means calcium is not available for absorption in the small intestine. Ditto for magnesium and all the trace minerals your bones need to rebuild.[196]

If you're convinced that the PPI you've been taking is not your bones' friend, work with your doctor to *slowly* get off the drug. Gradually cutting your dose lessens your chances of experiencing the *rebound effect.*

What causes this rebound effect? PPIs cause chronic *hypergastrinemia*, which means excessive gastrin production. This occurs in all patients taking chronic PPIs.[197] Gastrin is a hormone produced by cells in the lowest section of the stomach, right above the pyloric sphincter, and the beginning of the small intestine.

Gastrin helps trigger our secretion of hydrochloric acid (HCl) into the stomach. When PPIs shut down stomach acid secretion, we produce more and more gastrin to try to correct this. When you stop taking the PPI, you're still producing extra gastrin, so you produce too much stomach acid. Once normal stomach acid production returns, your body will recognize that the extra gastrin is no longer needed. Gastrin overproduction, and therefore excessive stomach acid production, will cease. Slowly cutting back on the dose of PPI gives your body the chance to readjust back to normal.

Atrophic Gastritis, Hypochlorhydria, and SIBO

BONE ESSENTIALS

- Hypochlorhydria, insufficient production of stomach acid production, is typical as we age.
- Hypochlorhydria can be caused by chronic overgrowth of *Helicobacter pylori* or atrophic gastritis, chronic inflammation in the lining of the stomach.
- Atrophic gastritis affects 1 of every 3 older adults in the United States. H. pylori infection is estimated to be present in 40% to 60% of elders with no gastrointestinal symptoms and in more than 70% of elders with chronic gastrointestinal complaints.
- Hypochlorhydria can cause deficiencies of vitamin B12, vitamin C, vitamin D, folate, and calcium.

Even without the *help* of a proton pump inhibitor, lack of adequate stomach acid production—called *hypochlorhydria*—is a serious problem for your bones and an all-too-common state of affairs in the aging gut.

Unhappy changes in the gastrointestinal tract are *typical* with aging. One of the most common and damaging to our bones is the development of *atrophic gastritis*, which is medical jargon for chronic inflammation in the lining of the stomach. Atrophic gastritis, which affects about a third of older adults in the United States, results in a loss of parietal cells, the cells that secrete stomach acid:

- When you don't secrete enough stomach acid, you can't release and absorb the minerals and vitamins your bones require from your food or supplements.
- Insufficient stomach acid production promotes small intestinal bacterial overgrowth (SIBO) and impairs our ability to absorb many minerals and vitamins, including calcium, iron, vitamin K, vitamin D, folate, and B12.

Atrophic gastritis is often caused by chronic overgrowth of *Helicobacter pylori*, which is surprisingly common! *H. pylori* overgrowth is estimated to be present in 40% to 60% of elders who have *no* symptoms of gastrointestinal disease and in more than 70% of elders who do. [198] [199] [200]

How damaging is H. pylori? Well, in Japan, where the incidence of osteoporosis is far lower than in the U.S., Canada, or Europe, overgrowth of *H. pylori* increases the risk for osteoporosis by 300%.[201] [202]

Irritable Bowel Disease (Crohn's Disease, Ulcerative Colitis) and Irritable Bowel Syndrome

BONE ESSENTIALS

- Irritable bowel disease (IBD) involves inflammation in the mucosal lining of the digestive tract significant enough to result in ulcerations, the appearance of blood in the stools, and elevated levels of calprotectin (an intestinal inflammation marker).
- Those suffering from IBD disorders, which include Crohn's disease and ulcerative colitis, face a 7 times greater risk of vertebral fracture.
- Irritable bowel syndrome (IBS) is considered a *functional* condition affecting the activity of the muscles in the intestines. While IBS does not cause bloody stools or anemia as seen in IBD, both conditions lead to chronic inflammation in the GI tract and nutrient malabsorption due to an impaired ability to reabsorb bile.
- Both IBD and IBS are often accompanied by an increase in cortisol levels and deficiencies of vitamin D and omega-3s.

Both Crohn's disease and ulcerative colitis make you almost 7 times more likely to experience a vertebral fracture. Patients with IBS, which is considered less serious than IBD, still had a 95% higher risk of osteoporosis in a meta-analysis of 5 studies involving 526,633 participants. In 3 of those studies, patients with IBS also had a 58% higher risk of osteoporotic fracture.[203]

What's driving the huge increase in fracture risk seen with IBD and IBS? Inflammation in the lining of the digestive tract, often accompanied by an increase in cortisol levels and deficiencies of vitamin D and omega-3s.

- IBD features elevated levels of pro-inflammatory cytokines, especially one called *tumor necrosis factor-α* (TNF-α) which is especially damaging. TNF-α increases the rate at which osteoblasts die, inhibits the production of new osteoblasts, and increases the production of osteoclasts.

- In both IBD and IBS, increased blood levels of cortisol directly suppress osteoblast development and inhibit the production of growth hormone, estrogen, and testosterone, further accelerating bone loss.[204]

- Deficiencies of vitamin D and EPA/DHA are very common in both IBD and IBS patients. In a study including 316 IBS patients, 39% were deficient in vitamin D in the summer and 57% during the winter.[205] A study that compared fatty acid levels in 30 women with IBS to those in 39 healthy women found those with IBS had far lower levels of total omega-3s and DHA.[206] [207] [208]

Why are IBD and IBS patients more likely to be deficient in vitamin D and the omega-3s? Because their ability to reabsorb bile is impaired. We need bile to form the little transporters (called *micelles*) that enable us to absorb vitamin D, other fat-soluble vitamins, and dietary fat (including the omega-3s, which are essential fatty acids). So, individuals with IBS are at higher risk of deficiencies of both the vitamin D needed to absorb calcium and sufficient EPA/DHA.[209] [210] [211]

BONE-HEALTHY ACTION ITEMS

- Note that selective serotonin reuptake inhibitors (SSRIs), commonly prescribed to manage IBS, promote bone loss because they increase gut-derived serotonin, which binds to a receptor on the surface of newly forming osteoblasts and stops their development.[212] [213]

- Tests detecting calprotectin in stools can be used to monitor the severity of IBD, avoiding the use of a more invasive colonoscopy. However, this test will not detect IBS.

- Safe, effective treatment for gastrointestinal conditions is available. An excellent, authoritative resource is Digestive Wellness, 5th Edition by Elizabeth Lipski, Ph.D. (McGraw Hill: NY, 2020).

Hypothyroidism and Hyperthyroidism

BONE ESSENTIALS

- Hypothyroidism promotes bone loss because when the thyroid's production of hormones isn't up to speed, everything slows down, including our ability to rebuild our bones.
- Hypothyroidism is treated by providing supplemental thyroid hormone. If the dose is too low, you remain hypothyroid. If too high, you become hyperthyroid, which is even worse for your bones.
- Check your thyroid function annually and that your dose of medication is correct. The blood test should include your levels of TSH, free T4, and free T3.

Hypothyroidism—or low thyroid function—is an increasingly common problem as we age. If not identified and *properly* treated, hypothyroidism promotes bone loss.[214][215]

- Our thyroid hormones regulate our metabolic rate. When our metabolism slows down, so does our ability to rebuild our bones.[216]
- Hypothyroidism is treated by providing supplemental thyroid hormone. Finding the proper dosage can be challenging and dosage needs can change over time. In 25% of patients, the dose of levothyroxine prescribed is slightly higher than what is actually needed.
- Too much thyroid hormone produces a state of hyperthyroidism, an overactive thyroid that is even worse for our bones. Osteoclasts go into overdrive, far too rapidly demolishing bone, and slower-working osteoblasts cannot keep up. Think about it this way: A demolition team can tear down a building in a matter of hours. Replacing that building takes months![217]

You want to be right in the sweet spot—which is called *euthyroid* (meaning healthy thyroid function). Either hypo- or hyperthyroidism promotes bone loss.[218]

If you have osteopenia or osteoporosis and other symptoms, such as bone loss, hair loss, dry skin, water retention, and constipation (see box below), ask your doctor about running the blood test needed to check your thyroid function. (See Labs, Chapter 10.)

Hypothyroidism Signs and Symptoms

- Weakness, fatigue
- Dry skin
- Cool extremities
- Puffy face, hands
- Difficulty hearing
- Alopecia (hair loss)
- Paresthesia
- Bradycardia (slow heart-beat, under 60 beats per minute)

- Menorrhagia (loss of menstrual periods if premenopausal)
- Poor concentration
- Edema in the arms and legs
- Poor memory
- Delayed tendon reflex relaxation (tested in knee joint or Achilles tendon)

- Constipation
- Carpal tunnel syndrome
- Weight gain
- Dyspnea (difficulty breathing)
- Hoarse voice

Hyperparathyroidism

BONE ESSENTIALS

- Hyperparathyroidism—an overactive parathyroid gland (or glands)—is the most common cause of chronically high blood levels of calcium in postmenopausal women.

- Hyperactive parathyroid glands secrete too much parathyroid hormone (PTH), which causes bone loss by over-activating osteoclasts.

- Primary hyperparathyroidism shows up as high blood levels of calcium along with high or even normal levels of PTH. When calcium is high, PTH should be very low.

- Secondary hyperparathyroidism is not due to a problem with your parathyroid glands. It's the parathyroid glands' normal protective response to chronically low levels of calcium in the bloodstream.

- Secondary hyperparathyroidism shows up as low blood levels of calcium along with elevated levels of PTH.

Hyperparathyroidism, an overactive parathyroid gland (or glands), is the most common cause of chronically high blood levels of calcium in postmenopausal women.[219] [220] The four tiny parathyroid glands in your neck—each about the size of a grain of rice—have a big job. They maintain an adequate supply of calcium in your blood, both to maintain your bones and facilitate other essential body functions.[221]

When you have enough calcium circulating in your bloodstream, your parathyroid glands should be *asleep*. When they sense blood levels of calcium dropping too low, they *wake up* and trigger the secretion of parathyroid hormone (PTH), which is sent into your bloodstream and increases your blood levels of calcium by:

- Telling the kidneys to decrease excretion and to resorb more calcium
- Increasing the conversion of vitamin D into its active form that helps us actively absorb calcium
- Activating osteoclasts, which break down bone, releasing its calcium into the bloodstream

These effects of PTH do not promote bone loss—*unless* your parathyroid glands become *hyperactive* and start constantly dumping PTH into the bloodstream. Then, you have a big problem because:

- PTH activates osteoclasts, increasing the risk for osteoporosis.
- PTH causes the kidneys to retain more calcium, increasing the risk for kidney stone formation.

Because PTH boosts the amount of calcium in the bloodstream, hyperparathyroidism can show up as high levels of calcium in your blood (hypercalcemia) or your urine (hypercalciuria) as your body attempts to normalize blood levels of calcium by peeing it away.

Two Types of Hyperparathyroidism

Primary hyperparathyroidism, typically due to a benign tumor on the parathyroid glands, causes 90% of all chronically elevated blood levels of calcium. Primary hyperparathyroidism shows up as high blood levels of calcium along with high or even normal levels of PTH. A high calcium without a *very* low PTH indicates primary hyperparathyroidism.

Like so many other diseases, primary hyperparathyroidism is becoming increasingly common. A big study conducted in Southern California found that the incidence of primary hyperparathyroidism tripled between 1995 and 2010.[222]

The answer may be vitamin D, as not getting a sufficient amount over time increases the risk of abnormal enlargement of these glands (parathyroid gland hyperplasia). Have your blood levels of vitamin D tested to make sure you are getting enough. For Caucasians, Hispanics, or Asians an optimal blood level is 60 to 80 ng/mL. For African Americans, who utilize vitamin D more efficiently, an optimal level is 40 to 60 ng/mL. While African American's better use of vitamin D makes them less prone to osteoporosis, current research shows a far higher occurrence of hyperparathyroidism in African American men and women making testing especially important.

Secondary hyperparathyroidism is not due to a problem with your parathyroid glands. It's a *normal* protective response to chronically *low* levels of calcium in the bloodstream. *What could cause low blood levels of calcium?*

- **Not consuming enough calcium**: You need at least 1,200 mg but not more than 1,500 mg each day, *combined* from food, supplements, and calcium-containing medications. The typical diet of postmenopausal women (ages 51 to 70) in the U.S. provides about 700 mg of calcium daily. (See Calcium, Chapter 5.)

- **Not consuming enough vitamin D3** to keep your blood levels of 25(OH)D in the optimal range described above.

- **Not producing enough stomach acid**, which is surprisingly common after age 50 and is further compounded by acid-blocking medications, like proton pump inhibitors and H2 blockers.[223]

- **Malabsorption of calcium and other minerals**, often caused by *hidden* gluten sensitivity, celiac disease, infection with *Helicobacter pylori* or other gut pathogens, or digestive disorders like SIBO, irritable bowel syndrome, or Crohn's disease. Significant lifelong malabsorption is also a *normal* outcome of gastric bypass surgery. Malabsorption also promotes high levels of PTH and bone alkaline phosphatase (bone ALP or B-ALP),, a marker of increased bone remodeling. (See Lab Tests, Chapter 10.)

- **Obesity:** Obesity can cause secondary hyperparathyroidism as it is often accompanied by vitamin D deficiency. Those of us who are significantly overweight or obese need as much as 3 times more vitamin D.

- **Chronic liver or kidney disease:** Vitamin D3 must first be converted to 25(OH)D in the liver and then to 1,25-D in the kidneys before it can help us absorb calcium. If your liver or kidney is not able to do its job, your ability to absorb calcium will be greatly reduced.

- **Two classes of drugs**: Calcineurin inhibitors and diuretics can cause secondary hyperparathyroidism.

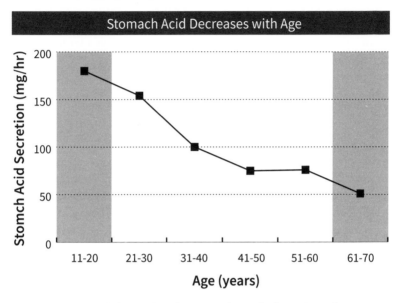

Contrary to popular belief, stomach acid secretions drop with advancing age, those age 61 to 70 having nearly half that of those age 31 to 40 and just 33% of those age 21 to 30.

Source: Why Stomach Acid Is Good for You...[224]

If you have *a low serum calcium and your PTH level is elevated,* check all these potential causes of secondary hyperparathyroidism. Once you're sure none apply to you, the next step is to look into whether you have primary hyperparathyroidism.

A key point: in all instances of secondary hyperparathyroidism, the blood level of calcium is *low.* If the calcium level is *high,* then the cause of the PTH elevation is a parathyroid tumor. A high calcium level without a *very low* PTH level indicates primary hyperparathyroidism.

Someone who has had gastric bypass surgery (or has Crohn's disease, celiac disease, or chronic diarrhea due to any cause) can still develop not just secondary hyperparathyroidism due to malabsorption, but also primary hyperparathyroidism due to a parathyroid tumor or tumors.

BONE-HEALTHY ACTION ITEMS

- Get enough vitamin D3 to maintain a blood level of 60 to 80 ng/mL (for Caucasians, Hispanics, or Asians) or 40 to 60 ng/mL (if you are African American).
- If you have high blood calcium, don't take more vitamin D! The low vitamin-D level is the body's way of preventing you from absorbing even more calcium and overloading your bloodstream.

Metabolic Syndrome/ Type 2 Diabetes

BONE ESSENTIALS

- MetS is a group of unhealthy conditions that typically appear together: insulin resistance, central (abdominal) obesity, high blood sugar, high blood pressure, and *dyslipidemia* (high triglycerides and LDL cholesterol plus low levels of HDL cholesterol). Each of the components of MetS promotes bone loss in different ways.
- T2D is a condition in which the body has lost blood sugar control. This typically includes resistance to insulin, a hormone secreted by the pancreas that enables sugar (glucose) to get into our cells, and eventually loss of our pancreas' ability to secrete insulin. Blood sugar stays elevated, increasing AGEs and cortisol levels, both of which cause serious problems for your bones.
- Osteoporosis in T2D is characterized by low bone turnover, greatly decreased bone formation, and increased risk of hip and vertebral fragility fractures.
- Because bone mineral density (BMD) is increased in T2D, the assessments usually relied upon to check fracture risk—DEXA and FRAX—are not reliable. Trabecular bone score (TBS), which checks bone quality, is a far better indicator of risk.
- Diabetes treatment can increase or decrease fracture risk. Metformin and sulfonylureas may slightly decrease, while the thiazolidinediones (TZDs and glitazones) increase fracture risk.

Metabolic Syndrome

Metabolic syndrome (MetS) is a bunch of unhealthy conditions that typically appear together: central (abdominal) obesity, high blood sugar, high blood pressure, and dyslipidemia, which is the medical term for abnormal levels of cholesterol and other lipids (fats) in the blood. In MetS, what's usually seen are high triglycerides and low HDL cholesterol levels.[225]

How does MetS cause bone loss? Each of the unhealthy components of MetS promotes bone loss in different ways.

- Abdominal fat produces chronic low-grade inflammation. Fat, especially belly fat, is not inert. It spews out inflammatory messenger molecules, including tumor necrosis factor-α (TNF-α), *interleukin-1β* (IL-1β), *interleukin-6* (IL-6), and *C-reactive protein* (CRP), all of which cause RANKL to bind to RANK. That binding triggers the production of osteoclasts and their bone-resorbing activity.

- Dyslipidemia increases the oxidation (free-radical damage) of cholesterol and other fats, which then stimulate a receptor on fat cells called PPAR-γ that tells the precursor cells for osteoblasts to become adipocytes (fat cells) instead.

- High blood sugar increases inflammation. When sugars remain in blood, they bind to proteins, deforming them and turning them into advanced glycosylated end products, aptly abbreviated as AGEs. AGEs age us prematurely. They don't work like normal proteins. Bones that contain AGE-deformed collagen are weak. AGEs also cause the precursor cells for osteoblasts to commit suicide (apoptosis).

- High blood sugar damages the kidneys, lessening their ability to reabsorb calcium. Blood levels of calcium drop, so the parathyroid gland secretes PTH, which activates osteoclasts.

- The processed foods consumed by most Americans deliver too much salt and too much sugar. Both increase blood levels of the stress hormone *cortisol*, which, when chronically elevated—either from salt and sugar or from glucocorticoid medications—promotes obesity and causes bone loss.

Type 2 Diabetes

Type 2 diabetes (T2D) is a condition in which the body loses control of blood sugar. As cells become resistant to insulin, a hormone secreted by the pancreas that enables sugar (glucose) to get into our cells, the pancreas has to increase insulin secretion to overcome the resistance. Normally, when your blood-sugar levels are low, such as having not eaten in a while, your liver breaks down stored glycogen, releasing glucose to keep your blood sugar within a normal range. In type 2 diabetes, cells become insulin resistant, so this process doesn't work properly. Instead of moving into your cells, sugar builds up in your bloodstream. Blood-sugar levels increase, triggering your pancreas to produce more insulin to drive the sugar into your cells. When constantly overworked, however, the beta-cells in your pancreas, which produce insulin, become exhausted and can't make enough to keep up with the increased demand. Blood sugar stays elevated, and this causes serious problems for your bones.

Individuals with T2D have an increased risk of fragility fractures, despite having normal or even increased bone mineral density. Fracture risk is greatest in those who are experiencing complications of T2D also caused by chronically elevated blood-sugar levels, such as retinopathy and chronic kidney disease. Meta-analyses report T2D increases the risk of hip fracture by 130% to 210% and other fractures by 120%. [226][227][228]

Until very recently, it was thought that while risk of hip and femur fractures increased, risk of vertebral fractures did not. Unfortunately, we now know this is not true. Vertebral fractures occur in at least 30% of individuals with T2D with good metabolic control and no diabetic complications. The reason vertebral fractures occur so often is that, as mentioned in our discussion of MetS, the high blood-sugar levels present in T2D cause an increase in cortisol secretion. Even slight chronic elevation in cortisol harms trabecular bone, the primary form of bone in our vertebrae. Such small but chronic elevations in cortisol are increasingly recognized as a cause of postmenopausal osteoporosis in everyone, not just in those with T2D.[229][230][231]

Because bone mineral density (BMD) is increased in T2D, the assessments usually relied upon to check fracture risk, DEXA and FRAX®, are not reliable. Trabecular bone score (TBS) is a far better indicator of risk.[232] (See Lab Tests, Chapter 10.)

Why does T2D increase fracture risk? Because bone quality drops. In type 2 diabetes, large amounts of glucose remain in the bloodstream, where they bind to (*glycosolate*) proteins, forming advanced glycation end products or AGEs, which are deformed proteins that no longer function properly. Within our bones, AGE-d collagen replaces healthy collagen. *Healthy collagen* is tough but flexible, enabling bone to endure strain without breaking. *AGE-d collagen* is stiff and inflexible, so bones break with far less strain.[233] [234]

If you have type 2 diabetes, you can get an idea of your risk for fracture by having a test run to check the amount of Hemoglobin A1c and/or pentosidine in your urine. Both are markers for the presence of AGEs. Higher levels are associated with a higher risk of vertebral fracture—even in postmenopausal women who do not have type 2 diabetes. (See Lab Tests, Chapter 10.)

Chronically elevated blood sugar also causes a slight, but chronic elevation in cortisol as mentioned above. Cortisol depletes vitamin D3 and causes osteoblasts to commit suicide, while osteoclast numbers remain unchanged or increase.[235] [236]

Bone renewal slows in T2D. Markers of bone resorption (CTx and NTx) *and* bone formation (PINP) both drop in T2D. Osteoporosis in T2D is characterized by low bone turnover with a normal or even slightly decreased bone resorption and greatly decreased bone formation.[237]

Diabetes treatment can increase or decrease fracture risk. Metformin and sulfonylureas don't increase and may even slightly reduce fracture risk. (Examples of first-generation sulfonylureas are chlorpropamide and tolbutamide. Second-generation sulfonylureas include glipizide, glyburide, and glimepiride.)

Treatment with the thiazolidinediones (TZDs and glitazones), however, increases fracture risk. TZDs activate a cellular receptor called *peroxisome proliferator-activated receptor gamma* (PPARγ). PPARγ decreases insulin resistance, which is beneficial, but PPARγ also suppresses insulin-like growth factor-1 (IGF-1) and causes mesenchymal stem cells to develop into fat cells (adipocytes) rather than osteoblasts.

IGF-1 is an anabolic hormone that plays a major role in building muscles and bones, including triggering osteoblast production and activities. So, it's not surprising that the use of thiazolidinediones is associated with greatly increased fracture risk. The ADOPT study reported double the incidence of fractures with rosiglitazone (15.1%) compared to metformin (7.3%).[238]

BONE-HEALTHY ACTION ITEMS

- Stop eating processed foods! The same healthful diet we keep talking about of minimally processed organically grown foods combined with regular weight-bearing exercise reverses both MetS and type 2 diabetes.
- Check your vitamin D level and, if indicated, adjust your supplement dosage to ensure your vitamin D level is optimal. (See Vitamin D, Chapter 5.)

Non-Alcoholic Fatty Liver Disease (NAFLD)

BONE ESSENTIALS

- Non-alcoholic fatty liver disease disrupts the body's ability to convert vitamin D3 into 25(OH)D, the form in which vitamin D circulates in the bloodstream.
- NAFLD impairs the liver's ability to detoxify harmful compounds, increasing their inflammatory effects.
- Now present in about 55% of women over age 60, NAFLD negatively affects many proteins involved in bone metabolism.
- NAFLD is caused by insulin resistance, the result of a diet loaded with pro-inflammatory fats and refined carbohydrates (i.e., the standard American diet).

Non-alcoholic fatty liver disease (NAFLD), as its name implies, is infiltration of the liver by fat that is not caused by excessive alcohol consumption. Specifically, NAFLD is said to be present when at least 5% of the liver's cells (called hepatocytes) are stuffed with fat.

Once a rare condition, NAFLD is now the leading cause of chronic liver disease, having doubled between 1988 and 2008, according to

NHANES data. From 1988 to 1994, NAFLD accounted for 46.8% of cases; from 1988 to 1994, that increased to 75.1% of chronic liver disease. Current USA projections indicate that by 2030, 33.5% of the U.S. population will have fatty livers. [239 240 241]

NAFLD and chronic kidney disease (CKD) fuel one another. The liver is supposed to be clearing out toxins for us. When it can't do so, those toxins cause inflammation. NAFLD is accompanied by insulin resistance, high cholesterol, oxidative stress, and high blood pressure. High blood pressure activates the renin-angiotensin system, promoting CKD. And unhappy kidneys return the favor, aggravating the liver with uremic toxins and a leaky gut. (See CDK, Chapter 4).

NAFLD often accompanies metabolic syndrome (MetS), which includes insulin resistance and elevated blood sugar, blood pressure, and LDL (potentially harmful) cholesterol, along with abdominal obesity (belly fat). Belly fat is a key trigger for NAFLD, which can occur in apparently thin people with too much belly (visceral) fat. *Why?* Because visceral adipose tissue (belly fat) is actively spewing out inflammatory signaling molecules. But even if your belly is flat, having cardiovascular disease, diabetes, or chronic kidney disease puts you at increased risk of having NAFLD.

Why does NAFLD cause bone loss? In addition to clearing out inflammatory toxins, your liver converts vitamin D3 into 25(OH)D, the form in which vitamin D circulates in your bloodstream. If your liver is unable to complete this initial conversion, your kidneys can't complete the second, final one: converting 25(OH)D into its active hormonal form (1,25-D) that helps us absorb calcium. So, a dysfunctional liver (or kidneys) impairs vitamin D's activation, calcium absorption, and bone health.

In NAFLD, belly fat secretes pro-inflammatory cytokines like tumor necrosis factor-α (TNF-α), *interleukin-1* (IL-1), and IL-6. These agents of inflammation inhibit insulin receptor signaling and suppress insulin sensitivity in the liver and skeletal muscles, promoting even more fat accumulation in both. More fat and less muscle are not only not what you want to see when you don that bikini, both increase risk for osteoporotic fractures.

In addition, NAFLD affects many proteins involved in bone metabolism—badly. Blood levels of adiponectin, ghrelin, osteocalcin, klotho, and *osteoprotegerin* (OPG) all drop, while those of RANKL increase.

This is the opposite of what you want to happen! Here's why:

- *Adiponectin* is involved in our use of glucose and fat in energy metabolism but also plays a role in bone metabolism, stimulating osteoblast development and bone mineralization, and inhibiting bone resorption.

- *Ghrelin* controls appetite, food intake, and body weight. Plus, ghrelin enhances the proliferation and differentiation of osteoblasts. Lower blood levels of ghrelin are associated with insulin resistance (and thus increased inflammation) in patients with NAFLD.

- *Osteocalcin* is produced by osteoblasts and, once activated by vitamin K2, pulls calcium into your bones. When it's not activated, osteocalcin promotes insulin secretion and protects against inflammation in fat tissue and muscles.

- *Klotho* was first identified as an anti-aging protein because mice who produce less active versions age a whole lot faster. Klotho is mainly expressed in the kidneys. Its cleavage from inside kidney tubules releases klotho into body fluids where it acts as a circulating anti-aging hormone. Clinical studies reveal that even in early CKD, klotho levels drop in the kidneys, serum, and urine, and lower levels correlate with CKD severity and progression. In the liver, klotho is secreted in response to fasting and promotes lipolysis (the breakdown of fats for use in energy production). Loss of klotho production promotes fatty liver. Klotho is also expressed in bone by osteocytes. In bone, Klotho acts as a Wnt (sclerostin) inhibitor, promoting new bone formation.

- RANKL starts the signaling that activates osteoclasts.

Factors that Cause NAFLD

The standard American diet's highly processed, chemically grown foods overload the liver with triglycerides, which leads to NAFLD.

What raises triglycerides? Consuming too much quickly available energy/calories. Triglycerides are the main form in which we store excess energy. We consume triglycerides directly in fats, and we also form triglycerides in our intestines, liver, and fat tissue from excess calories. When our needs for fuel are not met, the liver liberates triglycerides from fat tissue and oxidizes them, to produce glucose.

On the other hand, when our needs for fuel are met, the liver converts excess carbohydrates, fats, or proteins into free fatty acids and then to triglycerides for storage. Carbohydrates are first stored in the form of glycogen. After a carbohydrate-rich meal, however, our glycogen reserves are quickly filled, so the excess carbohydrates are converted by our liver cells, first into fatty acids and then into triglycerides, which are sent to fat cells for storage.[242]

Highly processed carbohydrates along with too much saturated fat raise triglyceride production. In the SAD, fructose and saturated fat are the worst offenders.[243]

- Fructose reduces insulin secretion. Insulin triggers the activity of lipoprotein lipase, the enzyme that breaks down triglycerides stored in fat for use as energy. Lower insulin secretion also results in increased delivery of free fatty acids (FFAs) to the liver, increasing the liver's creation of triglycerides and the most harmful form of cholesterol, very low-density cholesterol (VLDL), which then gets packed with triglycerides. When calories are consumed in the form of fructose or glucose, the liver will preferentially convert fructose to fat production and use glucose for energy production.

- Saturated fats increase postprandial (after meal) triglyceride production. All other fats lessen it.

What can you do to support your liver?

Consume a diet that lowers triglyceride production. Start by consuming more PUFAs (polyunsaturated fatty acids), the type of fats found in nuts, seeds, vegetable oils, and cold-water fish. PUFAs lower triglycerides by reducing the liver's production of fats, increasing the oxidation of fatty acids for energy production, and increasing the presence of lipoprotein lipase in fat cells.

Eat more soluble fiber. It lowers triglycerides by forming a thick gel in the gut, which slows gastric emptying and the rate at which fat is emulsified and encapsulated into micelles for absorption. Plus, soluble fiber can be fermented by the beneficial gut microbiota to release short-chain fatty acids (butyrate, acetate, propionate, isobutyrate), which increase the activity of genes [PPARα and PGC-1α] involved in our metabolism of lipids (fats). Insoluble fiber also helps lower triglycerides, but less than soluble fiber because insoluble fiber, as its name indicates, is less soluble in water and less fermentable than soluble fiber.

Eat whey protein, which lowers triglycerides, while other animal proteins raise them. Whey protein has a higher content of branched-chain amino acids, which are quickly digested and absorbed, stimulating the release of insulin. Insulin then increases the activity of lipoprotein lipase, which breaks down fat for use in energy production.

Eat a Mediterranean-type diet. You know the drill here: organically grown, minimally processed vegetables, fruit, legumes, nuts, and seeds; wild-caught cold-water fish; dairy products from pastured cows; eggs from free-range chickens; leaner meats from pastured animals; and small amounts of whole grains like millet, quinoa, and rice (but not wheat; see Wheat, Chapter 1).

Exercise! A recent meta-analysis of six studies revealed that exercise alone (in comparison to a non-exercise control group) without any dietary intervention caused a significant decrease in liver fat, even with minimal weight loss or in the absence of any change in weight.[244]

Physical inactivity is well known to promote both osteoporosis and *sarcopenia*, a progressive loss of muscle mass associated with aging. A recently discovered myokine (a signaling molecule released by muscle cells during exercise) called *irisin* increases calorie burn and has positive effects on adipocytes (fat cells) and osteoblasts.

Irisin causes white (inactive) fat to turn into brown (energy-burning) fat, plus irisin induces the production of osteoblasts. One recent study reported that higher blood levels of irisin were associated with lower amounts of triglycerides in liver cells in obese adults with NAFLD, independent of other metabolic factors. Due to irisin's beneficial effects on energy metabolism, glucose use, insulin resistance, and obesity, irisin may be a key player in the complex web of communications among the liver, muscle, and bone. And you can have irisin working for you if you just work out![245]

BONE-HEALTHY ACTION ITEMS

- Consume a diet that lowers triglyceride production, including more fiber (especially soluble), polyunsaturated fatty acids, and whey protein.
- Consider following a Mediterranean-type diet
- Get regular exercise, which has been associated with a significant decrease in liver fat.

Obesity and Bariatric Surgeries

BONE ESSENTIALS

- Abdominal obesity (measured by *waist circumference* or *waist-hip ratio*) increases the risk of hip fracture by 24% to 40%.
- Visceral adipose tissue (VAT) or belly fat is angry, highly inflammatory fat, especially destructive of trabecular bone.
- Bariatric surgeries do provide benefits but also cause immediate, significant, and relentless bone loss.
- Bariatric surgeries greatly reduce the amount of food that can be consumed and the digestive tract's ability to absorb bone-critical nutrients, including calcium, fat-soluble vitamins (D, K, E, and A), and omega-3 fatty acids.
- After bariatric surgery, 50% of patients are deficient in vitamin D within two years, and 65% are deficient four years after surgery.

Obesity now afflicts more people worldwide than any other chronic debilitating condition. Close to half (42.4%) of Americans are now considered obese. Almost one in every ten (9.2%) is morbidly obese—100 pounds or more above their ideal body weight or having a body mass index (BMI) of 40 or greater.

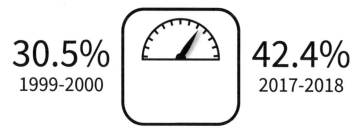

Obesity Increases Among U.S. Adults, 1999 to 2018

30.5%
1999-2000

42.4%
2017-2018

Source: Prevalence of Obesity and Severe Obesity Among Adults... [246]

We used to think obesity didn't harm bone. Or that carrying around all that extra weight made bones stronger. Now we know, it ain't so. Waist circumference—or waist-hip ratio—increases the risk of hip fracture:[247]

- A meta-analysis including 295,674 apparently healthy individuals 40 or older found that abdominal obesity increased the risk of hip fracture between 24% to 40%.[248]

- Another meta-analysis found individuals with the greatest waist circumference had a 58% greater risk for hip fracture, while those with the largest waist-hip ratio had a 32% increased risk.[249]

Why does the size of your waist affect your risk for hip fracture? The larger your waist, the more belly fat you carry. Belly fat (in medical jargon, visceral adipose tissue or VAT) doesn't just prevent you from zipping up your pants. VAT is angry fat, constantly spewing out inflammatory messenger molecules (cytokines like TNF-α, IL-1, and IL-6), which increase osteoclast and suppress osteoblast activity.

Belly fat's anger causes levels of *high sensitivity C-reactive protein* (hs-CRP), a marker of whole-body inflammation, to rise. Increased inflammation has nasty effects on trabecular bone, the type of bone found primarily in our vertebrae and at the ends of our long bones, like the femur. When hs-CRP is high, trabecular bone quality is low. Also, a belly that's bigger than your hips causes instability and impairs balance, increasing the risk for falls that cause fractures.

As Obesity Increases, So Have Bariatric Surgeries

Bariatric surgeries do provide benefits, offering rapid and significant weight loss. They can improve or even resolve obesity-related problems, such as heart disease, high blood pressure, obstructive sleep apnea, type 2 diabetes, non-alcoholic fatty liver disease (NAFLD), gastroesophageal reflux disease (GERD), and osteoarthritis (joint pain).

However, bariatric surgery also causes immediate, significant, and relentless bone loss. Between 1 to 2 years after bariatric surgery, BMD drops 5% to 9% in the lumbar spine and 10 to 14% at the hip, according to a review published in 2020. Earlier research showed a rapid loss in bone quality as well as quantity, along with a significant increase in fracture risk 2 years or less after surgery.[250]

- BMD in the total hip, measured by DEXA scans, dropped by 2% to 5% at 6 months and by 6% to 10.5% seen at 9 to 12 months. Trabecular bone score (TBS), which measures bone quality, found a 6% to 7% decrease in the lumbar spine 6 to 12 months post-surgery. Studies also report significant drops in BMD and TBS at the radius (wrist) and tibia (shin).

- Data from a review of 15 studies revealed that during the first year after a gastric bypass, declines in BMD of as much as 15% were seen in the hip. BMD in the femur neck, where most hip fractures occur, dropped an average of 9.2% to 10.9%.[251]

The significant bone harm resulting from bariatric surgery is common knowledge among medical professionals. Yet, shockingly, this is not widely shared with the public. Check out the websites for bariatric surgery centers. Look for the *adverse effects of bariatric surgery* section, and chances are bone loss won't even be mentioned.[252]

Why does bariatric surgery cause bone loss? Let's look at the most commonly performed bariatric procedures, the sleeve gastrectomy and Roux-en-Y gastric bypass (RYGB). Both greatly reduce not just the size of the stomach and thus the amount of food that can be consumed but also the digestive tract's ability to absorb nutrients.[253]

- **The sleeve gastrectomy removes 85% of the stomach**, including the area where stomach acid, intrinsic factor, and pepsin are produced. Stomach acid is required to digest food and prepare minerals for absorption. Intrinsic factor is required for B12 absorption, and pepsin is an enzyme responsible for digesting proteins.[254]

- **The Roux-en-Y Gastric Bypass (RYGB) removes 95% of the stomach**, duplicating the problems caused by sleeve gastrectomy. Then, it adds to them by bypassing the first two sections of the small intestine—the duodenum and proximal jejunum—where virtually all active calcium absorption occurs, along with absorption of the fat-soluble vitamins (D, K, E, and A), the omega-3 essential fatty acids (ALA, EPA, and DHA), iron, and folate.

After either procedure, 50% of patients are deficient in vitamin D within two years, and 65% are deficient four years after surgery. Along with vitamin D insufficiency, fractional calcium absorption (the amount of calcium consumed that a person actually absorbs) plummets. This causes parathyroid hormone (PTH) levels to rise, resulting in secondary hyperparathyroidism.[255] (See Hyperparathyroidism, Chapter 4.)

BONE-HEALTHY ACTION ITEMS

If you've had or are considering bariatric surgery, protect your bones:

- Make every bite count. Since you can consume far less food at a meal, choose foods that concentrate bone-building nutrients: calcium, magnesium, boron, and other trace minerals, vitamin C, B vitamins, and more.
- Eat organic! Organically grown plant foods and foods derived from pastured animals, free-range eggs, and wild-caught fish, deliver way more of the healthy nutrients our bones require.
- Take supplemental hydrochloric acid with betaine to help release nutrients from food.
- Consume 1,500 mg of calcium total from food and supplements daily, with no more than 500 mg at once.
- Use sublingual supplements for your fat-soluble vitamins (D3, K2, A, and E), and your B vitamins, especially B12. Sublinguals are placed under the tongue and are absorbed directly into your bloodstream, bypassing the nutrient absorption problems caused by bariatric surgeries.
- Choose a plant-derived calcium supplement that also naturally contains magnesium and the trace minerals your bones require.
- Take an omega-3 supplement that provides EPA and DHA in an emulsion.

- Get your hormone levels checked—not just estrogen, progesterone, and testosterone but also DHEA, thyroid, and adrenal hormones. Consider bioidentical hormones if necessary. (See Lab Tests, Chapter 10.)
- Enjoy regular weight-bearing exercise, one hour daily, to wake up your osteocytes, the cells within your bones that respond to mechanical loading by initiating bone renewal.

Sarcopenia

BONE ESSENTIALS

- Sarcopenia, the progressive replacement of muscle by fat typically seen with aging, is bad for bones because muscle contractions trigger bone renewal.
- When muscle precursor cells are told to turn into fat cells, so are the precursor cells for osteoblasts, the cells that build bone.
- If you have osteopenia or osteoporosis, you are likely to have sarcopenia. Sarcopenia was found in 25% of postmenopausal women with osteopenia and 50% of those with osteoporosis.
- After age 50, we can lose 1% to 2% of muscle mass each year, with 30% or more of our muscle mass and strength vanishing by age 80.
- You can be apparently slim and still have sarcopenia. What matters is not just what you weigh, but how much of that is muscle versus how much is fat.

Sarcopenia, from the Greek *sarx* for flesh and *penia* for lack or deficiency, is the medical term for the progressive loss of muscle mass typically seen with aging. Sarcopenia is all too common, affecting up to 29% of adults 50 or older. Due to sarcopenia, almost 20% of women and 10% of men 65 or older cannot lift a 10-pound weight or get back up without assistance after kneeling down.[256]

In sarcopenia, muscle is replaced by fat, and that's bad for your bones. Muscle contractions trigger bone renewal. Plus, bone and muscle interact not just anatomically but also chemically and metabolically. When the precursor cells for muscle, called *myoblasts*, are increasingly being sent signals that instruct them to develop into fat cells (adipocytes) rather than muscle cells (*myocytes*), the same signaling is being sent to the mesenchymal stem cells that are the precursors for osteoblasts. The result is that these precursor cells grow up to be fat cells instead of bone-building osteoblasts. Fat infiltration into muscle and bone is a common trait of both osteoporosis and sarcopenia.

If you have osteopenia or osteoporosis, chances are you have sarcopenia:

- A report of more than 300 women in Italy with hip fractures found that 58% were also sarcopenic.

- Another study from England indicated that in postmenopausal women, sarcopenia was present in 25% of those with osteopenia and 50% of those with osteoporosis.

- A study conducted in Australia involving 680 older individuals with a history of falls found almost 40% were *osteosarcopenic*, a new term coined because both problems are recognized to appear together.

Peak bone mass is reached by the end of 30 years of age; after which, do nothing and it's all downhill. If you don't actively combat bone loss with a healthy diet, targeted supplements, regular weight-bearing exercise, and toxin avoidance, you'll lose about 30% of your bone mass between your 40s and 70s.

Muscle mass reaches its peak earlier, around the age of 25. Muscle mass remains fairly stable. Just a slight 5% reduction in the number of muscle fibers occurs until age 50. After that, once again, if you don't take the very same actions that preserve your bones, you'll lose 1% to 2% of your muscle mass each year, resulting in 30% of your muscle mass and strength vanishing by the age of 80.[257]

You can be apparently slim and still have sarcopenia. What matters is not just how much you weigh, but how much of you is muscle and bone, and how much of you is fat. You can also be overweight or obese and not just over-fat but under-muscled, a recently identified condition called *sarcopenic obesity*.

Causes Of Sarcopenia

- Insufficient protein intake
- Micronutrient deficiency
- Inflammaging
- Low activity, sedentary lifestyle
- Malabsorption and other gastrointestinal conditions
- Thyroid diseases (hyperthyroidism, hypothyroidism, subclinical hypothyroidism)[258 259]

- Bone and joint diseases
- Type 2 diabetes [260]
- NAFLD [261]
- Chronic kidney disease [262]
- Drug related (aromatase inhibitors, chemotherapy, anti-diabetic drugs, metformin, sulfonylureas, glinide, glibenclamide) [263 264]

Source: Sarcopenia. Review Lancet...[265]

Here's How Exercise and Protein Can Help

You can take steps to help maintain your muscle and strong bones. The key is exercising regularly and ensuring optimal protein intake:

- **Exercise inhibits *myostatin,* a protein produced and released by muscle cells (myocytes) that inhibits their proliferation and growth**. Plus, exercise stimulates the production and release of muscle-building hormones, like growth hormone and testosterone.[266]

- **Your muscles are made of protein.** When you lift weights—or even the weight of your own body—this resistance exercise creates micro-tears in your muscles. Your body uses protein to repair these tears and to grow your muscles, increasing their strength to ensure you're able to meet the next challenge.

The catch here is that our aging muscle cells develop *anabolic resistance* (less responsiveness to protein). That means elders need more protein than younger folks to get the job done. At each meal, older adults need 0.4 grams of protein per kg of body weight or 30 to 45 grams of protein, which is 67% more than young adults do, to fully get their muscle rebuilding effort in gear. Elders need 1.2 to 1.5 grams/kg/bw daily to maintain muscle mass. Yet, data collected between 2005 and 2014 shows that 45% of adults do not consume even the (inadequate for elders) current 0.8 grams/kg/bw RDA for protein. Thus, sarcopenia is rampant in folks over age 50.[267]

Which protein sources build elders' muscles best? Animal proteins, whey, or pea protein are the most effective sources of muscle-building protein for elders. *The reason?* Each is high in *leucine*, one of the three branched-chain amino acids (BCAAs), which plays a key role in muscle synthesis.[268]

Leucine is metabolized into a derivative called β-*hydroxy-β-methylbutyrate (HMB)*, which is where the leucine muscle-building *tire meets the road*. HMB stimulates muscle-building signaling pathways and inhibits muscle breakdown. Research shows consuming leucine-rich foods supplying 2.5 to 3.0 grams of leucine at each meal greatly boosts muscle synthesis. In addition, you want to consume those leucine-rich foods as whole foods. Research shows muscle protein synthesis is greater when whole eggs or whole milk (not just egg whites or fat-free milk) is consumed.

Are you getting enough of the most effective types of protein? Keep a diet diary for 3 to 5 days using the table below. Based on available evidence, we recommend that adults aged 50 and older:

- Prioritize high-quality, nutrient-dense sources of protein (like eggs, milk, beef, fish, leucine-rich plant sources and supplements).

- Consume more protein spread throughout the day; specifically, increase the frequency of meals providing 30 to 45 grams of protein that contains 2.5 to 3.0 grams of leucine.

- Engage in regular weight-bearing resistance exercise to amplify the response to protein-containing meals.

Foods Rich in Leucine	
Food (Serving size: 100 grams)	Leucine (grams)
Whey protein concentrate, dry powder	10 to 12
Soy protein concentrate, dry powder	7.5 to 8.5
Soybeans, mature seeds, roasted, salted	2.87
Hemp seed, hulled	2.16
Beef, round, top round, raw	1.76
Peanuts	1.67
Fish, salmon, pink, raw	1.62
Wheat germ	1.57
Almonds	1.49
Chicken, broilers or fryers, thigh, raw	1.48
Chicken egg, yolk, raw	1.40
Oats	1.28
Edamame (soybeans, green, raw)	0.93

Source: National Nutrient Database for Standard Reference. U.S. Dept. of Agriculture. March 2015

Here are some other strategies to support the health of your muscles:

Ensure your vitamin D (25[OH]D) level is optimal (60 to 80 ng/ mL). Vitamin D plays key roles in skeletal muscle cell production and growth. When vitamin D binds to the vitamin D receptor (VDR) on our cells, it increases the expression of genes that regulate cell proliferation and development. As we age, our cells produce fewer VDRs, which combined with low levels of vitamin D, promote sarcopenia. Individuals with sarcopenia are typically found to have lower levels of vitamin D. This is an easy fix. Supplementing vitamin D increases the expression of the VDR in skeletal muscle cells.[269]

Ensure optimal EPA/DHA status. Quite a few recently conducted studies have shown that muscle mass is greater in elders consuming fish several times a week and/or whose blood levels of fish-oil-derived EPA/ DHA are higher.[270] [271]

EPA/DHA also activates a cellular signaling pathway called the *mTOR pathway*, which ramps up skeletal muscle production. In human studies, after just 8 weeks of EPA/DHA supplementation, activation of the mTOR pathway increases, boosting the rate of muscle protein synthesis. In elders with sarcopenia, a minimum daily intake of 4 to 4.59 grams of EPA/DHA is recommended.

Make sure you're getting bone-building minerals daily. Optimal nutrition involves not just protein and vitamin D, but vitamin K2, the B vitamins, calcium, magnesium, the essential fatty acids EPA and DHA, and at least 14 trace minerals.[272] [273]

BONE-HEALTHY ACTION ITEMS

- Get regular exercise to stimulate the production and release of muscle-building hormones.
- Ensure optimal nutrition: protein, vitamin D, vitamin K2, the B vitamins, calcium, magnesium, trace minerals, and the essential fatty acids EPA and DHA.
- Ensure optimal intake of protein (1.2 to 1.5 grams of protein per kilogram of body weight or 30 to 45 grams of protein at each of 3 meals).
- Get enough omega-3s, EPA and DHA; the minimum recommended daily intake for elders is 4 to 4.59 grams of EPA/DHA.
- Eat foods rich in leucine and consider taking supplements

of leucine and its derivative HMB. Dosages shown safe and effective in research are 3.8 grams/d of leucine and 3 grams/d of HMB.[274][275]

Subclinical Hypercortisolism

BONE ESSENTIALS

- Subclinical hypercortisolism, in which cortisol is slightly but chronically elevated, shows up on your DEXA as a loss of BMD in your spine, while your hip and femur remain stable or even improve—the opposite of what normally happens.
- Typically, new bone is laid down more quickly in the spine because the spine is primarily trabecular bone, which turns over 5 to 10 times faster than cortical bone, the type of bone that predominates in the hip.
- Chronically producing too much cortisol causes bone loss by decreasing osteoblast production and activity, increasing osteoclast production and activity, and decreasing calcium absorption.
- Subclinical hypercortisolism is caused by the growth of a non-cancerous tumor on the adrenal glands, called an *adrenal incidentaloma* as these are usually discovered incidentally when a scan is run for some other reason.
- Adrenal incidentalomas are present in up to 10% of older people. In as many as 4 of every 100 people with osteoporosis, the cause is slight cortisol excess.

Subclinical hypercortisolism is a recently identified disorder in which cortisol is slightly but chronically elevated. The result shows up on your DEXA as a loss of bone mineral density in your spine, while your hip and femur remain stable or even improve.

You may have heard of Cushing's syndrome (also called Cushing's disease), in which chronically, significantly elevated cortisol causes bone loss.[276] Subclinical hypercortisolism is a far less severe version of Cushing's that doesn't show up with the classical signs and symptoms, so it's easy for doctors to miss.

A loss of bone mineral density in your spine, while your hip and femur remain stable or even improve, is the opposite of what normally occurs. Typically, new bone is laid down more quickly in the spine than in the hip or femur.

Why? Because the hip/femur is primarily cortical bone, while spine is primarily trabecular bone, which is far more metabolically active. Trabecular bone turns over at a rate 5 to 10 times faster than cortical bone, so problems show up faster in the area richest in trabecular bone, your spine.[277] [278]

How does too much cortisol cause bone loss? Chronically producing too much of the stress hormone, cortisol—even a little too much—definitely adds stress to your bones! Cortisol has been shown to:

- Inhibit osteoblasts' development from mesenchymal stem cells, which develop into adipocytes (fat cells) instead
- Inactivate already mature osteoblasts
- Reduce the rate at which osteoclasts commit *apoptosis*, the self-destruct sequence cells normally initiate when they are old or damaged, thus extending osteoclasts' lifespan
- Promote the rate at which osteoblasts and osteocytes enter apoptosis, shortening their lifespan
- Reduce the production of growth factors and bone matrix proteins
- Decrease calcium absorption

These effects are why the use of the glucocorticoid medications, like cortisone and prednisone, so rapidly cause an increase in osteoclasts and bone resorption, along with a decrease in osteoblast development and activity—a deadly-to-bone combination that swiftly produces rapid bone loss and increased risk of fracture. Furthermore, when estrogen is lacking, as it is in postmenopausal women or in anyone taking an aromatase inhibitor, bones become more sensitive to harm from even slight elevations in cortisol.

Glucocorticoid medications are the most common cause of excessive cortisol production, followed by Cushing's disease, but subclinical hypercortisolism is becoming more common. It's caused by a non-cancerous tumor-like growth on the adrenal glands, called an adrenal incidentaloma—*incidental* because these growths produce no overt clinical symptoms and are discovered incidentally during an unrelated computed tomography (CT), magnetic resonance imaging scan (MRI), or ultrasonography scan.

Adrenal incidentalomas only affect about 3% of the general population, but the likelihood of having one increases significantly with age—their occurrence increases to up to 10% in older people.[279]

Higher vertebral fracture risks. Although adrenal incidentalomas are benign (non-cancerous tumors), they can still produce significant health problems for your bones, especially your spine. A recent population study linked higher risk of fracture with adrenal adenomas classified as *non-functioning* (not hormone secreting) or those with mild cortisol secretion.[280] Vertebral fractures are a hallmark of subclinical hypercortisolism, occurring in up to 82.4% of individuals with this condition:

- Individuals with an adrenal incidentaloma were found to be more than 7 times as likely to have had an asymptomatic vertebral fracture—regardless of their age, bone mineral density, menopausal status, or gender.[281]

- The same research group revealed that individuals with subclinical hypercortisolism had a 12-fold higher risk of having already had a vertebral fracture and then of having additional vertebral fractures.[282]

- In two studies of patients referred to an outpatient clinic for osteoporosis, between 11% and 18% of those who had already experienced a fragility fracture were found to have subclinical hypercortisolism. In other words, somewhere between 1 and 2 people out of 10.

Researchers now believe that in as many as 4% of patients with apparent primary osteoporosis—so 4 of every 100 people with osteoporosis—the cause is a slight cortisol excess.[283]

Is subclinical hypercortisolism causing bone loss in YOU? The latest papers are alerting doctors to check for subclinical hypercortisolism in osteoporotic patients with vertebral fractures, particularly when bone mineral density in cortical-rich bones, like the hip and femur, is not decreasing.

Measuring the levels of cortisol in the urine, saliva, or blood after taking a drug called dexamethasone—in the absence of possible interfering medications and/or disease—identifies patients likely to have an adrenal incidentaloma. Further lab tests are needed to confirm the diagnosis.

Experts stress that a DEXA scan alone is not an adequate indicator of fracture risk in individuals with subclinical hypercortisolism. *Why?* Because its adverse effects are primarily seen in trabecular bone microarchitecture, not just in bone density, so the degree of bone mineral density reduction is not a very good indicator of fracture risk.

What matters most here is bone quality (i.e., bone microarchitecture), and this is what a *trabecular bone score* evaluates. So, it's important that your doctor orders a TBS for you, not just a DEXA! (See Lab Tests, Chapter 10.)

The good news is that treating the underlying cause of subclinical hypercortisolism alleviates the condition in most individuals. If it's due to medications, these can often be slowly stopped. If caused by a tumor, it may be treated with surgery, chemotherapy, and/or radiation. If you are found to have subclinical hypercortisolism, the removal of an adrenal incidentaloma can quickly stop bone loss and speed your recovery of healthy bones.[284]

BONE-HEALTHY ACTION ITEMS

- Since subclinical hypercortisolism primarily affects trabecular bone microarchitecture, DEXA alone is not an adequate indicator of fracture risk. Order a trabecular bone score with your DEXA scan.
- If you are found to have subclinical hypercortisolism, removal of the adrenal incidentaloma can quickly stop bone loss and speed your recovery of healthy bones.

Conclusion Part One

The standard American diet is awash in bone-destructive refined sugars and carbohydrates, sodium, excessive amounts of animal protein, pro-inflammatory fats, pro-inflammatory chemicals, bone-damaging additives, and contaminants (e.g., phosphates and pesticide residues). The SAD is also deficient in virtually all the nutrients your bones require for healthy remodeling.

This, by itself, would be destructive enough, but we can add to these perils our daily exposure to heavy metals (e.g., lead, cadmium, and mercury), fluoride, and numerous persistent organic pollutants (POPs), all of which destroy bone and are abundantly present in our environment. In combination, these factors increase our risk for chronic degenerative diseases that have become all too common, produce chronic inflammation, and further promote bone loss. These are the true underlying causes driving our current epidemic of osteoporosis, not simply the drop in estrogen that occurs with menopause.

The good news is that we can completely avoid or at least greatly lessen the impact of every single one of these bone-destroying factors. The fact that the majority of us over age 50 are still standing upright is testimony to the resilience of our human physiology. If we can lessen the impact of as many of these bone-damaging factors as possible and provide our bones with an adequate supply of the nutrients they need to rebuild, our bones are programmed to maintain their own health. We'll show you how to give your bones the nutritional support they need in Part Two.

PART TWO

Nutrients Your Bones Need to Rebuild

Your body comes programmed to create healthy bones. Specialized cells (osteocytes, osteoblasts, osteoclasts, and bone lining cells) work to break down old bone and build strong new bone. Over the past decade, research has improved our understanding of this process and revealed nutrients our cells need as they interact and communicate throughout the body. This is quite an intricate dance, one in which a single poor performance can seriously hamper the entire production. Nonetheless, we now have deep insight into what our bodies require to optimize our personal choreography in a holistic and natural way.

You need more than *just* calcium and vitamin D, the two key players discussed first here! No single nutrient can or will ever be enough on its own, but if you minimize your exposure to the harmful factors discussed in Part One and provide the right materials, your body will automatically produce healthy bones for you. This is the *only* effective way to restore and maintain bone health. In this section, we'll share the latest scientific findings on the optimal amounts of critical vitamins, minerals, and healthy fats your body needs to build and support strong, healthy bones!

CHAPTER 5

Team Calcium and Other Key Players

When Team Calcium takes the field, some other star players really stand out. Vitamin D allows for most of calcium's absorption in the body. Vitamin K1 has powerful anti-inflammatory actions, while vitamin K2 directs calcium to your bones and away from soft tissue, like your blood vessels. Magnesium balances the effects of calcium in the body, while also fighting inflammation and supporting calcium absorption. Finally, the proper ratio of omega-6 to omega-3 essential oils prevents the chronic inflammation that continuously activates osteoclasts to break down bone.

We'll share how these nutrients work together along with practical strategies to determine how much you need, what forms are best, and where to get what you need from diet and/or supplements to ensure Team Calcium is at the top of its game.

Calcium

BONE ESSENTIALS

- A total of 1,200 to 1,500 mg/day of calcium, from food and supplements combined, is essential for healthy bones.
- Calcium is a *Team Player:* Effective absorption and healthful use of calcium requires both vitamin D3 and vitamin K2.
- Calcium helps you excrete more fat, burn more fat, and feel satiated longer.
- Calcium may cause constipation when supplies of magnesium are not adequate.
- Dairy products are good for our bones and do not increase fracture risk, with one exception: cow's milk.

Calcium is the most abundant mineral in the body, accounting for as much as 2% of an adult human's entire body weight. Calcium is definitely a *major* mineral within us and for good reason—actually, many good reasons. Without calcium, we couldn't build (or maintain) our bones (or teeth). Almost all (99%) of the calcium in our bodies serves as the key structural component in our skeleton, where it's also used as a calcium *bank account* from which withdrawals can be made to release calcium into our bloodstream when blood levels of calcium drop too low.

Just 1% of the calcium in our bodies is circulating in our bloodstream or working inside our cells, but this tiny amount plays critical roles in essential-to-life physiological processes, including:

- helping blood to clot, so we don't bleed out from something as minor as a paper cut
- enabling nerves to send impulses and muscles, including our heart, to contract, as in our heartbeat
- regulating the permeability of our cell membranes, so our cells can allow what they need to enter and send out their cellular trash

Because these activities enable us to remain alive, the body tightly monitors the amount of calcium in the blood and ensures enough remains available. Losing bone takes many years to kill you. Losing your heartbeat will terminate you within minutes. Therefore, your bones—not your bloodstream—will be robbed when you're not getting the calcium you need.

Are You Getting All the Calcium You Need for Healthy Bones?

Probably not, unless you're taking a calcium supplement. Data from the National Health and Nutrition Examination Survey (NHANES) shows that Americans of all ages are not getting anywhere near enough calcium from food. Ironically, the two age groups who need calcium most are the ones likely to be lacking:

- Children age 9 to 18 need 1,300 mg/d but are actually getting only 935 mg/d, about 70% of what they need to produce their adult teeth and bones.

- Women age 40 to 59 need 1,200 to 1,500 mg/d, but their average dietary intake is only 882 mg/d, just a little more than half the amount of calcium required to maintain a healthy skeleton, especially as they go through perimenopause and menopause.

- Average dietary calcium intake in women age 60 and above is even lower: 842 mg/d.[285]

Forty percent of total lifetime bone mass is accumulated during adolescence. Not getting adequate calcium as a teenager can result in a woman being osteopenic by her late 30s or early 40s, well before menopause. The teens you love may need your help getting this message. Teen brains are not yet fully wired to appreciate the potential long-term consequences of their actions, and adequate nutrition is not typically at the top of a teenage girl's priority list.[286] [287] [288]

Osteopenia by age 30 is not an outcome parents want for their daughters. Ensuring adequate calcium intake during adolescence and in one's early 20s when bone accretion (i.e., gradual growth) is still occurring is a key factor in the prevention of osteoporosis.[289]

Calcium requirements increase in perimenopausal women. During our perimenopausal years, dropping estrogen levels lead to an increase in bone resorption. By the time we're postmenopausal, in addition to estrogen deficiency, our calcium needs increase due to: (1) reduced efficiency to absorb calcium from our intestines, and (2) decreased ability of our kidneys to conserve and reabsorb calcium.

By age 65, calcium absorption is only 50% of adolescent absorption levels, in both men and women. The male version of menopause, andropause, also begins in the 50s and is accompanied by the same drops in calcium's intestinal absorption and reabsorption from the kidneys seen in women. You need to ensure you (and your man) are getting *at least* 1,200 mg/d from your diet and supplements combined.[290 291 292]

Why do we need more calcium as we age? Of the calcium we eat, our bodies only absorb a portion, described as our Fractional Calcium Absorption (FCA). For example, the FCA of a healthy, pre-menopausal adult woman is expected to be about 37.8%. After consuming 200 mg of calcium from food or supplements, she'll absorb just 75.6 mg. For 300 mg of calcium, the FCA is a bit less (33.9%) with 101 mg absorbed. The remainder will pass through her intestines and be excreted in stools.

Beginning at around age 40, our ability to absorb calcium decreases (by 0.21%/year). At menopause, an additional decrease in calcium absorption of 2.2% occurs. Between age 40 and 60, the combined effect of age and menopause results in a 20% to 25% decrease in absorption efficiency. By age 65, your FCA will be just 50% that of your adolescent levels.

Our reduced ability to absorb calcium as we age is thought to be due to:

- **the drop in estrogen**. Estrogen increases the activity of an enzyme in our kidneys called *renal hydroxylase*, which converts 25(OH)D (the form in which vitamin D circulates in the bloodstream) into 1,25-D (the hormonal form of vitamin D that helps us absorb calcium from the intestines).

- **faster elimination of 1,25-D from our bodies**. Estrogen decreases how quickly we break down and eliminate 1,25-D. Less estrogen means faster elimination of 1,25(OH)D, so again, less calcium is absorbed. Interestingly, the trace mineral boron can help us keep 1,25-D around longer. (See Boron, Chapter 6.)

- **decreased production of receptors in our intestines for 1,25-D**.

- **decreased kidney function**, including a drop in their ability to reabsorb calcium instead of excreting it in urine.[293 294 295]

Can Supplemental Calcium Alone (or with Vitamin D) Increase Bone Mineral Density?

By itself, no. Supplemental calcium can only slow bone loss, not outpace it. That's true even when it's accompanied by vitamin D. Be aware that many studies citing an *increase* are often doing so in comparison to a control group. Even if the participants taking calcium *lose less bone* than those taking a placebo, that's still not an overall gain. Large meta-analyses have shown that calcium, even accompanied by vitamin D, at best merely reduce the rate of bone loss:

Meta-Analysis 1 involved 63,897 subjects (age 50 and older) most of whom were healthy postmenopausal women (average age 67.8 years):

- Calcium, or calcium plus vitamin D, was associated with a reduced rate of bone loss of 0.54% at the hip and 1.19% in the spine.
- Instead of losing the typical 1% of BMD each year seen in women after menopause (which increases to 2% per year or more during the 10 years of the menopausal transition), study subjects continued to lose bone, though at a slower rate.[296]

Meta-Analysis 2 looked at 32 randomized trials of calcium supplementation involving 3,169 postmenopausal women:

- Bone loss occurred much faster in the women whose total calcium intake, from both diet and supplements, fell below 1,150 mg/d and was slowest in the women whose calcium intake was more than 1,350 mg/d.
- Those who did not receive calcium supplementation lost bone at an average rate of -1.07% per year, while those consuming at least 700 mg/d of supplemental calcium also lost bone though far less (average of -0.27% per year).

No one nutrient is a silver bullet! No matter how important calcium or any single nutrient is, our bones still need the full team of nutrients to remain strong, resilient, and fracture-free throughout our lives. The good news is that the combination of the right nutrients can provide a true increase in BMD.

In fact, one type of calcium supplement has shown an increase in new bone creation—actually *building more bone than is being lost.* That is AlgaeCal Plus, which contains 4 different types of plant-derived calcium *and* other key nutrients bones require to rebuild. We'll talk more about

AlgaeCal when discussing calcium supplement options. The key point to understand right now is that outpacing bone loss requires more than just calcium and vitamin D.[297 298 299]

When researchers ignore this fact, they sometimes come to erroneous conclusions that are unfortunately amplified in the general press. One example is a review called *Calcium Intake and Risk of Fracture: Systematic Review* by Bolland MJ et al.[300]

Media Misinformation: *Calcium Has No Meaningful Effect on Fracture Risk*

In September 2015, the *British Medical Journal* published a report that calcium, even with vitamin D, has no meaningful effect on your risk for fracture. You probably heard about it, as the media jumped on the claim by M.J. Bolland and his co-authors repeated *ad nauseam* that calcium supplements are useless. This misinformation continues to be cited as gospel. Don't believe it!

The fact is calcium supplementation, either alone or with vitamin D, lowered the risk of fracture in every single one of the studies in the Bolland et al. review. Healthy bones require adequate supplies of calcium, which is seriously lacking in our modern diet. However, the positive results seen could have been much better if the studies accounted for the two nutritional *elephants* missing from the room:

- **Inadequate vitamin D supplementation**. Vitamin D is essential for our active absorption of calcium. Without enough, we absorb only 10% to 15% of the calcium we consume.[301]

- **No vitamin K2 supplementation**. Vitamin K2 activates *osteocalcin*, the protein tasked with delivering calcium to our bones, and *matrix Gla protein*, the protein that prevents calcium from depositing in our soft tissues, like our arteries, heart, and kidneys.

Not a single one of the studies reviewed by Bolland even mentioned, much less utilized, vitamin K2. And with just one exception, the studies provided vitamin D in amounts so inadequate as to have a negligible effect on calcium absorption. This shows the challenge of trying to isolate the effect of a single nutrient and calls the conclusions regarding fracture risk into question.[302 303 304]

Team Calcium: Think of Bone Building as a Team Sport

In the real world in which your bones live, all of the nutrients are *players* who serve key roles. Imagine calcium is the football. Vitamin D is the quarterback. Vitamin K2, or more specifically the vitamin K-dependent proteins (osteocalcin and matrix Gla protein), are the wide receivers.

- If plenty of K2-activated receivers are on the field, vitamin D can easily pass the calcium football, either to osteocalcin for a bone-building touchdown or to matrix-Gla protein to prevent the calcium football from ending up in your arteries or kidneys.

- When K2 is lacking, our vitamin D quarterback still has to offload the calcium football but has no K2 receivers ready to accept a pass. Osteocalcin and matrix Gla protein are sitting on the bench, inactive. Vitamin D is forced to throw a wild pass. The calcium football flies out and lands somewhere off the field (i.e., floats unchaperoned in your bloodstream or gets excreted in urine or stools). Drive over. No first down.

- Or even worse, the pass gets intercepted. Our calcium football gets picked up by a player on the opposing (unhealthful use of calcium) team, who scores a goal in your arteries, brain, or kidneys.[305][306]

We'll revisit the idea of *Team Calcium* as a recurring theme, especially in the chapters where we discuss vitamin D and vitamin K2, who are certainly star players. For now, the key takeaways are that healthy bones require at least 1,200 mg of calcium (preferably 1,350 to 1,500 mg) each and every day. In addition, you need to get vitamin D and vitamin K2 in sufficient amounts.

Calcium Diary: See How Much Calcium Your Diet is Providing

Your diet alone is unlikely to provide all of the calcium you need. Data from many studies show that a significant number of Americans don't even get the Institute of Medicine's recommendations for Estimated Average Requirements (EAR) for calcium. The EAR is the amount estimated to meet the needs of just 50% of individuals in a life stage and gender group. (That means the EAR is not enough for the other 50%). (See table below.)

What We Eat in America, NHANES 2009-2010 showed that 42% of Americans were not meeting EAR recommendations.

Things have not improved since. The *2015-2020 Dietary Guidelines for Americans* reports on a number of shortfall nutrients, including calcium, where 58% of women and 26% of men get below the EAR in their diets. Even among those of us taking calcium supplements, 41% of women and 21% of men still fall short of the EAR.[307]

Calcium Daily Reference Intakes			
Age	Estimated Average Requirements	Recommended Dietary Allowance	Upper Level
19 to 50 years old	800 mg	1,000 mg	2,500 mg
51 to 70 years old	1,000 mg (women) 800 mg (men)	1,200 mg (women) 1,000 mg (men)	2,000 mg
>70 years old	1,000 mg	1,200 mg	2,000 mg

Source: Institute of Medicine Dietary Reference Intakes for Calcium and Vitamin D, Nov. 2010 nap. edu/resource/13050/Vitamin-D-and-Calcium-2010-Report-Brief.pdf

Calculate how much calcium you're getting. Understanding what your diet provides is critical to identifying your shortfall and what level of supplementation you need. An easy way to do this is by keeping a food diary for 5 to 7 days. We've provided a table below listing the best food sources of calcium. Simply add up the total calcium in the food or beverages you've consumed (noting your number of servings). Then, divide that total calcium (in milligrams) by the number of days you've kept your diary. The result is the average daily amount of calcium your diet provides. *How does this match up with the minimum 1,200 to 1,500 mg/d recommended for your bones?*

We're going to nag you to keep your diary. Most of us will find we need at least 700 mg of *additional* calcium daily. It's really worth taking a few minutes to do this for yourself.

Best Food Sources of Calcium		
Food	Serving Size	Calcium (mg)
Cow's milk*, 2% fat	1 cup	297
Yogurt, low-fat	1 cup	447
Cottage cheese, 1% fat	1 cup	100
Mozzarella cheese, part-skim	1 ounce	183
Swiss cheese	1 ounce	265
Goat milk	1 cup	326
Salmon, canned	4 ounces	300
Sardines, canned with bones	2 ounces	240
Spinach, steamed	1 cup	245
Collard greens, steamed	1 cup	226
Kale, steamed	1 cup	94
Romaine lettuce	2 cups	40
Broccoli, steamed	1 cup	75
Green beans	1 cup	57
Cabbage, shredded, steamed	1 cup	46
Sesame Seeds	¼ cup	351
Tofu	4 ounces	100
Orange	1 raw	52
Almonds (about 20 nuts)	1 ounce	70
Green beans	1 cup	57
Orange	1 raw	52
Cabbage, shredded, steamed	1 cup	46
Romaine lettuce	2 cups	40

Source: National Institutes of Health, Office of Dietary Supplements, Calcium-Health Professional Fact Sheet: ods.od.nih.gov/factsheets/Calcium-HealthProfessional/#en1; Institute of Medicine
(IOM). Food and Nutrition Board. Dietary Reference Intakes: Calcium, Phosphorus, Magnesium,
Vitamin D and Fluoride. Washington, DC: National Academy Press, 1997; Calcium World's Healthiest Foods www.whfoods.org/genpage.php?tname=nutrient&dbid=45

Calcium's safe UL (upper limit) is at least 2,000 mg/d across all age groups. Thus, an intake of 1,350 to 1,500 mg/d should be safe—provided, as explained previously, you're also getting adequate vitamin K2.[308]

Dairy foods are a great source of calcium and protein, but could cow's milk increase fracture risk? Dairy products, such as cheese, cottage cheese, yogurt, and kefir, are protective for our bones. However, drinking 2 or more glasses of cow's milk daily could increase your risk for fracture. *Why is that?*[309]

Cow's milk contains *lactose*, a sugar our bodies digest (for those of us who produce the enzyme, lactase) into two sugars: *glucose* and *D-galactose*. D-galactose is a sugar so inflammatory that it's used in animal studies to cause rapid, premature aging. As you know, chronic inflammation activates osteoclasts, the cells that break down bone. Therefore, drinking several glasses of cow's milk every day can contribute to bone loss. One glass of cow's milk contains about 5 grams of D-galactose; 6 to 10 grams could cause people trouble, based on equivalent dosages in animal studies.[310]

Understanding this finally makes sense of the conflicting results of the research on dairy products and explains why women with a higher intake of cheese or yogurt—but not milk—have a 25% to 32% lower risk of hip fracture.[311] Cheese, particularly hard, aged cheeses, and fermented dairy products (like yogurt, cottage cheese, and kefir) contain virtually no lactose, so we don't produce D-galactose from them. And these dairy foods contain 18 of 22 essential nutrients, including significant amounts of the protein, calcium, and vitamin D our bones require.

Lactose-free milk does not spare you from D-galactose—it's just predigested from lactose into these sugars. However, the amount of lactose in some lactose-free milk is reduced before it's pre-digested to avoid excess free glucose that would make the milk unpleasantly sweet.[312] This *ultra-filtered* milk does contain less D-galactose. However, we have several concerns about some brands offering ultra-filtered milk that is not derived from pastured cows and uses GMO grains from some of their supplying farms. For an in-depth scoop on the science-backed facts and actual costs of GMO farming, read *FOOD FIX*, written by Dr. Mark Hyman (Little, Brown Spark, NY, 2020).

Lastly, many ultra-filtered milk products are reduced fat. Both forms of vitamin K (K1 and K2) as well as vitamins A, D, and E are fat-soluble. When the fat is removed from milk, so are they. If you're going to drink milk, make it organic whole milk from pastured cows and consume no more than 1 glass daily.

Alternatives to Cow's Milk for Calcium

Is orange juice or soy milk, fortified with calcium, a good choice? Unfortunately, these beverages cannot be relied upon as a good source of calcium. Depending on the fortification system used, calcium can precipitate out. Have you ever gotten to the bottom of a container of calcium-fortified OJ or non-dairy milk and found a bunch of thickened goop? That's the calcium that dropped out.

Researchers compared the degree to which calcium settled out of 14 calcium-fortified beverages to the amount that settled out in fat-free cow's milk. In all the soy and rice beverages tested, 82% to 89% of the total calcium had separated from the solution. In calcium-fortified orange juice, as much as 50.4% of the calcium separated out. Even in the cow's milk, about 11% of the calcium had separated. *What can you do about this?* Give your milk or orange juice container a good shake before pouring yourself a serving. You'll redistribute the calcium from the bottom of the container back into the milk or orange juice.[313]

Calcium-rich mineral water: a surprisingly good calcium-rich alternative to milk—and it's calorie-free! Reaching our calcium goals can be especially difficult for those who are lactose-intolerant, vegan, or allergic to dairy products. Fortunately, studies have now shown that calcium-rich mineral waters can provide an effective alternative to cow's milk. A meta-analysis of four studies found that calcium *bioavailability* (how much is absorbed and utilized) from mineral waters was at least as good as, and possibly better than, that from dairy products. Not only did biomarkers indicate significant calcium absorption, but markers of bone resorption decreased. And calcium-rich mineral water is naturally calorie-free, certainly a much healthier alternative to sodas—especially for all of us who want to fit into our skinny jeans! *Pellegrino anyone?*[314]

Which Calcium Supplement is Best for You?

If you've completed your food diary and are like most people, you'll find your diet doesn't provide the full 1,200 mg of calcium (and preferably 1,350 to 1,500 mg) you need for healthy bones. To make up the difference, you can take a calcium supplement available in several forms, including calcium carbonate, calcium citrate, and algae-derived calcium.

Different forms vary in their percentage of elemental calcium. That's important as it indicates the actual amount of calcium available versus the other elements with which the calcium is bound. Other differences include what the calcium is derived from.

Calcium Supplements to Avoid

Before we describe the pros and cons of calcium forms to consider, let's briefly go over some additional forms you may see that we don't recommend:

- **Calcium from bone meal** fell out of favor back in the 1980s, when bone-meal derived supplements were found to be heavily contaminated with lead, arsenic, mercury, and cadmium—all of which are heavy metal poisons that destroy bone. Obviously, you don't want this!

- **Calcium lactate and calcium gluconate** are still available, though not widely because they deliver far less calcium per tablet or capsule than calcium carbonate (which contains the most elemental calcium per pill), calcium citrate, or algae-derived calcium. The percentages of elemental calcium in calcium lactate (13%) and calcium gluconate (9%) are so low as to make them impractical. One popular brand of calcium lactate contained only 255 mg of elemental calcium in 3 tablets. To get 750 mg of supplemental elemental calcium, you'd have to swallow 9 tablets daily.[315]

- **Hydroxyapatite** is a mineral complex derived from cow bones in which calcium is joined with phosphorus to form calcium phosphate, the principal storage form of calcium in bone. While this sounds helpful, hydroxyapatite is unlikely to be your best choice. Hydroxyapatite is marketed as a form of calcium readymade to go into your bones, but this is hype. The calcium we consume is going to be disassociated (or liberated) in our digestive tract from *any* compound to which it has been bound before it is absorbed. In other words, the calcium ions will be separated from the phosphorus, just like calcium will be separated from the citrate in calcium citrate or the carbonate in calcium carbonate.

  And we certainly don't need supplemental phosphorus! As explained in Part One, phosphate additives in processed foods and sodas are increasing our risk for heart attack, kidney disease, osteoporosis, and death from virtually all causes. Lara wrote about this in a review entitled, *Canaries in the Phosphate-Toxicity Coal Mines*, which you can access on PubMed (an online database of biomedical literature). We are the canaries.[316]

Furthermore, hydroxyapatite is the most expensive form of calcium and its effectiveness in building bone has very little scientific support. Few studies have been done on whether it's worth the added cost. One study, published in 2014, involved 100 postmenopausal women (average age of 71) randomly given 1,000 mg/d supplementation of different forms of calcium or a placebo for three months. Hydroxyapatite was not as well absorbed and did no better than calcium carbonate or calcium citrate.[317]

- **Ossein-hydroxyapatite (OHC)** is a version of hydroxyapatite that contains other factors in addition to calcium and phosphorus. A study comparing OHC to calcium carbonate over 1 to 3 years showed that BMD continued to drop, just not as much, remaining 1.02% higher on average in those given OHC. In other words, OHC taken alone or with vitamin D slows bone loss a bit more effectively than calcium carbonate. Note that the doses of OHC ranged from 3,320 to 6,640 mg/d, which is equivalent to 8.3 to 16.6 capsules per day for OHC sold in the U.S. By comparison, the calcium carbonate dosage ranged from 2,000 to 3,500 mg/d, exceeding the safe upper limit and required 6 to 10 capsules daily, if taken in 350 mg doses optimal for absorption.[318] [319]

Calcium Supplements to Consider: Carbonate, Citrate, and Algae-Derived

Once you exclude the above calcium supplements, three common forms of supplemental calcium remain. *How do they compare?*

Calcium carbonate and calcium citrate supplements are derived from rock. Each provides calcium in one form. Algae-derived calcium (AlgaeCal) is derived from the sea plant *Lithothamnion superpositum*, the richest plant source of calcium yet identified. It contains 4 different types of calcium: calcium hydroxide, calcium chloride, calcium sulfate, and calcium carbonate.

Calcium carbonate supplements are 40% elemental calcium. Calcium citrate supplements are 21% elemental calcium. AlgaeCal falls somewhere in the middle, with 28 to 31% elemental calcium. The big difference is that this calcium makes up part of a naturally balanced mineral matrix, containing 2% to 4% elemental magnesium and every trace mineral the marine algae species uses to build its bony structure. That's important because humans need the same minerals to build bone. Today's chemically grown plant foods no longer provide them in anywhere near adequate amounts.

Calcium carbonate is the most common form used in supplements. You can also find it in many over-the-counter antacids, largely because it's inexpensive. You'll find the supplemental calcium (and all other minerals) in the form of a *salt*, which contains both the mineral and a stabilizing partner, in this case *carbonate*. (This type of mineral salt is not what we typically consider *salty*, since it doesn't contain sodium.) As with most calcium salts, calcium carbonate requires an acidic environment in the stomach for the calcium to disassociate from the compound to which it is bound, so it can be absorbed. That's why calcium supplements should be taken with a little food—even a cup of coffee will do—in response to which our stomachs produce the stomach acid (hydrochloric acid) needed to release and solubilize the calcium.[320]

Calcium citrate, unlike other forms, works without the need for stomach acid. This is the one calcium compound that does not require acid to break it down. Therefore, you can take it either with or without food. However, calcium citrate is more expensive and contains less elemental calcium per tablet, so you need to take more pills.

Calcium citrate can be helpful for individuals unable to produce stomach acid. That includes specific conditions (i.e., hypochlorhydria), medications that prevent stomach acid production (histamine-2 blockers or proton-pump inhibitors for those with gastroesophageal reflux (GERD), and gastric bypass surgery, since the stomach acid-producing parts of the stomach have been removed.[321 322 323 324]

Only AlgaeCal has been clinically associated with *actual* increases in BMD. When taking calcium carbonate or calcium citrate, even if accompanied by vitamin D, you can expect a yearly age-related decline of at least -0.1% in bone mineral density (which increases to 2% per year or more during the menopausal transition). In contrast, AlgaeCal is the *only* calcium supplement shown to build more new bone than we lose through normal life-long bone remodeling. Four research studies, all published in the peer-reviewed medical literature on PubMed, have confirmed this.

In Vitro Study: The first study was *in vitro* (a cell study) in which human osteoblast cells (the cells that build new bone) were treated with either AlgaeCal, calcium citrate, or calcium carbonate—with or without vitamin D3 being present. After 4 days, the AlgaeCal treated cells showed differences in some key bone-remodeling markers:

- *Bone alkaline phosphatase* (BAP), an enzyme involved in the production of new osteoblasts and their mineralization of bone. AlgaeCal increased BAP activity 400%, compared to 200% for calcium carbonate and 150% for calcium citrate.

- *Proliferating cell nuclear antigen* (PCNA), a protein involved in DNA synthesis and repair: The levels of PCNA in the AlgaeCal treated cells were 3-fold greater compared to calcium carbonate and 4-fold greater compared to calcium citrate treated cells.

- Oxidative stress (free radical damage): AlgaeCal reduced oxidative stress in human osteoblasts by 4-fold compared to controls (untreated cells), 2-fold compared to calcium carbonate, and 2.5-fold compared to calcium citrate.

- The end result: far more calcium was deposited in AlgaeCal-treated cells, 2-fold more than controls, 1-fold more than calcium carbonate, and 4-fold more than calcium citrate-treated cells. When vitamin D3 was added along with AlgaeCal to the treated osteoblasts, the results were even better.[325]

Human Studies Demonstrate *Actual* Increases in BMD

The very promising results in the in vitro study led to three human studies conducted using AlgaeCal:

Human Study No. 1: A 6-month trial evaluated the bone-building effects of AlgaeCal, along with different combinations of other important bone-building nutrients. Two groups were followed for 6 months, one of 158 adults and a second group of 58 adults both using AlgaeCal, though with slightly varied nutrient combinations. Both groups experienced significantly higher BMD over that time period than would be otherwise expected—what scientists call a *mean annualized percent* *change* (MAPC). The first formulation resulted in a MAPC of 1.15%, while the second group fared far better with a MAPC of 2.79%. No adverse side-effects were seen.[326]

We want to stress that these were *positive* gains in BMD. When calcium studies report an *increase* in bone density, that is often misleading. Rather than an outright increase, reporting often compares subjects to an untreated control group, whose BMD is declining at the typical rate for their age, sex, and other factors. This landmark result showed a *real* increase in BMD, not a relative increase compared to a placebo group whose members are also losing BMD.

Human Study No. 2: Following these results, researchers followed 414 postmenopausal women over a year to compare three different versions of an AlgaeCal bone-health supplement program. Each of the three AlgaeCal Plans differed in the amounts of vitamin D3, magnesium, and other minerals. In addition, Plan 1 tried out vitamin K2 in the form of MK-4, while Plan 2 used MK-7 and also added 50 mg of vitamin C.

No adverse effects were seen in any of the plans and all 3 produced BMD increases of at least 1.3%. Plans 2 and Plan 3, which both included strontium citrate, fared best, with BMD increases of 2% and 4.1% respectively.[327] Note that the current formula for AlgaeCal Plus is based largely on Plan 3, though without strontium citrate, which is offered as a separate companion product (Strontium Boost). (See table below.)

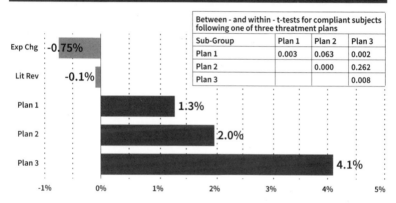

Annualized % BMD Change in Human Study No. 2

Between - and within - t-tests for compliant subjects following one of three threatment plans			
Sub-Group	Plan 1	Plan 2	Plan 3
Plan 1	0.003	0.063	0.002
Plan 2		0.000	0.262
Plan 3			0.008

Exp Chg: -0.75%
Lit Rev: -0.1%
Plan 1: 1.3%
Plan 2: 2.0%
Plan 3: 4.1%

Exp Chg: Age-adjusted expected change without treatment intervention
Lit Rev: Age-adjusted expected changes from non-plant calcium/Vit D3 supplements (derived from literature review)
Plan 1: Annualized changes in BDM after taking the plant-sourced form of calcium with Vitamin D3
Plan 2: Changes for all subjects following the 3-compound bone-health plan
Plan 3: Changes for all subjects following the 3-compound bone-health plan

A 1-year test of AlgaeCal shows a gain in bone mineral density of 1.3% to 4.1% in postmenopausal women depending on the specific formulation used. This group (adjusted for age) would normally expect bone losses: -0.75% without treatment or -0.10% from non-plant calcium with vitamin D supplements. See below table for specific formulations tested.

Source: International Journal of Medical Sciences, March 2011 (www.ncbi.nlm.nih.gov/pmc/articles/PMC3053489)

AlgaeCal Formulations Used in Human Study No. 2			
Components or ingredients	Plan 1	Plan 2	Plan 3
Plant-sourced Calcium (mg)	750	720	756
Trace Minerals in AlgaeCal (mg)	1,771	1,608	1,692
Magnesium (mg)*	65	72	350
Vitamin D-3 (IUs of Cholecalciferol)	1,000	800	1,600
Vitamin K-2 as MK-4 (mg)	0	1.5	0
Vitamin K-7 as MK-7 (mgc)	0	0	100
Boron (mg)	0	0	3
Vitamin C (mg)	0	0	50
Strontium Citrate (mg)	0	680	680
Pedometer based activity program	No	Yes	Yes
Health Literacy Information	No	Yes	Yes

While all 3 plans produced BMD increases of at least 1.3%, Plan 2 and Plan 3 resulted in BMD increases of 2% and 4.1% respectively. Note that the current formula for AlgaeCal Plus is based largely on Plan 3, though without strontium citrate, which is offered as a separate companion product (Strontium Boost).

*72 mg naturally occurring plus magnesium carbonate

Source: International Journal of Medical Sciences 2011; 8(3):180-191 (www.ncbi.nlm.nih.gov/pmc/articles/PMC3714389/)

- **Human Study No. 3**: The first two human studies had shown that postmenopausal women significantly increased BMD in as little as 6 months and definitely within one year when using AlgaeCal. This third human study looked at longer-term use and demonstrated an increase in BMD every year for 7 years (see chart below). In this study, 172 postmenopausal women in their mid-60s gained 7.3% more bone, adding about 1% to their BMD each year—instead of what typically happens, a loss of at least 1% per year.[328]

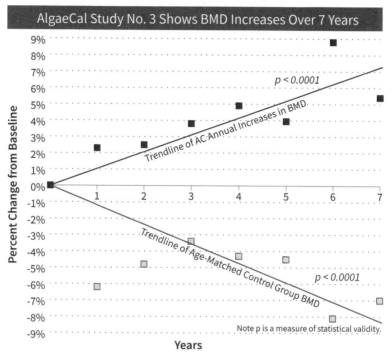

Trendline comparisons over 7 years show an annual 1% gain in bone mineral density for study participants on AlgaeCal Plus compared to the expected loss of 1% per year for an age-matched control group.

Source: American College of Nutrition, February 2016 (pubmed.ncbi.nlm.nih.gov/26885697)

In addition, long-term safety was well established by a panel of 45 blood chemistries drawn at the start and end of the study. This is important given recent papers, like the one mentioned earlier by Bolland, suggested traditional calcium supplements might increase the risk of heart attack or stroke. Therefore, cardiovascular risk was a focus in this 7-year AlgaeCal study, and the results were excellent, as you can see from the data in the graphic below.

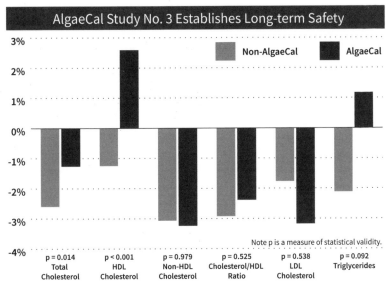

In this study of AlgaeCal, no evidence was found of increased cardiovascular risk as measured by adverse changes in blood lipids. This is notable as other studies have suggested traditional calcium supplements may increase the risk of heart attack or stroke.

Source: American College of Nutrition, February 2016 (pubmed.ncbi.nlm.nih.gov/26885697)

What makes AlgaeCal different? Remember our Team Calcium example from earlier? AlgaeCal contains the full roster of players—vitamin D3, K2, and magnesium—plus a variety of trace minerals.

Trace minerals have largely vanished from our food supply due to chemically grown foods. Nitrogen fertilizers lack these minerals and do not replenish the soil, with the exception of phosphorus, which we don't need more of. (See Phosphate Additives, Chapter 2.) Even when eating a *healthy* diet, we're unlikely to get the nutrients our bones require from diet alone. Our bones need these trace minerals, and AlgaeCal is an excellent source of many! I'll share the research showing the important roles of these nutrients in upcoming chapters devoted to them.[329][330][331]

Team Calcium includes more key players. *Lithothamnion superpositum* naturally contains a mix of plant-derived calcium salts, magnesium, and important trace minerals. The manufacturer of AlgaeCal mills the whole, live-harvested sea algae into a powder. For their AlgaeCal Plus product, the dosages of vitamins and minerals shown in the research to be effective for healthy bones are matched by adding additional vitamins and minerals:

- Vitamin D in its D3 (cholecalciferol) form, rather than its much less effective D2 (ergocalciferol) form. (See Vitamin D, Chapter 5.)

- Vitamin K2 in its MK-7 form rather than its much less effective MK-4 form. (See Vitamin K, Chapter 5.)

- Plus, vitamin C, additional magnesium (to achieve the recommended calcium to magnesium ratio of 2:1), and additional boron (in the 3 mg/d dose required for its beneficial effects on bone).

The Truth About Calcium Bioavailability

Does bioavailability differ among various types of calcium? The different forms of calcium are only effective to the extent that calcium ions can be released from their stabilizing partners (e.g., calcium from carbonate), so they can be used in your body. Many papers have clearly demonstrated that when calcium supplements are taken with a meal—or even a snack—the various forms of calcium are all comparably bioavailable.

You may have heard that calcium citrate is more easily absorbed than other forms of calcium. It's simply not true. What is true is that calcium will disassociate from citrate even if no stomach acid is present, but once disassociated from whatever compound it has linked up with—and calcium will happily form a salt with quite a few other elements in the periodic table—all forms of calcium are equally well absorbed.

We've also been told that older folks might be better off taking calcium citrate because, as we age, stomach acid production declines in about half of us. We believed this for a long time—until Lara dug into the research upon which this claim is based: one very small study published in 1985. In this study, calcium carbonate was given to elders with achlorhydria under fasting conditions (which means their stomachs produced virtually no stomach acid when no food was present). These individuals could absorb the calcium from calcium citrate better than from calcium carbonate.[332] That's not surprising, since no food was present!

What's not reported is that the study participants absorbed calcium with no problem when calcium carbonate was administered as part of a normal breakfast. Again, not surprising since food initiates the production of stomach acid, necessary for breaking down forms of calcium other than calcium citrate. Other research has shown similar findings:

- In a more recent study of elderly subjects, when calcium carbonate and calcium citrate were used to fortify skim milk and orange juice, calcium carbonate was found to be just as bioavailable as calcium citrate.[333]

- Another study, published in the *Journal of the American College of Nutrition* in 2001, compared the bioavailability of calcium citrate to calcium carbonate in 24 postmenopausal women. Both types of calcium supplement produced identical 24-hour increases in blood levels of calcium. In other words, the calcium from either source was equally well absorbed and had equivalent bioavailability.[334]

With very few exceptions, calcium bioavailability is a non-issue! However, calcium citrate can be beneficial in individuals who:

- **have had gastric bypass surgery.** Gastric bypass surgery involves removal of the fundus, the part of the stomach where hydrochloric acid is produced. Therefore, the use of calcium citrate eliminates the need for stomach acid to release calcium from the compound with which it is combined.[335] (See Obesity, Chapter 4.)

- **take acid-blocking drugs.** Those who regularly take stomach acid-suppressing medications, such as proton pump inhibitors or H2 blockers, to manage symptoms of GERD (gastroesophageal reflux disease) produce little stomach acid, so they may be better off with calcium citrate.[336][337] (See GERD, Chapter 4.)

Optimize Your Ability to Absorb Calcium

Certain steps can help you absorb calcium, whether from food or supplementation (or likely a combination of both). Here are some strategies:

Ensure that you are getting adequate vitamin D to meet YOUR needs. Active absorption in the first part of our small intestine (the duodenum) accounts for 85% to 90% of the calcium absorbed and depends on your vitamin D status. Passive absorption in the final portion of the small intestine (the ileum) provides only a small fraction of our calcium. Individuals who are vitamin D deficient absorb only 10% to 15% of the calcium they consume.[338][339]

- A study looking at blood levels of 25(OH)D (the form in which vitamin D circulates in the bloodstream) found absorption rates were

65% higher at blood levels of 34.6 ng/mL than at levels of less than 20 ng/mL. And 34.6 ng/mL is well below optimal 25(OH)D status, which is closer to 60 to 80 ng/mL. You can easily find out your blood levels of 25(OH)D with a simple blood draw or finger prick test, a test often covered by health insurance.[340][341] (See Lab Tests, Chapter 10.)

Take your calcium supplement in doses of about 350 mg twice daily. Lower doses improved absorption in a study of 37 healthy men and women given either calcium carbonate or calcium citrate. Subjects taking either form of calcium at a 300 mg dose absorbed 36%, while those taking 1,000 mg at once absorbed just 28.4%. The researchers determined 500 mg as a maximum dose of elemental calcium and suggested about 350 mg taken twice daily would likely provide the best absorption. (As a side note, the absorption of calcium carbonate and calcium citrate were again found to be equivalent when taken with a meal.)[342][343]

Having some unabsorbed calcium pass through our digestive tract has important benefits. The calcium we don't absorb combines with potentially harmful substances in our digestive tract after a meal, such as oxalic acid, unabsorbed fatty acids, and bile acids. That is one of the reasons why calcium helps us excrete more fat.[344]

Another Bone Protective Benefit: Calcium Helps us Burn Fat (and Produce Less)

Calcium's relationship to body fat has been a topic of research since 1980. Both animal studies and human placebo-controlled trials have shown daily consumption of calcium to be inversely related to body fat. Calcium promotes fat loss.[345]

This is important for your bones because excess fat, particularly *visceral adipose tissue* (VAT) doesn't just prevent you from zipping up your jeans! VAT is highly inflammatory, constantly spewing out pro-inflammatory cytokines that increase osteoclast activation. And for those of us who find ourselves trying to take off a few extra pounds, here's some really good news: Supplementing with calcium and vitamin D has been shown in several recent studies to greatly increase the amount of fat loss when calories are restricted while dieting.[346]

The latest studies have focused on figuring out why these happy events happen. Here's what we know so far:

- Calcium causes more fat to be excreted in stools. In a study, subjects took supplemental calcium while restricting their calories to 500 below what was needed to maintain their ideal weight. The subjects lost 5 grams of fat in stools per day—more than twice the 2 grams a person typically loses each day.

- Calcium promotes the release of insulin (the hormone that delivers sugar to our cells), so the calories we consume are used to produce energy rather than stored away as fat.

- Calcium, particularly when accompanied by vitamin D and protein, increases satiety, so we eat less.

For more details on how calcium helps us lose fat, see the below box. To find out how many calories a 500-calorie deficit would leave for you, here's a link to a simple, but accurate, calorie calculator you can use: www.calculator.net/calorie-calculator.html.

Mechanisms Through Which Calcium Helps Us Lose Fat

Calcium's role in increasing fat loss is due, in part, to its effects on two peptides produced in our digestive tract that stimulate insulin's release from the pancreas. GIP and GLP are secreted by special cells in our gastrointestinal tract and later broken down by an enzyme called dipeptidyl peptidase-IV (DPP-IV). *What triggers our secretion of GIP and GLP?* Calcium, when its concentration in the digestive tract increases and wakes up the calcium-sensing receptors. The insulin-secretion actions of GIP and GLP are further increased by the presence of amino acids (i.e., protein). It turns out that the peptides that make up the amino acids in protein, and especially milk protein, inhibit DPP-IV from breaking down GIP and GLP.[347]

When calcium and protein are both present in our digestive tract, the two nutrients act synergistically to enhance concentrations of GIP and GLP, boosting our secretion of insulin and our cells' use of the sugar in our bloodstream to produce energy. Plus, when calcium is consumed, both GIP and GLP also boost *lipolysis*—the breakdown of fat. Calcium also decreases fat absorption, which is why we excrete more fat in our stools.[348]

Lastly, calcium stimulates the *mitochondria* (our cellular energy production factories) in brown fat to join up with other nearby mitochondria—even the white fat mitochondria that normally store rather than burn off excess fat—to increase their energy-burning and heat-producing ability (thermogenic capacity).[349] Calcium also delays gastric emptying, so we feel full sooner and for longer. Put this all together and it spells weight loss—and even better, weight loss due to fat loss.[350]

We also produce less fat when we consume more calcium. Low levels of calcium circulating in our bloodstream trigger the release of parathyroid hormone (PTH), whose jobs are to (1) activate osteoclasts to release calcium from bone and (2) ramp up the kidney's production of 1,25-D, the form in which vitamin D increases our absorption of calcium from the intestines and our reabsorption of calcium from the kidneys.

Since vitamin D receptors (VDRs) are also present in fat cells, the actions of PTH cause calcium to be brought into our fat cells, which then trigger changes in our metabolism that cause us to produce more fat. This fat-cell calcium increases the activity of an enzyme called *fatty acid synthase*, which as its name implies, synthesizes more fat. This enzyme also inhibits *lipolysis*, the breakdown of fats in our mitochondria. In other words, when we don't get enough calcium, we produce more fat and block its use as a source of energy. Insufficient calcium makes us fat and tired. Now the good news: consuming 1,200 mg/d of calcium (total from diet and supplements) decreases our production of fatty acid synthase and causes a drop in lipogenesis (new fat production).

Plus, calcium increases fat burning (oxidation). In one study, when calcium intake (1,400 mg/d, total from diet and supplements) was combined with lowered calories (600 calories less than needed to maintain subjects' current weight) and exercise (1 hour/d), 24-hour fat burning went up more than 30%! Calcium helps you get more fat-burning bang for your exercise buck!

Another group of researchers found a significant increase in lipid oxidation (i.e., fat burning) following a 12-week placebo-controlled trial of calcium (900 mg/d through dairy products or supplementation) along with a diet that resulted in a 500-calorie deficit per day. Not only did subjects lose more fat, they lost belly fat—the worst kind of inflammatory fat. In addition, blood levels of PTH decreased. And we want PTH levels to stay low to keep calcium out of our fat cells.

To maximize calcium's fat-burning effect, take supplemental calcium and vitamin D with breakfast. Research shows that higher calcium and vitamin D intake at breakfast increases the rate at which fat is burned over the next 2 meals, and also reduces how much food you eat in the subsequent 24-hour period (i.e., until breakfast the following day).

The results of all these studies tell us that not getting enough calcium not only promotes bone loss, but also changes our metabolism in ways that make us gain more inflammation-producing fat and lessen our ability to burn fat for energy. So, now, in addition to maintaining healthy bones, you have more reasons to ensure you're getting 1,200 to 1,500 mg of calcium every day from your food and supplements combined.

Calcium Safety

Health authorities set calcium's safe upper limit (UL) based on a person's life stage. For adults, both men and women age 19 to 50, the calcium UL is 2,500 mg per day. At age 51 and above, it drops to 2,000 mg per day. Consuming more than the UL can result in *hypercalcemia*, a condition in which your blood levels of calcium are elevated. Hypercalcemia, particularly when insufficient vitamin K2 is available, can lead to kidney stone formation and the calcification of soft tissues, including the arteries, heart, breasts, and brain.

Does calcium supplementation increase my risk of a heart attack or kidney stones? No, not when the key Team Calcium players—including vitamin D3 and vitamin K2—are *all on the field*. Your doctor may not be aware of this teamwork. Yet, more than 30 years of research and dozens of studies published in the peer-reviewed medical literature confirm that our use of calcium requires both vitamin D (for calcium's absorption) and vitamin K2 (for calcium's delivery to bone and prevention of calcium deposition in our heart, blood vessels and kidneys).

You don't need to be a medical Einstein to know that our healthful use of calcium requires K2—*especially when taken with vitamin D*, which greatly increases our absorption of calcium. Interestingly, when we take vitamin D, our body automatically increases production of the vitamin K-dependent proteins we need to chaperone the calcium we're now absorbing, so it gets to the right places. Of course, with no vitamin K2 around, these proteins can't do their job.

Ignoring these basic realities of human physiology continues to cause much *needless* harm. *Consumer Reports* sent out an ALERT! in November 2015, citing a study that calcium supplements (again, calcium taken by itself) increase the risk for kidney stones. The research, presented that month at the American Society of Nephrology's Kidney Week conference, was unpublished, meaning it lacked the critical analysis of peer-review. As usual in *research* linking calcium supplementation with increased risk of unhealthy calcification, the authors of this report didn't consider vitamin K2.[351]

By now, you can guess why supplementing with only calcium, or even worse only calcium and vitamin D, might not be a good idea. *Reality check:* Effective absorption and healthful use of calcium require *both* vitamin D3 *and* vitamin K2.

Could my calcium supplement be causing constipation? Yes, taking a supplement that provides too much calcium in a single dose can cause constipation, particularly if calcium is not properly balanced by magnesium. One woman who wrote to me (Lara) was getting 1,000 mg of elemental calcium in just one dose of her supplement! Yikes, this is way too much! As discussed earlier, stick to about 350 mg twice daily. Take large doses and the excess will either be excreted or remain in your intestines increasing your risk of constipation, particularly if you're not getting enough magnesium.

Balance your calcium supplement with magnesium. The best bone-health supplements already include magnesium, ideally half as much magnesium as the amount of calcium they provide. If your supplement provides both calcium and magnesium and you are still suffering from constipation, then you may need a bit more magnesium or may not be effectively absorbing magnesium. (See Magnesium, Chapter 6.)

Calcium and magnesium work together in *many* cellular activities and need to be in a 2:1 balance for optimal function. Calcium generally constricts tissues (like our blood vessels and intestines) while magnesium relaxes them. In the heart, for example, calcium is involved in making the heart muscle contract; magnesium in its relaxation and release. In your intestines, the same principle applies. For this reason, insufficient magnesium in relation to calcium can promote constipation (and is why milk of magnesia can help relieve it). When you take calcium, especially coupled with vitamin D, which promotes its absorption, you need to be consuming enough magnesium to maintain proper balance.

Though the recommended ratio of calcium to magnesium is 2:1, you may need a bit more magnesium. Stress depletes magnesium as does exercise (since we lose magnesium through sweat). Then, there's estrogen's effect on magnesium. In premenopausal women, estrogen levels rise during the first half of the menstrual cycle and continue to accumulate until menses occurs. Estrogen pulls magnesium into bone. [352 353 354 355 356] (See Magnesium, Chapter 5.)

Note from Lara: While I'm postmenopausal, I work out at least an hour daily to both relieve stress and send my bones the signal to remain strong, so I need extra magnesium! Given the fast pace of our lives and relentless stress we all experience, you may too.

If you're getting sufficient magnesium and taking less than 500 mg (optimally around 350 mg) of calcium per dose (taken twice daily), your calcium supplement should not cause constipation or bloating. If you're still constipated, you may not be producing sufficient stomach acid (See Hypochlorhydria, Chapter 4.) or your diet may be lacking in fiber or fluids. Make sure you are consuming plenty of clean water and organically grown fiber-rich vegetables, fruits, whole grains (except wheat), nuts, and seeds.

Calcium-Drug Interactions

Calcium must be taken separately from certain drugs, as it reduces their absorption by forming insoluble complexes:[357]

- **Levothyroxine**: Take levothyroxine on an empty stomach at least one hour before consuming calcium-rich foods or calcium supplements.
- **Tetracyclines**: Take tetracyclines 2 hours before or 4 to 6 hours after calcium-rich food or calcium supplements.

- **Quinolone antibiotics:** Take quinolone antibiotics at least 2 hours before or 4 to 6 hours after consumption of calcium-rich foods or a calcium supplement.

- **Bisphosphonates**: Bisphosphonates cannot be taken with food, beverages, or supplements, including calcium, as they will create complexes that cannot be absorbed. In an attempt to make these drugs easier to use, the oral bisphosphonate (risedronate) is now available combined with a calcium chelator (a compound that locks onto calcium and prevents absorption), so the drug can be taken without fasting.[358]

Some drugs have other methods of decreasing calcium's absorption. Plus, be aware of one which can decrease calcium's excretion in a way that can be dangerous:

- **H2 blockers and proton-pump inhibitors** decrease calcium absorption by preventing the stomach from secreting stomach acid, which is necessary for the absorption of most forms of calcium (plus vitamin B12 and numerous other nutrients). If you must take one of the acid-suppressing drugs, take calcium citrate as it does not require stomach acid for absorption.

- **Corticosteroids**: In doses of 7.5 mg/d or more, corticosteroids cause significant bone loss; they decrease calcium absorption, increase calcium excretion, and inhibit bone formation.

- **Anticonvulsants** (i.e., phenytoin, fosphenytoin, carbamazepine, and phenobarbital) decrease calcium absorption by increasing the elimination of vitamin D.

- **Thiazide diuretics:** Thiazide diuretics decrease the normal rate of calcium excretion, so these drugs increase the risk of *milk-alkali syndrome*, high blood calcium caused by taking in too much calcium and absorbable alkali. Common sources of calcium and alkali are antacids and calcium hydroxide supplements. If untreated, milk-alkali syndrome may lead to kidney failure or death. Serum calcium and PTH levels should be monitored regularly in anyone taking thiazide diuretics.

Calcium-Food Interactions

Excessive salt (sodium) intake increases urinary excretion of calcium and markers of bone turnover—a lot. In the most recent study, serum (blood) levels of CTX-I (*C-terminal telopeptide*, a peptide sequence cleaved by osteoclasts during bone resorption) were 21.3% higher in the women with the highest dietary salt intake.[359 360 361]

Eat more phytate-rich foods! Once thought to decrease calcium absorption, *phytates*—compounds concentrated in legumes and whole grains—have been revealed in the latest research to lessen bone loss and protect against osteoporosis.[362]

Don't worry about caffeine. Caffeine's effect on urinary excretion of calcium is negligible, small enough to be fully offset by as little as 1 to 2 tablespoons of milk. There is no evidence that caffeine has any harmful effect on bone status or on calcium in individuals who ingest the currently recommended daily allowances of calcium.[363]

BONE-HEALTHY ACTION ITEMS

- Get a total of 1,200 to 1,500 mg/day of calcium, from food and supplements combined.
- Take calcium supplements with food and split into doses of 500 mg or less to improve absorption.
- If you don't produce adequate stomach acid or need to take calcium without food, calcium citrate is best as it does not require stomach acid.
- Get sufficient vitamin D to maintain a 25(OH)D level of 60 to 80 ng/mL to optimize your ability to absorb calcium.
- Be sure to take K2, essential to direct calcium into bones. Consider taking AlgaeCal, which contains K2 along with other vitamins and minerals, *plus* has been shown to provide *actual* improvements in bone mineral density.
- Take calcium in a 2:1 ratio with magnesium to avoid constipation (though some people need additional magnesium).

Magnesium

BONE ESSENTIALS

- The majority of Americans are deficient in magnesium. More than half of people over age 50 are not consuming the Estimated Average Requirement, an amount already too low for half the population.
- Low magnesium disables your ability to absorb calcium by impairing your parathyroid hormone secretion and the ability of your kidneys to convert vitamin D into its active form.
- Besides helping us keep our bones, magnesium relaxes muscles and blood vessels, and combats tension and anxiety.
- Stress causes us to use up magnesium more quickly, and magnesium insufficiency increases stress—a vicious cycle.

Looking for an oasis of calm? Then, magnesium's your mineral! When magnesium's around, you can simply relax—literally. Your muscles, including your heart, relax; your blood vessels relax; your lungs relax; even the environment in your brain becomes one of calm. If your cells are having a Type-A, hyper-reactive kind of day, they settle down and calmly go about their business. No cellular temper tantrums or rioting when magnesium is in charge, just efficient energy production with a minimum of free radicals allowed.

Magnesium stabilizes cellular membranes, providing a calm, soothing environment in which the job gets done. Actually, 350+ jobs because magnesium is the cofactor for at least 350 enzymes. Without magnesium, these enzymes, many of which play roles in bone formation, don't work. Without magnesium, we cannot produce *adenosine triphosphate* (ATP), the energy currency of all cells in your body, including those in your bones. Magnesium also plays critical roles in lipid, protein, and DNA synthesis, balances the actions of calcium, and functions as a cellular signal transducer—and there's a whole lot of signaling going on every second in your cells.[364]

Magnesium and Calcium Balance Each Other Out

Magnesium and calcium are like partners in a good cop, bad cop routine. Both are absolutely necessary, but it's essential to your cellular drama that their opposing character roles are kept in balance. When magnesium is too low, calcium takes over and runs the show unopposed—and in terms of your cellular metabolism, calcium is an uptight kind of mineral. Too much calcium unchecked by magnesium triggers the release of stress hormones and other substances that constrict blood vessels and cause the blood to clot more easily. Calcium elevates your blood pressure and contracts muscles—a good thing when you're working out, but not constantly, 24/7.

When magnesium levels are low, which recent NHANES data indicates is *situation normal* for most of us, you get nervous. Literally, your brain cells (neurons) get trigger-happy, hyperactive, and prone to a special kind of brain cell unhappiness called *spreading depression (SD)*, which is the first phase of a migraine attack. All of your cells get uptight, in large part because magnesium is what prevents calcium from overloading your cells.

In addition to osteoporosis, not getting enough magnesium to balance calcium may contribute to cardiovascular disease, fibromyalgia, type 2 diabetes, chronic fatigue syndrome, asthma and migraine headaches—to name a few. [365] [366] [367] [368] [369] [370]

What Magnesium Does for Your Bones

Approximately 60% of the magnesium in the human body is found in bone, mainly in cortical bone (the hard outer layer of our bones) where magnesium is part of the apatite crystals that make up the bone matrix and where it's accessible for magnesium's many other uses in bone cells and in the rest of the body. Bones serve as a bank account for magnesium, just as they do for calcium. Plus, magnesium is required for our production of osteoblasts, the cells that build bone, and for osteoblasts' maturation and bone-building activities. [371] [372]

Magnesium affects the two master regulators of calcium balance: parathyroid hormone (PTH) and 1,25-D (the active hormonal form of vitamin D). This gets a bit complex, though bear with us here. Magnesium is the punchline for how both sides of this entire scenario work:

- **Parathyroid hormone** ensures that you always have enough calcium readily available in your bloodstream. Your parathyroid gland contains a special *calcium-sensing receptor* (CaSR) that constantly samples how much calcium is passing by in your bloodstream. When calcium levels drop too low, the CaSR triggers the secretion of PTH, which boosts production of the active form of vitamin D (1,25-D).

- **The activated vitamin D (1,25-D)** enables active absorption of calcium from your intestines and its reabsorption in your kidneys. Magnesium plays an essential role as the cofactor of the enzyme (25(OH) D-1α hydroxylase), the enzyme that converts 25(OH)D into 1,25-D.

Restoring blood calcium levels quickly is critical for our survival. Therefore, PTH takes further steps to secure calcium by triggering its release from your bones:

- First, it signals osteoblasts (bone-building cells) to produce *RANKL,* a signaling molecule that binds to a receptor on bone cells called *RANK,* which triggers osteoclast (bone-clearing cells) activity.

- Next, PTH reduces your osteoblasts' production of a compound called *osteoprotegerin,* a decoy molecule that also binds to RANKL, preventing it from binding to RANK. Without osteoprotegerin in the mix, virtually all the RANKL secreted by your osteoblasts will bind to RANK, activate osteoclasts, and cause calcium to be released from your bones.

So how does magnesium fit in with the RANKL/RANK/osteoprotegerin process? All this PTH signaling to the kidneys starts with a messenger molecule called *cyclic adenosine monophosphate (cAMP)*. The increased production of cAMP occurs through the activation of an enzyme called *adenylate cyclase,* which requires magnesium to do its job.[373]

Low Magnesium Results in Low Calcium Absorption

As you can see from the last few paragraphs, absorbing calcium is a pachinko game in which magnesium is an essential player. When you're low in magnesium, your calcium-absorbing ability is nuked. PTH secretion is impaired; the kidneys don't react to PTH signals, and the enzyme in the kidneys that converts 25(OH)D to 1,25-D doesn't work. The end result: 25(OH)D does not get converted to 1,25-D, your kidneys do not increase their reabsorption of calcium, and active absorption of calcium does not occur in your small intestine.

Since active absorption is responsible for 85% to 90% of our absorption of calcium, this means that your blood levels of calcium will plummet. When this happens, PTH will continue to be secreted, and calcium will continue to be withdrawn from your bones for its other immediately critical jobs, like enabling your heart muscle to contract.

In postmenopausal women with osteoporosis, magnesium deficiency is also associated with low blood levels of PTH. You don't want consistently high levels of PTH as this will result in too much RANKL-RANK binding and too much osteoclast activity, but you don't want too little PTH either! You need enough PTH secretion to ensure your kidneys get the message to resorb calcium and convert 25(OH)D to 1,25-D. Just supplementing postmenopausal women with low PTH with magnesium (thus restoring calcium absorption) has been shown to improve bone mineral density.[374][375]

How Magnesium Insufficiency Affects Bones

When magnesium is not in good supply, it will be pulled from bone for its many other uses throughout the body. When you become deficient, your bones lose 30% to 40% of their magnesium content. That affects the strength and health of our bones in an impressive number of ways. Here are just a few:

* **Magnesium directly affects the bone-building mineralization process.** Here's a case where size—that of the mineral crystals being produced in your bone matrix—definitely matters! But in this case, bigger is not better. Smaller crystals, and more of them, make strong bones. When bone-apatite crystals are too large, bones are brittle and unable to bear a normal load. When magnesium is in good supply, smaller crystals are produced; when magnesium's not around, you get the big, brittle ones.[376][377][378][379]

* **Magnesium insufficiency** produces highly damaging free radicals (*peroxynitrite* and *superoxide*, two of the body's most frightening berserkers) run rampant. *Substance P* (which stands for *pain*) gets released from immune cells and at bone nerve endings and ramps up osteoclast activity and bone resorption. Restoring magnesium sufficiency saves the day.[380][381]

How Much Magnesium Do You Need for Healthy Bones?

Sufficient magnesium is critical for proper absorption of calcium. The exact amount is a balancing act that takes into account your calcium intake, your vitamin D consumption (which enables you to actively absorb the calcium), and factors that more quickly deplete magnesium (discussed shortly).

In general, you want a 2:1 ratio of calcium to magnesium. In other words, you should be consuming half as much magnesium as calcium. To balance a daily intake of 1,200 mg/d of calcium (RDA for women over age 50 and men over age 70), you need at least 600 mg/d of magnesium per day. If consuming 1,500 mg/d of calcium, then 750 mg/d of magnesium is needed.

The RDA for magnesium is not sufficient! That becomes clear when you see the recommended magnesium amounts (for adults over age 30), which are only 320 mg for women and 420 mg for men, far below what is needed for a healthy 2:1 (calcium to magnesium) balance. Do not rely on the RDIs for magnesium for your bones' health!

Magnesium intake is far from optimal in the U.S. general population. An analysis of data from the National Health and Nutrition Examination Survey (NHANES) of 2005-2006 found that a majority of Americans of all ages consume less magnesium from food than their respective EARs (Estimated Average Requirement)—an amount thought to be *adequate* (not optimal) for only 50% of us. It's estimated that 55% of women and 58% of men age 51 to 70 years, and 70% of women and 80% of men over age 70 are not even meeting the EAR.[382]

However, consuming too much magnesium will also upset this balance and that's not good for you either. Data from the Women's Health Initiative studies revealed that excess magnesium in relation to calcium is harmful to bone and increases fracture risk. In China, where people tend to consume more magnesium and less calcium (they eat more vegetables and virtually no dairy), consuming too little calcium in relation to magnesium (a ratio of <1.7:1) increased women's risks of all-cause mortality and death due to cardiovascular disease and colorectal cancer.[383]

Comparison of Magnesium and Calcium Recommended Dietary Allowances				
Age	Women*		Men	
	Magnesium	Calcium	Magnesium	Calcium
9 to 13 years	240 mg	1,300 mg	240 mg	1,300 mg
14 to 18 years	360 mg	1,300 mg	410 mg	1,300 mg
19 to 30 years	310 mg	1,000 mg	400 mg	1,000 mg
31 to 50 years	320 mg	1,000 mg	420 mg	1,000 mg
51 to 70 years	320 mg	1,200 mg	420 mg	1,000 mg

*Excludes women who are pregnant or lactating

Source: Institute of Medicine (IOM). Food and Nutrition Board. Dietary Reference Intakes: Calcium, Phosphorus, Magnesium, Vitamin D and Fluoride. Washington, DC: National Academy Press, 1997

Factors that Increase Your Magnesium Needs

If you're stressed out (stress depletes our magnesium far more quickly) or work out a lot (we lose some magnesium in sweat), you should seek to get more either through diet or supplementation. Other factors can lead to our requirements for magnesium increasing:

- **When we lose estrogen, our bones lose magnesium.** In premenopausal women, estrogen levels rise during the first half of the menstrual cycle and continue to accumulate until menses occurs. Estrogen pulls magnesium into bone, which is helpful, but can also lead to menstrual cramps because less magnesium is available to relax the smooth muscle lining the uterus and lessen production of the prostaglandins that cause menstrual pain. This helps explain those chocolate cravings before a woman's period: chocolate is very high in magnesium. If you're perimenopausal, the hot flashes you may be experiencing are estrogen surges, and they increase your need for magnesium. Be grateful for them; your body is stockpiling magnesium to help your bones transition through menopause safely.[384]

  When you're postmenopausal, unless you're taking BHRT (bio-identical hormone replacement), estrogen's assistance in getting magnesium into your bones is pretty much gone.[385 386 387 388 389 390]

  Note from Lara: I'm on BHRT and eat lots of magnesium-rich foods. However, given the fast pace of our lives in this day and age, the relentless stress we all experience, and the fact that I exercise at least an hour each day both to relieve stress and to send my bones the signal to remain strong, I need extra magnesium! You may, too, particularly if you are postmenopausal and not on BHRT.

- **Certain medications deplete magnesium**: See the Safety Section below, and discuss your increased magnesium needs with your doctor.

Getting the Most Magnesium Out of Your Diet and Supplements

Just as calcium is most effectively absorbed when a lower dose is taken twice daily instead of a large dose all at once, magnesium is best absorbed and utilized when taken in smaller doses over the course of your day.

Don't consume that 600 mg of magnesium all at once! Let's be frank here. If you take more magnesium than your cells are able and willing to absorb, your muscles won't be the only part of your anatomy to loosen up. You will feel crappy (pun intended). *Why?* Because ingesting too much magnesium at one time draws more water into the bowels than they find acceptable. Distension of the bowel occurs, followed by its forceful evacuation (a.k.a. osmotic diarrhea). This is how milk of magnesia works as a laxative.

Magnesium is best absorbed and utilized when taken in smaller doses over the course of your day. This happens naturally when magnesium is delivered at mealtimes in your food. Take a look at the table below and you'll see that many whole foods are rich in magnesium, so getting 200 to 300 mg from your diet should be fairly easy.

Best Food Sources of Magnesium		
Food	**Serving Size**	**Magnesium (mg)**
Pumpkin and squash seed kernels, roasted	1 ounce	151
Bran ready-to-eat cereal (100%)	1 ounce	103
Halibut, cooked	3 ounces	91
Quinoa, dry	¼ cup	89
Almonds	1 ounce	78
Spinach, cooked from fresh	½ cup	78
Buckwheat flour	¼ cup	75

Best Food Sources of Magnesium		
Food	Serving Size	Magnesium (mg)
Cashews, dry roasted	1 ounce	74
Soybeans, mature, cooked	½ cup	74
Pine nuts, dried	1 ounce	71
Mixed nuts, oil roasted, with peanuts	1 ounce	67
White beans, canned	½ cup	67
Black beans, cooked	½ cup	60
Bulgur, dry	¼ cup	57
Oat bran, raw	¼ cup	55
Edamame (soybeans, green), cooked	½ cup	54
Tuna, yellowfin, cooked	3 ounces	54
Artichoke hearts, cooked	½ cup	50
Peanuts, dry roasted	1 oz	50
Lima beans, baby, cooked from frozen	½ cup	50

Source: Nutrient values from Agricultural Research Service (ARS) Nutrient Database for Standard Reference, Release 17

A magnesium supplement can happily provide the remaining 300 to 400 mg of magnesium you need. Remember to split your dosage and further improve absorption with the following strategies:

- **Choose a supplement that contains magnesium oxide.** This form of supplemental magnesium contains the most elemental magnesium by far. Plus, the magnesium ions it provides are released more slowly and absorbed along the entire length of the digestive tract, so you don't experience diarrhea. Most other forms of supplemental magnesium will produce diarrhea after just 400 mg—or even less in those of us who release our magnesium quickly.[391][392]

- **Balance your magnesium with calcium**. Remember the 2:1 ratio discussed above. Ideally, you will be taking twice-daily doses of both 175 mg of magnesium oxide along with 350 mg of calcium for best absorption of both minerals. When properly balanced, your calcium supplement will not cause constipation, and your magnesium supplement will not cause diarrhea.

- **Consume at least 3 mg of boron daily**. Boron significantly improves both magnesium's absorption and its deposition in bone and becomes even more important for both actions when we are postmenopausal[393] (See Boron, Chapter 6.)

- **You may need pyridoxal-5-phosphate (P5P) to effectively absorb magnesium.** Like many other vitamins, vitamin B6 (pyridoxine) must be converted into its active form, P5P to be effective. One of P5P's functions is to bring magnesium inside our cells, where it does its work for us. (See box below.)

Many Have Difficulty Converting B6 into its Active Form (P5P)

Recent studies indicate about nearly 1 in 3 Americans produce a slow version of the enzyme that converts B6 to P5P. Lara is among this 30% who are not good at converting vitamin B6 into P5P, and therefore can not absorb magnesium as easily.[394][395][396][397][398]

Low levels of P5P are also associated with increased levels of a variety of markers of inflammation. That shows just how critical the active form of vitamin B6 is.[399] Fortunately, this is a really easy fix. Just take P5P (50 mg once daily) along with your magnesium supplement. P5P is inexpensive, and you should be able to find it at any good health food store or from reputable online nutritional supplement companies.

Magnesium Safety

Certain medications deplete magnesium. If you are regularly taking any of the following, please discuss your increased magnesium needs with your doctor:

- Antibiotics: such as gentamicin (causes magnesium wasting by inhibiting activation of B6 into P5P) and amphotericin (commonly prescribed antifungal drug that is highly toxic to the kidneys).[400][401]
- Cisplatin, a chemotherapy medication.[402]
- Cetuximab, an epidermal growth factor receptor blocking agent used in the treatment of colon cancer.[403]
- Diuretics, such as hydrochlorothiazide and furosemide.[404][405]
- Oral contraceptives (birth control pills) deplete magnesium, as well as many other nutrients: B6, folic acid, B2, B12, vitamin C, vitamin E, and the trace minerals selenium and zinc.[406]

- Proton pump inhibitors, such as omeprazole used to manage symptoms of GERD.[407]
- Transplant therapy drugs, such as cyclosporine and sirolimus.[408]

BONE-HEALTHY ACTION ITEMS

- Balance your calcium to magnesium in a 2:1 ratio. Ideally, you will be consuming a total of 1,200 mg of calcium and 600 mg of magnesium daily from your diet plus supplements.
- Supplements should be taken in twice-daily doses of 350 mg calcium balanced by 175 mg of magnesium.
- Choose a supplement that contains magnesium oxide, which has the most elemental magnesium and is less likely to cause diarrhea.
- Consume at least 3 mg of boron daily to significantly improve magnesium's absorption and deposition in bone.
- If supplemental magnesium gives you loose stools, consider taking 50 mg/d of supplemental P5P, the active form of vitamin B6.
- You may need extra magnesium if you are under stress or frequently exercise as these deplete magnesium.
- If you take any of the listed drugs, which may cause severe loss of magnesium, discuss your increased magnesium needs with your doctor.

Vitamin D

BONE ESSENTIALS

- Calcium's active absorption requires vitamin D. Without it, you will absorb only 10% to 15% of the calcium you consume.
- Vitamin D improves muscle strength and repair, helping us to avoid falls.
- Vitamin D builds muscle that helps build bone
- Vitamin D supports healthy immune function.

- The 3 forms of vitamin D include: the D3 we can produce in our skin in response to sun exposure; 25(OH)D, which circulates in the bloodstream; and 1,25-D, the hormonal form that produces vitamin D's beneficial effects.
- Converting vitamin D3 into 25(OH)D and then into 1,25-D relies upon a healthy liver and kidneys.

Vitamin D is a *Goldilocks* vitamin: **D**elightful but **D**emanding.

It's so essential to our well-being that we can make it when sunshine kisses our skin—but only when conditions are *just* right. It can't just be sunny. That sunlight has to be at the right wavelength, one that is not available north of the 35° latitude during the winter months. Actually, the wavelengths with vitamin D's *seal of approval* are not readily available for about 6 months out of the year. So, if you live in San Francisco, Denver, St. Louis, Richmond, VA, or anywhere north of these cities, even on a sunny day, you won't be producing your own vitamin D for most of the year.

And that's just the start of vitamin D's demands. The vitamin D produced in your skin, D3, is not yet in its active form. To get there, it has to travel first to your liver, where it's converted into 25(OH)D, the form that circulates in your bloodstream, and then to your kidneys, where it's again changed into 1,25-D, the hormonal form of vitamin D that gets all the work done in your body. If either your liver or kidneys are not working well, neither is your ability to produce 1,25-D. (We'll dive into the details of this a bit later.)

Vitamin D has other demands for you, too. A whole *to-do list* we'll cover here, so you'll know everything you need to meet all of vitamin D's requirements and get it working for you.

What Vitamin D Does for Your Bones

Vitamin D is required for our active absorption of calcium. Calcium is absorbed both actively and passively in our intestines. Active absorption accounts for 85% to 90%. Without adequate vitamin D, you will absorb only 10% to 15% of the calcium you consume, whether from your diet or a supplement.[409][410]

Vitamin D improves muscle strength and repair, helping to prevent falls. Vitamin D deficiency causes the loss of muscle along with bone. That's a key reason why sarcopenia, when muscles essentially turn to fat as we age, is typically present along with osteoporosis.[411] It's long been recognized that vitamin D deficiency increases the risk of fracture, in part due to muscle weakness and resulting falls.

- A meta-analysis of 8 randomized clinical trials, involving 2,426 individuals (average age of 65) has shown that vitamin D supplementation decreases the incidence of falls by 19%.[412]

- An analysis of the beneficial effect of vitamin D supplementation in preventing falls in older adults (aged 60 and older) in the United Kingdom found that providing even 800 IU per day of vitamin D3, over a 5-year period, would: (1) prevent in excess of 430,000 minor falls; (2) avoid 190,000 major falls; (3) prevent 1,579 acute deaths; (4) avoid 84,000 person-years of long-term care and (5) prevent 8,300 deaths associated with increased mortality in long-term care.

Vitamin D builds muscle to build bone. Bones provide rigid levers for muscles to pull against. When our muscles contract, the force generated on bone signals a network of special cells inside our bones called *osteocytes*, which then recruit our bone-building osteoblasts. This, and all of our muscles' other bone-building effects, require the help of 1,25-D.

Muscle mass and bone mass are linked by vitamin D-triggered crosstalk between muscle and bone cells. We now know that vitamin D:

- inhibits production of *myostatin*, a powerful inhibitor of muscle growth that also has strong negative effects on bone mass and fracture healing [413]

- increases formation and development of new *myocytes* (muscle cells)

- promotes production of *osteoglycin*, a protein made by muscle cells that regulates osteoblasts' bone-building activity and increases the rate of new bone formation

- enhances osteoblasts' ability to deposit minerals into newly forming bone

- helps regulate how quickly our muscles heal and regenerate after injury

- reduces muscle injury due to high-intensity exercise (Blood levels of 25(OH)D directly correlate with how quickly our muscles recover after exercise.)

- decreases levels of IL-6, an inflammatory *cytokine* (messenger molecule) produced following exercise that stimulates osteoclast formation and bone resorption

- regulates the production of *osteocalcin*, a protein secreted by our bone-building osteoblasts that, once activated by vitamin K2, brings calcium into our bones and starts the bone mineralization process. 414 415 416 417

Vitamin D improves immune function and lowers the risk of excessive osteoclast activation. With the help of vitamin D, our immune cells and cells in the lining of *barrier sites* produce antimicrobial peptides that kill and destroy infectious germs. (Barrier sites are the parts of the body in greatest need of defense against the dangers of the outside world, e.g., our respiratory tract, digestive tract, and skin.)

- These vitamin D-dependent, infection-fighting compounds (*cathelicidins*) are our most important class of antimicrobial agents. So, it's not surprising that an analysis of NHANES III data found people whose 25(OH)D levels were between 10 to 30 nanograms per milliliter (ng/mL) were 24% more likely to have had a recent respiratory tract infection than those with 25(OH)D levels greater than 30 ng/mL. 418 419 420

Vitamin D is Present in Your Body in 3 Forms: Vitamin D3, 25(OH)D, and 1,25-D

Understand vitamin D's different forms and you'll understand how vitamin D works in your body, and why you need to take vitamin D3 daily:

- **Vitamin D3** is the form we can synthesize in our skin when exposed to sunlight, or get from food, such as certain fatty fish (like salmon, sardines, tuna), free-range eggs, or fortified beverages. D3 only remains in your bloodstream for 1 to 2 days. To get enough vitamin D for healthy bones, virtually all of us require some supplemental vitamin D3.

- Your liver converts vitamin D3 into a form called ***25(OH)D***. This form circulates in your bloodstream far longer—2 to 3 weeks, so 25(OH)D is the form measured to check your vitamin D status.

- Your kidneys further convert *25(OH)D* into a form called ***1,25-D***. This is the final, fully activated form of vitamin D and is responsible for all of vitamin D's beneficial effects, including 85% of the calcium we absorb in our small intestine. 1,25-D is only available for a few hours.

- If you do not consume adequate vitamin D3 daily *or* your liver is unable to effectively convert D3 to 25(OH)D *or* your kidneys are unable to convert 25(OH)D to 1,25-D, you will not absorb calcium effectively or get vitamin D's muscle building or immune boosting effects.

Are You Getting the Vitamin D You Need for Healthy Bones?

Worldwide, few people are. *At least* 61% of Canadians and 36% of Americans are vitamin D-deficient, which means their 25(OH)D level is less than 20 ng/mL—far less than the 60 to 80 ng/mL most experts now believe is the optimal level.[421] [422] [423] [424]

The amount of vitamin D *you* need to reach this optimal level is not one size fits all. It depends on many factors: where you live, what you eat, and even your genetics. Here are the criteria that come into play:

- the latitude where you live
- your typical sun exposure
- your use of sunscreen
- the health of your liver and kidneys
- your weight (particularly, how much of you is fat)
- medications you take regularly
- the foods you eat (and how well you digest and absorb fat-soluble nutrients)
- your age
- your skin color
- your vitamin D-related genes
- whether your vitamin supplement provides D3 or D2
- if you take your vitamin D daily rather than weekly or monthly[425]

Location, location, location—it's not just key for real estate, but sun exposure! As mentioned earlier, the latitude where you live determines how many months of the year you can make your own vitamin D3. At latitudes below the 37th parallel, even winter sunshine has a vitamin D-producing attitude. (See illustration below.)

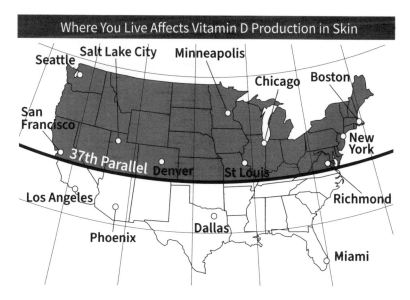

Those living in areas above the 37th parallel are at increased risk for vitamin D deficiency.

Source: www.health.harvard.edu/staying-healthy/time-for-more-vitamin-d

However, living in any of the areas above the 37th parallel, you are at increased risk for vitamin D deficiency. Obviously, Canadians and Alaskans are also not in the bone-building *sunshine zone*. But neither are those living in the northern part of sunny California. *Why?* Because producing vitamin D3 in your skin requires not just sunlight, but a specific wavelength of UVB radiation (290 to 315 nanometers)—one not available north of 35° latitude for 6 months out of the year. So, even on a sunny day, you won't be producing vitamin D.[426][427]

How much sun exposure do you typically get? Tell the truth here. If your skin is all covered by clothing or coated in sunscreen, you will not produce vitamin D, no matter where you live. Even an SPF 8 sunscreen reduces sunlight's ability to produce vitamin D3 in our skin by 95%. *Must you choose between increased risk for wrinkles and skin cancer or increased risk for osteoporosis?* Fortunately, no. In the summer, all you need is 20 to 30 minutes of mid-day sun exposure, during which time, as much as 10,000 to 25,000 IU of vitamin D can be produced in your skin.[428] And you don't need to expose all of your skin. For one thing, you could be arrested! A bikini would be optimal, but probably not acceptable lunch break attire. No worries. Just get outside, remove your suit jacket and let the sun shine on bare arms and legs. You can wrinkle-protect your face with a dab of sunscreen.

Even with supposedly adequate sun exposure, you still may not produce enough vitamin D. Researchers recruited 93 men and women (average age 24) from the University of Hawaii and a Honolulu skateboard shop, who met specific criteria for being outside over the prior 3 months. These young people averaged 22.4 hours outdoors each week with no sunscreen (40% reported never using sunscreen) and 6.5 additional hours with sunscreen. Despite all that, 51% of them had low blood levels of vitamin D. Less than 30 ng/mL indicates vitamin D deficiency, and this group's *average* blood level of 25(OH)D was just 31.6 ng/mL, meaning a bunch of them scored lower.[429]

Vitamin D relies upon the health of your liver and kidneys. As outlined earlier, only the active (1,25-D) version of vitamin D helps you absorb calcium effectively, in a multi-step process:

1. Vitamin D3 (a form called *cholecalciferol*) gets sent to your liver.

2. Your liver converts D3 into 25(OH)D3 (25-hydroxycholecalciferol aka *calcifediol* or *calcidiol*)—the form in which vitamin D circulates in the bloodstream. It's 5 times more potent than D3 but still not active.

3. Your kidneys receive 25(OH)D3 and further convert it into 1,25-D (1,25-dihydroxycholecalciferol or 1,25(OH)D3). This form is 10 times more potent than the vitamin D3 you made in your skin or took as a supplement and is the hormonal form of vitamin D that does all the work of vitamin D, including helping us absorb calcium.

What's the practical use of all of this? Get outdoors and get some sun on your (sunscreen-free) skin, but also get your blood levels of 25(OH)D checked. Furthermore, getting the vitamin D you need, in the right form, requires *both your liver and kidneys* to be functioning well. If not, all bets are off. The function of both organs normally declines with age and both liver and kidney dysfunction are increasingly common.[430][431] If you are taking vitamin D3 (plus the other nutrients discussed here), but are still not building bone, a liver or kidney problem could be causing your bone loss. (See NAFLD and CKD, Chapter 4.)

Vitamin D requirements increase with age. A review of recent studies compared older adults (age 65 and above) with younger adults, all with vitamin D blood levels less than 30 ng/mL. The findings: the older group needed more supplementary vitamin D3 (5,000 IU/day) compared to young adults (2,000 IU/day) to bring their 25(OH)D levels up into optimal range (60 to 80 ng/mL).[432]

Why? An age-associated decline in kidney function is one reason. The measure of kidney function (*glomerular filtration* rate) of a healthy 20-year-old man is about 140 ml/minute compared to about 90 ml/minute for a healthy 70-year-old man. This age-typical decline in kidney filtration function increases the amount of 25(OH)D needed in the blood to sustain adequate production of 1,25-D by more than half. Current Institute of Medicine recommendations, while still far too low to produce optimal health, recognize that people over age 70 may need three times more vitamin D than young adults.[433]

Your weight—particularly how much of you is fat—affects how much 25(OH)D you produce. A review of 94 studies examined how much supplemental vitamin D people of different body weights needed to bring their 25(OH)D levels into *adequate* range (30 ng/mL). A person weighing 110 pounds required 1,680 IU of D3/day. A person weighing 165 required 2,500 IU/day, and someone weighing 220 pounds needed 3,360 IU/day. And keep in mind that an optimal range for 25(OH)D is 60 to 80 ng/mL, not 30 ng/mL.

A meta-analysis looking at the research identifying the prevalence of vitamin D deficiency in the obese identified 15 studies involving 3,867 obese subjects and 9,342 normal-weight controls. European or American individuals had a 370% increased risk of vitamin D deficiency, while Asian individuals' likelihood was 343%. In other words, regardless of where you live, your age, nationality, or genetics, you're almost certainly vitamin D deficient if you are obese.[434][435]

Why does carrying too much fat promote vitamin D deficiency? Vitamin D is fat-soluble. Excess body fat hijacks D3 and sequesters it in fat cells before it can get to the liver to become 25(OH)D. After exposure to sunlight, obese individuals produce 53% less 25(OH)D than normal-weight people. A high *body mass index* or BMI (a measure of how much of your body is fat) doubles or even triples your vitamin D needs.

If this weren't bad enough, vitamin D deficiency causes parathyroid hormone levels to go up. That causes calcium to enter fat cells, which then tells these cells to produce more fat. In contrast, 1,25-D prevents fat cell precursors from maturing into grown-up fat cells (adipocytes). A lack of vitamin D can make you fatter, while having enough vitamin D helps you build muscle to burn calories even when you're not exercising.[436][437]

The Endocrine Society's weight-based recommendations: Vitamin D supplementation should be 1.5 times higher for overweight subjects and 2 to 3 times higher for obese subjects compared to normal-weight subjects. See table below.[438]

Vitamin D Supplementation Needs Based on BMI			
	Serum Level of 25(OH)D (ng/mL)		
Vitamin D (IU/day)	Normal weight	Overweight	Obese
1,000	35.2	32	28
2,000	39.6	36	31.2
4,000	47.2	42.8	36.4
10,000	60.4	56	48.4
20,000	65.2	61.2	54

The Endocrine Society offers these specific body-weight recommendations to achieve 25(OH)D targets. Remember, optimal levels of 25(OH)D are 60 to 80 ng/mL.

How much vitamin D does your diet typically provide? Unless you frequently eat salmon, halibut, or mushrooms specially exposed to UV light (and mushrooms produce D2, a far less effective form than D3), your diet is not going to provide you with enough vitamin D. See table below.

Best Food Sources of Vitamin D		
Food	Serving Size	Vitamin D (IU)
Mushrooms, Portabella exposed to UV light	3 ounces	1,135
Halibut, Alaskan	3 ounces	1,148
Salmon, King	3 ounces	1,052
Salmon, Sockeye, canned	3 ounces	761
Sardines, canned	3 ounces	190
Cow's milk, 2%	1 cup	120

Source: www.cronometer.com

Certain medications increase the amount of vitamin D you need. Anticonvulsants, glucocorticoids, and AIDS medications double or triple the amount of vitamin D required by normal-weight individuals to satisfy their body's vitamin D requirement. If you are taking one of these medications, discuss your increased vitamin D needs with your doctor.[439] For those who are obese, this is especially important.

Skin color may affect vitamin D requirements. Naturally dark skin contains a higher melanin content which protects against sunburn. However, it also reduces the ability to produce vitamin D3 from sun exposure, leading to African Americans having lower blood levels of vitamin D (both D3 and 25(OH)D produced from D3 in the liver) than Caucasians.[440]

Despite this, African Americans tend to have higher levels of the active form, 1,25-D, and better bone density. A study of 164 healthy post-menopausal women confirmed that while *total* 25(OH)D was lower in African American women (19.5 ng/mL) compared to Caucasian women (26.9 ng/mL), the amount of *free* 25(OH)D was identical in both (5.25 ng/mL). Furthermore, levels of parathyroid hormone (which increases our production of 1,25-D), 1,25-D, and bone density were higher in African Americans.[441]

What could explain this? Researchers point to a more effective form of *vitamin D-binding protein*, responsible for transporting vitamin D in the bloodstream. Also called *GC globulin*, vitamin D-binding protein comes in 3 different versions. GC1F, which has the strongest binding affinity for D3 and 25(OH)D, is the most abundant form in African Americans. GC1S, a less effective form, is the most abundant form in Caucasians. (GC2, which hardly anyone has, doesn't bind vitamin D well anyway.)[442]

In addition, African Americans produce less vitamin D-binding protein than Caucasians (probably because of the greater effectiveness of the GC1F form). Less vitamin D-binding protein results in more of the 25(OH)D produced in the liver being sent out into the bloodstream unbound. This free 25(OH)D can be converted into 1,25-D inside a variety of cells in our bodies, including our bones.

In contrast, 25(OH)D bound to vitamin D-binding protein can only be converted into 1,25-D in the kidney. So, even though they have lower *total* blood levels of 25(OH)D compared to Caucasians, African Americans have equal or greater blood levels of free 25(OH)D that can be converted to 1,25-D in our bones (as well as kidneys) and do a better job of getting that 25(OH)D to their kidneys for conversion to 1,25-D.[443]

Currently, lab tests measure only the level of *total* 25(OH)D but not how much is bound to vitamin D-binding protein and how much of it is free. Until testing is improved, we can't determine the optimal level of 25(OH)D for African Americans, though based on population studies, it's likely to be in the range of 40 to 60 ng/mL (compared to 60 to 80 ng/mL needed by Caucasians), not taking into account any other genetic variants that also affect our vitamin D needs. (See box below.)[444][445][446]

The Genes Related to Vitamin D Affect Your Needs

The genes we inherited from our parents impact our use of vitamin D and therefore our ability to build and maintain healthy bones. Gene variants, called *single nucleotide polymorphisms (SNPs,* pronounced *snips)* result in small changes in genetic instructions, so what gets made is slightly different from *normal* (also called *wild-type).*

For vitamin D, the most important and best studied SNPs are those that tell our cells how to make (1) vitamin D-binding proteins; (2) the enzymes *7-dehydrocholesterol-reductase* (DHCR7) and *vitamin D-25-hydroxylase* (CYP2R1); and (3) our vitamin D receptors.

SNPs affecting 7-dehydrocholesterol-reductase (DHCR7) and/or vitamin D-25-hydroxylase (CYP2R1). Sunlight acts upon the 7–dehydrocholesterol in our skin to form vitamin D3. However, the enzyme DHCR7 breaks down 7-dehydrocholesterol before it can be activated by sunlight. Those who have inherited an overactive version of this enzyme have difficulty producing vitamin D3 from sun exposure.

CYP2R1 is an enzyme in the liver that converts vitamin D3 into 25(OH)D. A SNP that produces a less active version of this enzyme results in less 25(OH)D produced, so you will have difficulty maintaining optimal blood levels.

If you've inherited a less effective vitamin D-binding protein, faster version of DHCR7 and slower version of CYP2R1—all of which are quite common—your risk for having blood levels of 25(OH)D lower than 30 ng/mL is increased by 247%.[447][448]

Fortunately, you can make up for all these SNPs. Get your blood levels of 25(OH)D checked and take extra supplemental vitamin D3 if needed to move your 25(OH)D into the optimal range of 60 to 80 ng/mL. If you have trouble reaching this level, you may have inherited a slow, as opposed to overactive, CYP2R1. This can also be easily corrected. Simply take your vitamin D3 in the form of a sublingual drop (under your tongue). That bypasses the normal digestive route to your liver and instead delivers vitamin D3 via the mucosal lining in your mouth directly into your bloodstream. That gives a longer opportunity for 25-hydroxylase, which is found in cells all over the body, to convert D3 into 25(OH)D.

An important word of caution here: you will need less vitamin D as a sublingual drop. The general rule of thumb is to take 5,000 IU of D3 for at least 8 weeks, then retest. However, if you are using a sublingual drop (the one Lara takes delivers 2,000 IU per drop), just one drop may be all you need because it will be more effectively utilized.

Vitamin D Receptor SNPs. Before vitamin D can help us, even in its fully active form of 1,25-D, it must first bind to VDRs, which are like docking stations on the outer membrane of our cells. Not all VDRs are equally good at binding 1,25-D. At least 4 different SNPs cause our genes to produce poorly formed receptors that don't bind vitamin D well. Lara has inherited the worst version of every one of them, resulting in lousy VDRs. The good news is she makes up for this by giving her VDRs plenty of vitamin D, so enough manages to bind to get the job done. That's why Lara still needs more vitamin D3 than *average* and takes some as a sublingual drop.[449 450 451]

Note from Lara: Malformed receptors are a key reason why my mother, aunt, and grandmother developed osteoporosis and died early from complications following hip fractures. Running genetic tests that revealed my malformed VDRs more than 25 years ago now was the first step (but definitely not the only one!) in my journey back from quickly advancing bone loss in my mid-40s to the beautiful bones I now enjoy at age 72.

How Can You Find the Right Vitamin D Supplementation Level?

The Endocrine Society recommends for normal-weight adults 1,500 to 2,000 IU of vitamin D3 daily. However, you can't assume that amount meets your specific requirements. Have your blood levels of 25(OH)D checked and supplement *daily* with sufficient vitamin D3 to bring your 25(OH)D level into optimal range (i.e., 60 to 80 ng/mL)—and keep it there. Be sure to check your 25(OH)D levels at least twice yearly (optimally, mid-winter and mid-spring). You may require more vitamin D3 during the winter and early spring than you do in the summer and early fall.

What 25(OH)D level is optimal? We've been told that 25(OH)D levels of 30 ng/mL are good enough. They're not. Humans evolved in a sun-rich environment and were outside most of every day (without sunscreen, which was not yet invented). Our ancestors (the ones who survived to produce offspring who also produced offspring and so on) maintained blood levels of 25(OH)D *higher* than 40 ng/mL. These higher levels are still common in people living at latitudes below the 37th parallel who spend, what is now an above-average amount of time outdoors (again, without sunscreen). Natural 25(OH)D concentrations (what you would produce simply from sun exposure) range at least as high as 68.4 ng/mL.

Studies indicate that a 25(OH)D status of 60 to 80 ng/mL is needed. Even a 25(OH)D level of 100 ng/mL is still within the normal range according to the Endocrine Society. Current research has not shown any benefit to having levels this high, but no ill effects have been seen at these levels either. However, a 25(OH)D level greater than 100 ng/mL is not advisable.[452 453 454 455]

Choose a Supplement with Vitamin D3, Not D2

Supplemental vitamin D is available in two forms: D3 and D2. Here's how they differ:

- **Vitamin D2 (*ergocalciferol*)** was first produced in the early 1920s from the UV irradiation of ergosterol, a steroid found in certain fungi, including mushrooms. Today, vitamin D2 is synthetically produced from irradiation of ergosterol derived from the mold ergot.

Vitamin D2 is the FDA-approved pharmaceutical form available in the U.S. and used in fortified foods such as margarine.

- **Vitamin D3 (cholecalciferol)** is produced in our skin by sunlight and can be found in egg yolks and oily fish. Synthetic production of vitamin D3 occurs similarly to the way it is naturally produced in human and animal skin, with 7-dehydrocholesterol produced from cholesterol and subsequent irradiation to its active D3 form. You'll find vitamin D3 in most single-vitamin supplements as well as calcium supplements containing vitamin D.[456][457]

Vitamin D2 is not as effective as vitamin D3 in producing and maintaining blood levels of 25(OH)D. Many studies have confirmed this:

- A study of 33 healthy adults given vitamin D in a dose of 50,000 IU per week for 12 weeks found vitamin D3 was 87% better than D2 at raising and maintaining blood levels of 25(OH)D.[458]

- Ninety-five healthy adults were divided into 3 groups and given 1,000 IU/day of either vitamin D3, vitamin D2, or a placebo. Daily supplementation with D3, but not D2, begun at the end of the summer maintained 25(OH)D levels during winter months. The average increase per 100 IU of vitamin D was almost 50% greater in the vitamin D3 group. In those taking vitamin D2, the winter drop in 25(OH)D was 2.5 times greater than the drop seen in subjects given a placebo; in other words, taking vitamin D2 was less helpful than taking no vitamin D![459]

- In a 14-day study of healthy middle-aged men and women, blood levels of 25(OH)D increased 70% more in those given 4,000 IU of vitamin D3/day compared to those receiving 4,000 IU of vitamin D2/day.[460]

- A meta-analysis of 7 studies found regardless of whether vitamin D supplementation was provided in small daily doses or in larger, infrequent bolus dosages, vitamin D3 was far superior to vitamin D2 in raising and maintaining blood levels of 25(OH)D.[461]

- In another systematic review and meta-analysis (22 randomized controlled trials with 30,716 participants), in which vitamin D2 or vitamin D3 was given alone versus placebo or no treatment, vitamin D3 *reduced* the mortality by 11%, whereas vitamin D2 *increased* mortality by 4%.[462]

In medical circles, Cochrane Reviews are known to be the best single source of scientific evidence about the effects of healthcare interventions.

A Cochrane Review looked for research on whether vitamin D supplementation lowers the risk of death and found 56 randomized trials including 95,286 participants. Vitamin D decreased mortality in all 56 trials, but when different forms of vitamin D were assessed, only vitamin D3 decreased mortality (a reduction in risk of 6%).[463]

Take your vitamin D3 daily. Taking vitamin D3 daily is much more effective than taking a large (bolus) dose less frequently. *Bolus* is the medical term for a large dose given all at once. Studies in which vitamin D has been given as a bolus dose once a week, month, every 3 to 4 months, or even once a year, have produced little or no beneficial effect. In contrast, studies using smaller doses of vitamin D, typically ranging from 1,000 to 6,000 IU/day, consistently show significant benefit and no adverse effects. This is not surprising. In fact, it's what you'd expect if you understand what happens to vitamin D3 in the human body.

When vitamin D3 enters your bloodstream—either by migrating into the central circulation from tiny capillaries in your skin after sun exposure or via the mucosal lining of your mouth if taken sublingually, or after it is absorbed from your intestines when you consume a vitamin D-rich food or supplement containing vitamin D—it immediately becomes *lightly* bound to vitamin D-binding protein. Vitamin D-binding protein carries D3 around your body in your bloodstream and eventually takes vitamin D3 to your liver, the primary place where 25(OH)D is produced. 25(OH)D, which gets *strongly* bound to vitamin D-binding protein, is then sent out into the bloodstream and delivered to the kidneys, where it is used to produce 1,25-D, the active form of vitamin D. 1,25-D gets very *lightly* bound to vitamin D-binding protein and is then sent from your kidneys into your bloodstream. When it reaches the lining of your small intestine, it helps you absorb calcium.

Admittedly, this can all get a bit technical. Here are the important takeaways here:

Point 1: The different forms of vitamin D—vitamin D3, 25(OH)D, and 1,25-D—are not all bound to vitamin D-binding protein with the same tightness. 25(OH)D binds more strongly than D3, and 1,25-D binds least strongly.

Point 2: How strongly each form of vitamin D binds to vitamin D-binding protein greatly affects how long each form remains available for your body to use:

- 25(OH)D can stay in your bloodstream for a couple of weeks.
- Vitamin D3 is available for only 1-2 days.
- 1,25-D is gone in just a few hours.

Point 3: How strongly each form of vitamin D binds to vitamin D-binding protein determines whether or not it can get from the bloodstream into your cells. Vitamin D3 is *lightly* bound to vitamin D-binding protein, so it can be brought from your bloodstream into your cells, while 25(OH)D cannot. 25(OH)D is very strongly bound to vitamin D-binding protein, and the resulting molecule is too big to get into your cells—except for the ones in your kidneys and parathyroid glands, which have a special system, called the *megalin-cubilin system*, set up to bring in these large *25(OH)D + vitamin D-binding protein* combinations. 1,25-D produced in your kidneys is *weakly* bound to vitamin D-binding protein, so 1,25-D can easily get inside your cells, but 1,25-D made in the kidneys is only available for a couple of hours and is primarily delivered to your intestines to help you absorb calcium.

Point 4: Vitamin D3, can be absorbed by cells all over the body and used inside them to produce 1,25-D, the active form of vitamin D. Researchers have recently discovered that tissues all over your body, not just your liver and kidneys, contain the enzymes needed to convert D3 to 25(OH)D, and 25(OH)D to 1,25-D. The lightly-bound vitamin D3 in your bloodstream is carried not just to your liver, but to tissues throughout your body, for example, your muscles.

In other words, vitamin D3 is the form that's doing the heavy lifting, so to speak, in your muscles to lower your risk of falling and inside the cells in your skin, organs, and immune system, where it is converted into 25(OH)D and then to 1,25-D to provide it's other beneficial functions.

The different forms of vitamin D remain available in your body for different amounts of time. Vitamin D3 produced in your skin moves into the bloodstream over the following 24 hours. In contrast, vitamin D3 consumed in foods or a supplement appears in your bloodstream more quickly, with levels peaking at 12 hours rather than 24 hours. In both cases, vitamin D3 is cleared quickly. Even large bolus doses of 50,000 to 100,000 IU are cleared from the body within 2 days. This has been known for at least 10 years. Vitamin D's rapid disappearance from the bloodstream was attributed to it being stored away in fat tissue for later release. We now know this doesn't happen. The vitamin D3 consumed in a bolus dose not used within 12 to 24 hours is simply excreted in bile, feces, and urine. For this reason, sustaining the needed amounts of vitamin D in the bloodstream requires either daily D3 supplementation and/or daily sunlight exposure (at the right UV wavelength).

Furthermore, we also now know that adults require at least 2,000 IU (possibly as much as 6,000 IU or even 10,000 IU) of vitamin D3 each day for extended periods to maintain 25(OH)D levels in optimal range. A dose of vitamin D3 of 400 IU/d will have no detectable effect on levels of 25(OH)D in the bloodstream. Daily dosing of 2,000 IU of vitamin D3 is far more likely to result in a slow, sustained rise in circulating 25(OH)D that will reach a steady state at 3 to 4 months. Large bolus dosing of vitamin D3 will not.

Despite these *facts* of human physiology, research has been conducted using vitamin D3 in bolus doses of 28,000 IU/week; 120,000 IU/month; 360,000 IU every 3 to 4 months; or even higher annual doses. The good news is that none of these extremely high doses caused adverse effects. None resulted in excessively high blood levels of calcium or excessive concentrations of calcium in the urine. The bad news—and the key point here—is that although weekly, monthly, or longer interval bolus dosing will result in surges of vitamin D3 in your bloodstream, no matter how big a bolus dose you take, vitamin D3 will vanish from your body in 1 to 2 days unless you take more.

If you take 100,000 IU of vitamin D3, it will go through your liver, and some will be used to produce 25(OH)D, whose levels will increase in your bloodstream by about 1 to 4 ng/mL about 24 hours later. But that's all—and within a maximum of three weeks later, all this 25(OH)D will have been cleared from your body.

Vitamin D Safety

A few uncommon health conditions may cause high blood levels of calcium (hypercalcemia) when taking vitamin D. These are sarcoidosis, Williams–Beuren syndrome, some lymphomas, and SNPs that result in the body producing an inactive version of the enzyme that breaks down 1,25-D, which is called 1,25-D, 24-hydroxylase (or CYP24A1). These SNPs are estimated to occur in at least 4% of the population.

If you do not have one of these very uncommon health conditions, you would have to take extremely high doses of vitamin D every day (e.g., at least 50,000 IU daily) for months to become vitamin D toxic. This is logical because the body tightly controls the conversion of 25(OH) D to 1,25-D, and it is 1,25-D that is responsible for regulating calcium metabolism by increasing intestinal calcium absorption and mobilizing calcium from the skeleton.

Drugs that inhibit your ability to digest and absorb fats can hinder vitamin D absorption. Vitamin D is fat-soluble, and research has shown that taking your vitamin D3 supplement with a meal containing some fat improves vitamin D's absorption and results in better increases in 25(OH)D. For the same reason, drugs that cause fat malabsorption may also impair your ability to absorb vitamin D. Orlistat and cholestyramine are two examples. Orlistat inhibits the activity of the lipase enzymes that break down fats. Cholestyramine is used to lower cholesterol levels by binding to bile in the digestive tract and preventing its reabsorption. Since bile is produced from cholesterol, your liver uses cholesterol from your bloodstream to make more bile, thus lowering cholesterol levels. But bile is also required for the digestion of fats in your small intestine, so a lack of bile can cause fat malabsorption, and consequently, vitamin D malabsorption. (And malabsorption of all the other fat-soluble vitamins, which include vitamin K, vitamin A, and vitamin E.)[464][465][466]

Drugs that lower cholesterol (the statins) can lessen our ability to produce vitamin D3 in our skin. The statins inhibit cholesterol production. Since vitamin D3 is synthesized in our skin from 7-dehydrocholesterol, statins may lessen our ability to produce vitamin D3. Many studies have reported that statin use is associated with *myalgia* (muscle pain), particularly in individuals who are vitamin D-insufficient. Ensuring vitamin D supplies are adequate can help reduce or prevent myopathy in those who take atorvastatin, simvastatin, fluvastatin, or lovastatin, though is less likely to reduce muscle pain in those taking pravastatin, rosuvastatin, or pitavastatin. Lastly, one statin, rosuvastatin, appears to even *increase* vitamin D levels in humans, and it's been proposed that rosuvastatin's beneficial effects are due, at least in part, to causing an increase in blood levels of vitamin D in subjects who were vitamin D-insufficient.[467][468]

Bariatric Surgery

Bariatric surgery greatly lessens your ability to digest your food and absorb its nutrients, including calcium and the fat-soluble vitamins, vitamins D, K, A, and E.

BONE-HEALTHY ACTION ITEMS

- The Endocrine Society recommends at least 1,500 to 2,000 IU/day of vitamin D for healthy adults whose blood levels are at least 30 ng/mL.
- *Optimal* levels of vitamin D (25(OH)D are 60 to 80 ng/mL. Stay below 100 ng/mL, the uppermost range of normal.
- Have your vitamin D level checked mid-winter and mid-summer. If your blood levels of 25(OH)D are not in the optimal range, take 5,000 IU/d for 3 months and then retest to adjust your daily dosage.
- We recommend supplementation with vitamin D3 rather than vitamin D2.
- Take vitamin D daily, rather than a large dose taken weekly or monthly. If your 25(OH)D level remains below optimal, try taking some vitamin D3 as a sublingual supplement.

Vitamin K

BONE ESSENTIALS

- Vitamin K comes in two different forms: vitamin K1 (phylloquinone) and vitamin K2 (menaquinone).
- Vitamin K1 helps prevent osteoclast activation and bone loss.
- Vitamin K2 is a family of vitamins, the menaquinones (MKs). Of the forms available as supplements, MK-7 is far more effective than MK-4.
- Vitamin K2, via the enzymes it activates, determines where calcium gets deposited in your body, sending it to bones and keeping it out of blood vessels, kidneys, breasts, and brain.

- Your intake of K2 needs to be in balance with your intake of vitamin D as both vitamins work together.
- Vitamin K2 supplements cannot be taken with warfarin, but can be used with the newer anticoagulant drugs: the Xa inhibitors and the direct thrombin inhibitors.

Vitamin K is not a single nutrient. It comes in two different forms, vitamin K1 or phylloquinone, and vitamin K2 or menaquinone, each of which plays different, though very important roles in the health of our bones.

Vitamin K1: Critical for Blood Clotting and Producing a Healthy Inflammatory Response

The scientific name for vitamin K1 is *phylloquinone*, so called because it's found in green leafy plants. *Phyllo* is Greek for leaf. *Quinone* refers to its chemical structure. Phylloquinone plays a major role in photosynthesis, which is the way plants make energy for themselves. In our bodies, phylloquinone (K1) plays at least 2 essential roles:

- **Enabling our blood to clot.** Vitamin K1 protects us from *death by paper cut* by being the co-factor in an enzyme called *gamma-glutamyl carboxylase*. Without vitamin K1, gamma-glutamyl carboxylase cannot activate the vitamin K-dependent proteins (also called the *GLA proteins*) involved in the blood clotting cascade.
- **Providing antioxidant effects by** lessening the production of signaling agents (cytokines including IL-6, TNF-α, and C-reactive protein) that increase the production and activity of osteoclasts, the cells that break down (resorb) bone.[469]

Of these two roles, enabling blood to clot—the more urgent for keeping us alive—takes precedence. Only once your short-term survival needs have been met will any remaining K1 be used for its anti-oxidant and bone-building purposes.[470]

I (Lara) admit I'm a klutz. When chopping vegetables, I cannot tell you how often I manage to nick a finger. This has become such a family joke that my daughter gave me stainless steel kitchen gloves for Christmas. Fortunately, I eat lots of vitamin K1-rich leafy greens, so my clotting factors are always ready to protect me from myself. Plus, any leftover

K1 helps reduce free radicals that can activate osteoclasts. This becomes especially important after menopause, as our production of cytokines increases.[471 472]

Insufficiency of vitamin K1 greatly increases risk of osteoporotic fracture. Research published in 1984 found that patients who suffered fragility fractures had vitamin K levels 70% lower than age-matched controls, an association that has been repeatedly confirmed. A study involving almost 900 men and women found a 65% greater risk of hip fracture in those with the lowest blood levels of K1 compared to those with the highest levels of the nutrient, who averaged a K1 intake of 254 mcg/d (well below the optimal 1,000 mcg/d.) In the U.S., we consume far less—only about 80 mcg/d in *both* K1 and K2 forms combined.[473 474]

How Much Vitamin K1 Do You Need and What Foods Provide It?

The Recommended Daily Allowance (RDA) for K1 is a paltry 80 mcg/d, developed in relation to activating clotting factors, not bone health. For comparison, the women in the above study showing decreased fracture risk were given 5,000 mcg daily. Remember, RDA recommendations are set at amounts deemed adequate to prevent *overt* disease in most people, not for the goal of promoting optimal health.

For healthy bones, your vitamin K1 intake should be *at least* 1,000 mcg (1 mg) per day, an amount you can *easily* consume with a healthy diet that includes lots of leafy greens.[475] K1 is present in the highest amounts in kale, spinach, Swiss chard, collards, parsley, and broccoli. It's also found in cold-pressed organic oils derived from plants, especially soybean and canola oils. See table. [476 477]

Best Food Sources of Vitamin K1		
Food	Serving Size	Vitamin K1 (mcg)
Swiss chard	3 ounces (1.25 cups, chopped)	706
Spinach, cooked from fresh	3 ounces (1.25 cups, chopped)	494
Spinach, raw	3 ounces (1.25 cups, chopped)	483
Kale, cooked from fresh	3 ounces (~ 0.5 cup)	817
Kale, raw	3 ounces (1.25 cups, chopped)	705
Parsley, fresh	1 cup, chopped	984
Collards, cooked from fresh	3 ounces (~ 0.5 cup)	407
Beet greens, cooked	3 ounces (~0.5 cup)	484
Broccoli, cooked	3 ounces (~0.5 cup)	86
Canola oil (not hydrogenated)	1 tablespoon	10
Soy* oil (not hydrogenated)	1 tablespoon	25
Olive oil, extra virgin, organic	1 tablespoon	3

*All soy products that you consume should be organic. If not organic, the soy will be GMO. Consumption of GMO foods has been found to promote inflammation, and chronic inflammation promotes bone loss.

Source: www.cronometer.com, responsibletechnology.org/, www.gmojudycarman.org/wp-content/uploads/2013/06/The-Full-Paper.pdf

Oils in most processed foods do not contain usable vitamin K1. In the standard American diet, few folks are eating leafy greens. Instead, their primary source of K1 comes from the soybean or canola oils found in processed, chemically-grown packaged foods. Unfortunately, virtually all of these oils are partially hydrogenated. That changes the K1 in these oils from its natural form, phylloquinone, into an unnatural form called dihydrophylloquinone, which is far less effective:

- Dihydrophylloquinone is not as well absorbed as phylloquinone.
- What does get absorbed has much lower biological activity and is more rapidly excreted.
- Dihydrophylloquinone has a greatly reduced ability to activate the liver proteins needed to form clotting factors, K1's primary job for our survival.

Plus, the healthy intestinal bacteria that would normally convert leftover phylloquinone in K2 ignore the altered dihydrophylloquinone form of K1. None of this is good news for your bones.

Dihydrophylloquinone is associated with reduced bone mass. Data collected on 2,544 participants (average age 58.5) in the Framingham Offspring Study showed that those with the highest intake of vitamin K1 from the oils used in processed and fast foods—in other words, dihydrophylloquinone—had the lowest BMD at the neck, hip, and spine.[478]

What Vitamin K2 Does for Your Bones

Vitamin K2 activates proteins that: 1) help pull calcium into bones, and 2) prevent calcium from depositing in soft tissues, like your cardiovascular system or kidneys. Similar to K1, vitamin K2 serves as the cofactor for the enzyme, gamma-glutamyl carboxylase, but K2 activates different proteins. All the vitamin K-dependent proteins are referred to as the *GLA proteins* because, once vitamin K has activated gamma-glutamyl carboxylase, it creates an area in each of these proteins that contains γ-*carboxyglutamate* (or GLA for short).

Why are the GLA proteins important for bones? Think of them as *glamorous proteins* because you owe your beautiful bones to their specific actions:

- **Osteocalcin** attracts calcium molecules and anchors them into the hydroxyapatite crystals that form our bone matrix. If no activated osteocalcin is around, the calcium molecules you absorb won't get pulled into your bones. If too little activated osteocalcin is around, only some of the available calcium will make it into your bones.

- **Matrix Gla protein** prevents calcium from depositing in and *calcifying* soft tissue. When K2 levels are too low, matrix-Gla protein remains off duty, so the calcium you want for your bones gets sidetracked and goes where you don't want it—into your heart, arteries, breasts, brain, and/or kidneys.

Vitamin K is the spark plug for your bones' glamorous proteins. Without K2, neither will work, and both are absolutely essential for healthy bones.

Vitamin K2 Forms: Differences Between MK-4 and MK-7

While more than a dozen forms of vitamin K2 have been identified, research has focused on two forms of vitamin K considered most important, MK-4 and MK-7. The MK-4 form of K2 is structurally similar to K1. Both have a side-chain of just 4 sections. In contrast, the MK-7 form of vitamin K2, as its name indicates, has a 7-section side-chain, and is called a *long-chain* menaquinone. While all forms of vitamin K are absorbed in your small intestine and sent to your liver, their differences in structure affect how they operate after that.[479] (See diagram below.)

Structural Differences in Forms of Vitamin K

The K1 form of vitamin K1 is structurally similar to the MK-4 version of vitamin K2. Both have a side-chain of just 4 sections. In contrast, the MK-7 form of vitamin K2, as its name indicates, has a 7-section side-chain, and is called a long-chain menaquinone.

- Vitamin K1 and MK-4 are first used to activate blood clotting proteins in the liver. (Remember, the body prioritizes blood clotting as their primary job.) If any extra is left, both are packaged inside triglycerides (little packages of fat bound to a glycerol sugar molecule) and sent out into the bloodstream, where they are either quickly used for fuel or stored in adipose (fat) tissue. In either case, the vitamin K1 or MK-4 they contain don't stick around long; they're cleared from the bloodstream within 6 to 8 hours.

- In contrast, MK-7 won't be used to activate the blood clotting proteins (unless you're seriously lacking vitamin K1 and MK-4). Instead, MK-7 is packaged up in LDL cholesterol and sent into your bloodstream. Since LDL cholesterol circulates around your body for several days, MK-7 also stays in your body for up to 4 days!

Staying in your bloodstream about 12 times longer—4 days versus about 8 hours—gives the MK-7 form an important advantage over MK-4.[480] You can maintain a steady blood level of vitamin K2 when you consume MK-7 regularly. It's like having a special vitamin K2 bank account. You can withdraw from it each day to continuously activate the osteocalcin and matrix Gla proteins that steer the calcium you consume in the right direction—into your bones and out of your arteries! We'll discuss other aspects of this later in the section on K2 supplementation.

Dietary Sources of Vitamin K2

Our bodies can process K1 into K2, but don't expect very much. After K1 serves its main roles, not much will remain. Any that does will move on to the intestine, where specific healthy bacteria (the *Bacteroides* species) can convert it into vitamin K2. Until very recently, this extra K1 was thought to be converted into the short-lived MK-4 form because this is what happens in rats. We now know that the converted K2 is actually the longer-lasting long-chain menaquinones: MK-7 through MK-13.[481]

But you'd need to eat *a lot* of leafy greens every day to have enough K1 left over for this because:

- K1 is tightly bound to chloroplast membranes in plant cells, from which it is released with low efficiency.
- K1 is cleared from your body within 6 to 8 hours.
- K1's conversion to K2 requires a healthy digestive tract containing plenty of the *Bacteroides* bacteria capable of doing the job.[482]

You can improve your absorption of the K1 in leafy greens by dressing them with a little oil. After eating spinach, for example, circulating levels of vitamin K1 may increase by at least 3-fold *if the greens are accompanied by a little vegetable oil.* (But be sure to use organic, cold-pressed canola or soy oil on your salad. Processed oils will have changed into the dihydrophylloquinone form that your intestinal bacteria will ignore.) Even if all goes well, your gut bacteria will at best produce only a few mcg of K2, while healthy bones require *at least* 100 mcg of the MK-7 form daily.[483]

Few sources provide vitamin K2 in quantities sufficient for our bones' health. One exception is an unusual food—and one that's unpalatable in the Western diet—a Japanese fermented soybean product called natto. Unfortunately, natto's slimy texture and aroma, reminiscent of dirty gym socks, renders it difficult to love. A single 1.4-ounce serving (and some eat much more) delivers 380 mcg of MK-7. In the U.S., natto is unlikely to be available at your grocery but, like virtually everything else in the known universe, can now be found on Amazon.[484]

Best Food Sources of Vitamin K2			
Food	Serving Size	Vitamin K2 (mcg)	Primary Type of K2 Provided
Natto	1.4 ounces	380	MK-7
Blue cheese	1 ounce	21	MK-9, MK-10
French Brie style cheese	1 ounce	16	MK-9
Chicken liver pan-fried	4 ounces	14.4	MK-4
Meat franks	4 ounces	11.2	MK-4
Chicken breast	4 ounces	10	MK-4
Beef, ground, medium fat	4 ounces	9.25	MK-4
Egg yolks, Netherlands	1 ounce (2 yolks)	9	MK-4
Eggs, pan-fried	3 eggs	9	MK-4
Eggs, hard boiled	3 eggs	7	MK-4
Emmentaler	1 ounce	6-19.5	MK-9
Norwegian Jarlsberg cheese	1 ounce	6-9.5	MK-9
Sauerkraut	3.5 ounces	4.8	Mixed
Egg yolk, U.S.	1 ounce (2 yolks)	4.4	MK-4
Cheddar cheese	1 ounce	2.9	MK-9
Whole milk	8 ounces	2.2	MK-4
Beef, ground, low fat	4 ounces	1.9	MK-4
Salmon	3 ounces	0.57	MK-4

Source: Quantitative measurement of vitamin K2...[485], Determination of phylloquinone...[486], Vitamin k contents...[487], Menaquinone Content...[488]

Certain cheeses can provide a tiny bit of vitamin K2, particularly English Stilton (blue cheese), Greek Feta, Swiss Emmental, and Norwegian Jarlsberg. These cheeses contain somewhere between 5.6 to 18.2 mcg per ounce, so 3 ounces spread over a day's meals can give you as much as 54.6 mcg of K2. Not enough, although the predominant forms of K2 in these cheeses are long-chain menaquinones, MK-8, MK-9, and MK-10, which, like MK-7, remain in the body for 3 to 4 days—a lot longer than the MK-4 form, which is cleared out within 6 to 8 hours.[489]

Why do certain cheeses, but not others, contain vitamin K2? It depends upon which type of bacteria is used to ferment the cheese. The *Leuconostoc species* and the *Lactococcus species* produce K2, but *Streptococcus thermophilus, Lactobacillus delbrueckii, or Bifidobacterium* do not, so neither do cheeses made with them. Also, neither do yogurt nor cottage cheese, while they are potentially good sources of other health-promoting bacteria, calcium, and protein. Enjoy the cheeses listed in the above table and ask your grocery store if they know or can find out for you which bacteria are used to produce your favorite cheeses.[490][491]

Liver, meat, and egg yolks contain tiny amounts of K2 and only in its short-lived MK-4 form. For example, 4 oz. of pan-fried chicken liver contains 14.4 mcg; 4 oz. of chicken breast supplies 10 mcg; 4 oz of medium-fat broiled ground beef delivers 9.25 mcg (for low-fat beef, reduce that to 1.9 mcg); 3 hard-boiled eggs contain 7.0 mcg. You can't rely upon these foods to provide the K2 your bones require.[492]

To meet your bones' vitamin K2 requirements, you need to take a supplement. In the U.S., our dietary intake of *all* forms of vitamin K combined (K1 and all types of K2) is only about 80 mcg/d. Even in the Netherlands, where they eat lots more vitamin K1-rich leafy greens and more K2-rich cheese than we do, vitamin K2 intake is far from optimal. The Rotterdam study found those consuming the highest amounts of vitamin K averaged 370 mcg/d of K1 and just 45 mcg/d of the long-chain menaquinones (MK-7, MK-8, MK-9, MK-10). And these people were eating 100 grams (about 3 ounces) of leafy greens and 100 grams of cheese every day.[493]

Which Supplemental Form of K2 is Best: MK-4 or MK-7?

Most of us will want to choose the MK-7 form of vitamin K2 as a supplement. While there are exceptions based on genetics (described below), the MK-7 form has been shown to offer most people the greatest benefits:

- **MK-7's incorporation into LDL translates to much more stable blood levels**. When taken each day, your MK-7 levels accumulate to

7- to 8-fold higher levels than vitamin K1 or MK-4. That helps build and maintain a nice balance in your K2 bank account so you can continuously activate the osteocalcin and matrix Gla protein to be *on the job* building bones or preventing calcium from depositing in your arteries or kidneys. Researchers found after just one day, MK-7 was 250% more available than MK-4, and after 4 days, 600% more available.[494]

- **MK-7's much longer availability allows for a very small dose.** As little as 100 mcg/d is typically all that is needed. In contrast, MK-4 is cleared from your body quickly, so you need large doses several times a day. The dose of MK-4 showing benefit for people with osteopenia or osteoporosis is 15 mg (15,000 mcg) three times daily (i.e., 45,000 mcg over the course of the day compared to as little as 100 mcg once per day for MK-7). Consuming 45,000 mcg of MK-4 from your diet is not possible. Even if you took a supplement containing 15,000 mcg of MK-4 every 6-8 hours, your blood levels would fluctuate, dropping too low to activate osteocalcin and matrix Gla protein, particularly if a dose is missed and when sleeping through the night.[495 496 497]

In many species, including humans, K1 (and MK-4) make up only a small amount of the vitamin K content of the liver. The majority of vitamin K in the liver is the long-chain menaquinones, MK-7 through MK-13. Typically, the ratio is about 90% long-chain menaquinones: 10% K1 and MK-4.[498] Plus, for some reason, our bodies quickly clear K1 and MK-4, but allow the longer-chain MKs to accumulate. Mother Nature has chosen to program our use of vitamin K in this way—another reason we would be wary of taking the unnaturally large doses of MK-4 required and rely instead upon the small dose of MK-7.[499]

Nonetheless, a small percentage of us do better on MK-4 than MK-7. The reason for this is the genes you inherited from your parents, which affect not just your physical appearance, but the way your body functions. Our genes encode instructions for how our bodies make proteins/enzymes, which are then employed to carry out all the other activities that keep us functioning, including how effectively we use vitamin K. A small percentage of us have inherited genetic variants (SNPs) that result in keeping vitamin K2 around longer than the average person. Others have inherited gene variations that result in using up vitamin K2 more quickly than average, so they need more vitamin K2. In those who keep vitamin K around longer, MK-7 may cause trouble falling or staying asleep because K2 boosts energy production in our brain cells. In those who keep MK-7 longer, their brain's energy level may remain high enough to interfere with sleep.[500][501] (See box for details on genetic variations.)

SNPs in 4 Genes Impact How Much Vitamin K You Need for Healthy Bones

These SNPs produce variations in Apolipoprotein E (APOE), the Vitamin K Epoxide Reductase enzyme (VKOR), the Gamma-Glutamyl Carboxylase enzyme, and the Cytochrome P450 4F2 (CYP4F2) enzyme. Following, we'll talk about each of these SNPs, how they impact your needs for vitamin K2, and how you can determine which ones you carry.

Apolipoprotein E (APOE) is a protein that binds to fat-containing *lipoproteins*, like cholesterol and the fat-soluble vitamins, including vitamin K (along with vitamins D, A, and E), so they can be carried throughout your body in the bloodstream. As you know, fat and water don't mix well—just think of the way oil and vinegar separate in salad dressing. Since our bloodstream is primarily water, APOE helps our lipoproteins circulate. APOE comes in 3 flavors or SNP variations, which affect how quickly we clear lipoproteins and the amount of K2 we need:

- **APOE2 SNP** (just 7% of us have inherited): If you have this SNP, you clear vitamin K-rich lipoproteins—and therefore K2—more slowly than average. Taking the *average* amount of MK-7 recommended may cause levels in your brain to accumulate and promote energy production in your brain cells so effectively that you have trouble sleeping. If taking MK-7 every day keeps you awake, try taking your MK-7 supplement every third day or supplementing with MK-4 instead.

- **APOE3 SNP** (78% of us carry): If like most of us, you have inherited this most common SNP, you clear cholesterol neither rapidly nor slowly. You'll likely do best with 100 mcg/d of MK-7. Of course, you may need a bit more based upon how much vitamin D you need to maintain optimal (60 to 80 ng/mL) blood levels of 25(OH)D.

- **APOE4 SNP** (14% of us carry): If you are among the one in seven with this SNP, you remove vitamin K-rich lipoproteins from your bloodstream more quickly than average and will therefore need more vitamin K2. You will want to take MK-7, though possibly an amount larger than the average 100 mcg/d dose.[502 503 504 505 506 507]

Vitamin K Epoxide Reductase (VKOR) is a special enzyme our bodies make just to recycle vitamin K, which tells you how important vitamin K is for us. SNPs in the VKOR gene affect how quickly this enzyme works.

- If your VKOR works efficiently and quickly, you will be very good at recycling vitamin K, so you can use it over and over before it's excreted. As a result, you'll need less K2 and may be able to use a lower dose of MK-7 than the *average* person. Or you might even be okay with MK-4.

- If your VKOR works slowly, you won't be very good at reusing your vitamin K. You will need MK-7, and you may need a higher dose than average.

- VKOR is the enzyme inhibited by warfarin, which explains why this medication increases risk of osteoporosis, vascular calcification and kidney disease.

Gamma-Glutamyl Carboxylase (GGCX) is the enzyme that activates all your vitamin K-dependent *glamorous* proteins, including osteocalcin and matrix-Gla protein. If you've inherited a slow GGCX, you need to ensure this enzyme is fully saturated with vitamin K to activate your glamourous proteins. That means you need more vitamin K available than *average*. [508 509]

CYP450 4F2 belongs to the *Cytochrome P450 system*, a family of enzymes found in your liver. CYP450 enzymes help you detoxify and clear out substances your body doesn't want hanging around, like used vitamins (including K) and hormones, plus drugs, environmental toxins, and much more. Humans excrete both K1 and K2 using a common prepare-for-elimination pathway in the liver, which begins with the action of the *Phase I* enzyme, CYP450 4F2.

After CYP4F2 works its magic, *Phase II* of detoxification sends the resulting products to undergo *glucuronidation,* a process that mainly uses *glucuronic acid* to make them water soluble. That allows vitamin K excretion via urine or bile (which goes into feces). So, now you know how your body eliminates used-up vitamin K.

By now, you won't be surprised to know that the CYP4F2 enzyme doesn't work at the same speed in all of us. A CYP4F2 enzyme that more slowly eliminates vitamin K means your vitamin K stays around longer. Therefore, carriers of this slow version are likely to require *less* vitamin K to maintain an equivalent vitamin K status. You may be able to take a lower-than-average dosage of MK-7 or find that MK-4 is a better fit. The slow version of the CYP4F2 enzyme is present in about 30% of Caucasians and Asians, but only around 7% of African Americans.

Lab testing can reveal which SNPs affect your vitamin K needs. Your doctor can run a blood test that tells you which APOE type you inherited. Another blood test, used to check your levels of uncarboxylated osteocalcin (ucOC), can show how well your VKOR enzyme is working and give you some idea of your GGCX activity. Another commonly run lab test, which checks your *prothrombin time* (a measure of blood clotting), can give you insight into your CYP4F2. (See Lab Tests, Chapter 10.)

Determining Your Dosage of Supplemental K2

Your genetic inheritance impacts your vitamin K2 needs. The majority of us (85% to 95%) will find vitamin K2 in its MK-7 form at a dose of 100 to 180 mcg/d is adequate; however, as discussed above, your genetic make-up can affect this:

- If you've inherited a SNP that causes you to use up vitamin K more quickly than average, you will benefit from a larger dose.
- If you've inherited a SNP that enables you to keep vitamin K around far longer than average or recycle it for re-use more quickly, you may find that you can take less MK-7 (45 mcg per day or every other day) or even that the MK-4 form of vitamin K2 (15 mg once or twice daily) works well for you.

Your best bet here is to see how you react to MK-7. If you find you have trouble falling asleep or staying asleep when taking this form of K2, try taking less per day, taking it every third day, or switching to MK-4. If you do try MK-4, you'll likely need less than the 15 mg every 6 to 8 hours (45 mg/d) used in the studies. We suggest starting out by taking 5 mg 3 times daily and after 3 to 4 weeks, checking your ucOC. (See Lab Tests, Chapter 10.)

Balance your intake of vitamin D and vitamin K2. Vitamin D and vitamin K work together. Vitamin D increases *both* your body's ability to absorb calcium *and* your body's production of the vitamin K-dependent proteins that regulate your healthful use of calcium. Because vitamin D increases the amount of vitamin K-dependent proteins, a higher intake of vitamin D results in the need for more vitamin K to activate them. Not increasing your vitamin K intake to balance your vitamin D intake can produce a functional deficiency of vitamin K. Also, if you currently have one of the diseases promoted by vitamin K insufficiency that results in calcium deposition in soft tissues (e.g., coronary artery disease, kidney disease), you're likely to require higher doses of vitamin K2. In recent studies, daily doses of at least 360 mcg of MK-7 have been safely used for this purpose.[510][511]

If you are supplementing with MK-7, you need to look at the intake of vitamin D that meets your needs. Your needs are met when blood levels of 25(OH)D remain in the optimal range of 60 to 80 ng/mL. If that optimal amount of vitamin D3 supplementation is:

- 1,000 to 2,000 IU/d, you are likely to only need 100 to 180 mcg of MK-7/d
- 3,000 to 4,000 IU/d, you may need more, 200 to 300 mcg of MK-7/d
- 5,000 or more IU/d, you may require 360 mcg of MK-7/d

If you are supplementing with MK-4, a dose of 45 mg per day (15,000 mg every 6 to 8 hours) is the dose shown in the research to produce beneficial effects on bone. This amount, although far greater than could be consumed from the diet, has been found to produce no adverse effects in many studies.[512] If you are among the few whose genetic inheritance enables them to keep vitamin K around longer, your needs may be met with less: 15 to 30 mg of MK-4 daily.

If you have a condition involving calcification of soft tissues (e.g., coronary artery disease or kidney disease), you may benefit from 360 mcg of MK-7/d. Doses of MK-7 ranging from 180 to 360 to 420 mcg/d (or as high as 1,080 mcg 3x/week, which averages out to 462 mcg/d) have now been used in recent studies. No adverse effects have been seen, except for mild stomach upset in a few hemodialysis patients receiving the highest dose. In Japan, people eating natto regularly consume 865 mcg of MK-7 daily, and researchers have used *reinforced natto* to deliver daily doses of MK-7 as high as 1,730 mcg with no adverse effects. [513] [514] [515] [516] [517] [518] [519] [520] [521]

Vitamin K2 Safety

Supplemental vitamin K2 is extremely safe for most people, except for those on prescribed oral anticoagulant (blood-thinning) medication (i.e., the coumarin drugs), which we'll detail below.

Other than those for those taking warfarin or similar anticoagulants, vitamin K is extremely safe. Studies looking at vitamin K2's use to decrease bone loss in postmenopausal women have been run using as much as 360 mcg/d without a single adverse event reported. As mentioned earlier, people in Japan who enjoy natto often consume more than 800 mcg/d. Furthermore, research showed no adverse effect on those who ate vitamin K2-enriched natto that provided 1,298 or 1,765 mcg in a 3-ounce serving.[522]

No toxicity symptoms have been documented for vitamin K2 intake from food and/or supplements. In animal studies, vitamin K in amounts as high as 25 micrograms per kilogram of body weight per day (the equivalent of 1,750 mcg of MK-7/day for a 154-pound adult human) has produced no toxicity. For these reasons, experts at the Institute of Medicine at the National Academy of Sciences chose not to set a Tolerable Upper Limit (UL) for vitamin K when publishing their health recommendations in 2010.

K2 has even been used safely at very high doses in hemodialysis patients, whose kidney function is so damaged they must have their blood filtered by machine. The large doses of K2 are intended to prevent further calcification in their kidneys, a well-known risk for such patients. In one recent study, 200 chronic hemodialysis patients randomly received 360, 720, or 1080 mcg of MK-7 three times a week for 8 weeks. No adverse effects were seen, just increased benefits as the dose of MK-7 was increased.[523] [524] [525] [526] [527]

Supplemental Vitamin K is Prohibited When Taking Any of the Coumarin Drugs

You must avoid all vitamin K supplements if you are taking commonly prescribed oral anticoagulant (blood-thinning) medications, e.g., the coumarin drugs (warfarin, acenocoumarol, phenprocoumon, and fluindione). These work by blocking the activity of the vitamin K epoxide reductase enzyme (VKOR), which recycles vitamin K. Since the coumarins work by inhibiting the recycling of vitamin K, adding more vitamin K to the body simply cancels out the drugs' effect of lowering the pool of available vitamin K.

Here's the problem. While these drugs lower the risk of excessive blood clot formation, they also prevent the activation of osteocalcin and matrix Gla protein, thus greatly increasing risk for osteoporosis, cardiovascular disease, and chronic kidney disease. Patients on coumarins have been repeatedly shown to have high levels of inactive (or undercarboxylated) matrix Gla protein (ucMGP).[528 529 530]

Medical researchers found that blood levels of ucMGP increase significantly with the use of warfarin, and decrease after supplementation with vitamin K. The vitamin K-antagonist drugs (the coumarins) also greatly increase your risk for a bleed inside the brain (intracerebral hemorrhage). This is one of the reasons monitoring the rate at which your blood clots—*international normalized ratio* (INR)—is so critical. Doctors look at the INR to check how high a dose of the coumarins is needed to prevent the available vitamin K from increasing.[531 532] (See Lab Tests, Chapter 10.)

Supplemental K2 is off-limits even in very low doses if you are taking warfarin. Doses of MK-7 as low as 10 to 20 mcg/d have been shown to decrease INR by 40 to 60% and to significantly increase blood clot formation by 20% and 30% in all patients tested. Even worse, these tiny doses of MK-7 had no beneficial effect on increasing activation of matrix Gla protein. Virtually all the MK-7 got side-tracked to activate blood clotting proteins. This makes sense: your body first uses vitamin K to ensure you don't bleed out from a tiny cut. Only after this need has been taken care of will any vitamin K be used to prevent your bones from breaking and your arteries, kidneys, breasts, and brain from calcifying.[533 534 535 536 537]

Small amounts of dietary K1 may still be safe. Vitamin K1 only affects the INR at a dose of 315 mcg/day. As this dosage causes just a small decrease in INR (from 2.0 to 1.5), even those taking warfarin can eat some leafy green vegetables *if their INR is frequently checked by their physician*, so their dose can be adjusted accordingly. What foods are rich enough in K1 to significantly decrease a person's INR? Leafy greens, though you'd have to eat a fair amount: 2.5 cups of spinach, 5 cups of lettuce, or a half-cup of kale, which delivers the most K1 (547 mcg/cup). Oils, even unrefined, should not be a problem as they provide so little K1: a tablespoon of soybean oil gives you just 25 mcg, canola oil only 17 mcg, and olive oil just 8 mcg.

Vitamin K2 Can Be Taken with New Classes of Anticoagulant Drugs

Vitamin K2 is safe to take with Factor Xa inhibitors (e.g., rivaroxaban and apixaban) or the direct thrombin inhibitor, dabigatran. Unlike coumarins, which interfere with vitamin K recycling to prevent blood clots, these new anticoagulant drugs work through a different mechanism.[538 539]

- The Factor Xa inhibitors block the activity of already produced Factor Xa, so vitamin K does not lessen their anti-clotting effects.

- The direct thrombin inhibitors, as their name implies, bind to already formed thrombin, directly blocking its clot-forming action, so again, vitamin K does not lessen their anti-clotting effects.

Neither the Factor Xa inhibitors nor the direct thrombin inhibitors require INR monitoring, and both types of medication need only be taken once daily. If you must take an anticoagulant medication and are currently taking one of the coumarins, please discuss switching to one of these newer anticoagulants with your doctor.[540 541 542 543 544]

BONE-HEALTHY ACTION ITEMS

- Get at least 1,000 mcg (1 mg) of vitamin K1 daily by eating a healthy diet that includes lots of leafy greens.
- You can also get smaller amounts of K1 in organic, cold-pressed oils. Avoid processed foods; they contain oils in which K1 has been altered into an unusable form.

- To meet your bones' needs for vitamin K2, you need to take a supplement. Almost always, the MK-7 form will be best.
- Balance your daily intake of vitamin K2 with your daily needs for vitamin D:
  - » If you need 1,000 to 2,000 IU of vitamin D3, you may need 100 to 180 mcg of MK-7.
  - » If you need 3,000 to 4,000 IU of D3, you may need 200 to 300 mcg of MK-7.
  - » If you need 5,000 IU or more D3, you may need 360 mcg of MK-7.
- To verify your vitamin K2 needs are being met, check your blood levels of ucOC, undercarboxylated (inactive) osteocalcin.

Omega-3 Essential Fatty Acids

BONE ESSENTIALS

- Both omega-3 and omega-6 are essential fatty acids, though maintaining balance between them is most important for our bone health.
- Omega-3s boost our production of bone-building osteoblasts by causing mesenchymal stem cells (MSCs) to develop into osteoblasts rather than fat cells. In contrast, omega-6s cause MSCs to become fat cells.
- The highly pro-inflammatory omega-6, arachidonic acid (AA) is present in greatest amounts in meats (e.g., beef, lamb, pork, chicken, duck, turkey), eggs, and farmed fish.
- The ratio of omega-6: omega-3 in the modern Western diet is 20:1 far from the minimally recommended 4:1—a key reason why the SAD promotes sarcopenia (the medical term for muscles' replacement by fat).
- You'll need an EPA/DHA supplement for 2 reasons:
  - » People (especially men) do a poor job of producing EPA/DHA from their precursor in plants, ALA.
  - » Omega-3-rich wild-caught fish contain mercury, and farmed fish contain too much omega-6.

Your osteoclasts are supposed to remove old and brittle or damaged bone—a job they do very quickly. Then, they're supposed to clear out, go on vacation and let our osteoblasts start on the more time-consuming job of building new, replacement bone.

However, when our bodies create too many free radicals, osteoclasts go on overtime. Too much osteoclast bone-demolishing activity results in bone thinning. By helping your body produce a healthy inflammatory response, your osteoclasts can take a break (and prevent a break due to excessive bone removal), while your osteoblasts are given time for bone formation.

Omega-3 Fatty Acids Promote Healthy Bones

The two common omega fatty acids in our diets are omega-3s and omega-6s. They're both essential to health, but maintaining the right balance between these two long-chain polyunsaturated fatty acids (PUFAs) is even more important. In Part One, we discussed how maintaining a balanced ratio of omega-6s: omega-3s (no more than 4:1) is critical for a healthy inflammatory response. Unfortunately, the standard American diet—which is closer to 20:1 omega-6s to omega-3s—produces chronic inflammation and encourages bone loss!

We'll dig deeper into the specific reasons that getting sufficient omega-3s is critical for your bones and how you can get what you need, either from food and supplements. First, it's important to understand that fatty acids are a *family* affair.

EPA and DHA can be derived from their *parent compounds*. *Alpha linoleic acid* (ALA) is the parent compound of the omega-3s, including EPA and DHA. Similarly, linoleic acid (LA) is the parent compound of the omega-6s, including arachidonic acid (AA). ALA and LA are considered essential fatty acids because they cannot be synthesized by humans. While our bodies can use these parent compounds found in plants to produce their offspring essential fatty acids, the conversion efficiency is low. In other words, consuming ALA is unlikely to give you the omega-3 EPA and DHA you need.

Omega-3 Fatty Acids Help You Build Bone Instead of Fat

The omega-3s help you build bone rather than fat by encouraging your mesenchymal stem cells (MSCs) to become bone-building osteoblasts, instead of adipocytes (fat cells).

Mesenchymal stem cells (MSCs) are precursor cells that live in your bone marrow and haven't yet made up their minds what they want to grow up to be. They can become osteoblasts and build new bone for you, or they can become adipocytes and store fat. Obviously, we'd prefer to build healthy bones rather than increase our fat stores. *How do our MSCs choose a bone-building rather than a fat-storage career path?* They meet with the body's MSC career counselors: the essential fatty acids (EFAs).

MSCs get their career counseling from both the omega-6 and the omega-3 essential fatty acids, starting with the parent compounds: the omega-6 linoleic acid (LA) and the omega-3 alpha-linolenic acid (ALA).

- The offspring of LA (the omega-6-ers), particularly AA (arachidonic acid), convince MSCs to become fat cells. AA almost always chooses to join a bone-demolition crew as its way of life. AA is an anarchist and loves to promote bone resorption.

- The offspring of ALA (the omega-3-ers) put MSCs on the path to a much more rewarding career for our bones: life as an osteoblast. Offspring EPA and DHA and their children (ALA's grandchildren: the resolvins, protectins, and maresins) are all peaceful folk who enjoy building new bone.

The omega-3 clan inhibits the production of osteoclasts, thus slowing the rate of bone removal, and encourages MSCs to become osteoblasts, thus increasing the available number of these cells that build new bone.[545 546]

As we age, if we lack omega-3s, we produce fat instead of bone. MSCs are very responsive to influences in their environment (such as who gets to give them career advice, an omega-6 or an omega-3). Recently, researchers have learned something else: MSCs in younger individuals are far less likely to become adipocytes (fat cells)—even in response to omega-6 career counseling—than are the MSCs in older folks.

Are we doomed to grow fat and lose our bones as we age? Absolutely not! We're not stuck with this unhappy version of aging! We can boost osteoblast production as we age by consuming enough omega-3s to balance our intake of omega-6s (which are way too plentiful in the typical modern diet). *Enough* omega-3s will range between 2 to 4 grams of EPA/DHA per day, depending upon your overall diet.[547][548]

Your Diet is Unlikely to Give You the EPA/DHA You Need

When enough EPA/DHA is consumed to result in a ratio of omega-6: omega-3 of no greater than 4:1, your metabolism shifts to one that favors a healthy inflammatory response. Plus, it puts a damper on the production of bone-resorbing osteoclasts and encourages your MSCs to become bone-building osteoblasts instead of fat cells.[549]

Unfortunately, the standard American diet (SAD) will not produce this ratio for you. It's loaded with the pro-inflammatory omega-6, arachidonic acid, which is found in meats (e.g., beef, lamb, pork, chicken, duck, and turkey), eggs, and fish, particularly farmed fish.[550]

What affects the amount of AA in animal and fish products? The diet of the animal or fish from which the meat or eggs, or fish was derived. A pastured cow has significantly lower AA than that of a feedlot animal. Research found AA content ranged from just 20 mg in a 3-ounce serving of rainbow trout fed a diet rich in flaxseed oil (high in ALA, the form of omega-3 in plants) to 138 mg in a 3-ounce serving of chicken fed a corn-based diet (high in omega-6), to 681 mg in a 3-ounce serving of rainbow trout fed a commercial grain/corn (omega-6-rich) feed mixture.

Pastured cows consume grasses rich in ALA, so the omega-3 content of their milk is far higher. Plus, cows eating grass produce a highly anti-inflammatory fatty acid called conjugated linoleic acid from the ALA they consume. Cows eating grains produce AA instead. Garbage in, garbage out. If you eat animal products, choose meat and dairy products from pastured animals, and eggs from free-range chickens. If you eat fish, choose wild-caught. Lastly, when consuming dairy products, for the best ratio of omega-6: omega-3, choose products made from whole milk. One cup of whole cow's milk contains 0.29 grams of omega-6 and 0.18 grams of omega-3, a healthy 2:1 ratio of omega-6: omega-3. One cup of 2% cow's milk contains 0.15 grams of omega-6 and only 0.2 grams of omega-3, an unhealthy ratio of 7.5:1. The yogurt and cheeses

derived from the milk will contain the same proportion of fatty acids.
551 552 553 554 555

Food sources of the parent omega-3, ALA, are few and less frequently eaten. The majority of our diet contains foods high in LA (the parent omega-6), such as vegetable oils used in processed foods, or its pro-inflammatory derivative AA, which is in the eggs, meat, and dairy products from farmed fish and animals fed corn and grains.

In contrast, few frequently eaten foods contain either ALA (the parent omega-3) or its anti-inflammatory derivatives EPA and DHA. ALA is found in the greatest amounts in flaxseed and its oil, Brussels sprouts, collard greens, spinach, and broccoli. While ALA is also found in walnuts, pumpkin seeds, soybean oil, canola oil, and corn oil, these foods contain more LA (the parent omega-6) than ALA (the parent omega-3), which results in little ALA being converted to EPA and DHA.

The enzyme COX-2 produces the offspring of both AA and EPA/DHA, prefers to work with AA. So, when we consume a food that contains more omega-6 than omega-3, the available COX-2 will first be used to produce pro-inflammatory compounds from AA, leaving little or even no COX-2 to produce anti-inflammatory compounds from the smaller amounts of ALA in the food.

Best Food Sources of Alpha-Linolenic Acid (ALA) Compared to Linoleic Acid (LA)			
Foods	Serving Size	ALA Omega-3 Content (mg)	LA Omega-6 Content (mg)
Walnuts	1 ounce	2,565	10,761
Pumpkin seeds	1 ounce	51.5	5,849
Brussels sprouts	1 cup	87.1	39.6
Collard greens,	1 cup	38.9	29.5
Spinach, raw	1 cup	41.4	7.8
Broccoli, raw	1 cup	19.1	15.5
Oils			
Flaxseed oil	1 tablespoon	7,196	1,715
Soybean oil	1 tablespoon	917	6,807
Canola oil	1 tablespoon	1,279	2,610
Corn oil	1 tablespoon	157	7,224

Source: nutritiondata.self.com/

Furthermore, humans produce only tiny amounts of EPA/DHA from ALA. Of the small amount of ALA in plant foods, humans can only convert tiny amounts into EPA and DHA. One study reported that only 6% of dietary ALA was converted to EPA and just 3.8% was converted to DHA in humans eating a diet high in saturated fat. Add in the fact that a diet high in any omega-6 rich vegetable oils (e.g., soy, corn, safflower, canola)—one that most of us eat—reduces ALA's conversion to EPA and DHA by 40% to 50%.[556 557 558 559]

Men do an especially poor job of converting ALA to EPA/DHA. Studies show that healthy young women convert 21% of the ALA they consume into EPA, of which 9% is further converted to DHA. Healthy young men convert only about 8% of the ALA they consume into EPA and convert at most 4% (just half as much as women) into DHA. And many men convert none of that EPA into DHA.[560 561]

Plus men typically eat far fewer foods rich in ALA. The richest food sources of ALA—which contain more omega-3 than omega-6—are flaxseed oil, Brussels sprouts, collard greens, and spinach. Newsflash: these are not foods most men eat frequently. OK, you already knew this, but now you can cite the research. Actual data analysis of what men and women typically eat when dining out shows that men subsist on pizza, chicken wings, bacon cheeseburgers, and fries. (Joe doesn't eat these but would gladly live on nachos—not an omega-3-rich option.) Women are more likely to order ALA-rich salads.[562]

Why are women better at converting ALA to EPA/DHA than men? The effects of estrogen boost the activity of the enzymes involved in changing ALA into EPA and then to DHA, which is essential for brain development and brain function. When a woman is pregnant or nursing, she must supply all the DHA required to her baby's brain. If she's not frequently eating cold-water fatty fish (or taking a supplement), that DHA has to come from the ALA she's getting from plants.[563]

Even women can't rely on converting ALA to get the EPA/DHA needed for healthy bones. Women can convert only between 5% and 10% of the ALA consumed into EPA/DHA. To reach a 2.6 gram daily dose of EPA/DHA, a woman would need to consume foods containing 52 grams of ALA. One tablespoon of cold-pressed flaxseed oil, the richest plant source of ALA contains up to 7,000 mg of ALA, so you would need 4 to 8 tablespoons of flaxseed oil—representing 400 to 800 extra calories per day. Forget the skinny jeans.

Ground flaxseeds would be no better. You'd need 34.6 tablespoons of flaxseed meal daily, which adds 1,038 calories. Plus, this is a seriously large amount of flaxseed—and fiber. You'd better be drinking *a lot* of water to get all that flaxseed moving through your digestive tract! Obviously, relying upon ALA-rich oil or flaxseed is not a practical way of getting the EPA/DHA your bones need. In today's world, in which the food supply is overloaded with omega-6, the tiny amounts of ALA in plant foods, even if eaten daily, cannot provide us with enough EPA and DHA to protect our bones.[564][565]

Can fish provide the long-chain omega-3s, EPA and DHA, we need?
The only good dietary sources of EPA and DHA are *wild-caught*, cold-water fatty fish, such as sardines, salmon, sablefish, halibut, and tuna. It's important that the fish be *wild-caught* because, as mentioned above, the amount of EPA and DHA is highly dependent on the fish's diet. Wild fish eat algae, sea plants, and other smaller fish that are rich in omega-3s, so they produce and store EPA and DHA in their tissue. Wild fish do not eat omega-6-rich grains or refined plant oils, so they consume and store very little LA and even less AA. In contrast, the farmed fish are given feed that is loaded with omega-6-rich oils, so farmed fish contain at least as much, and possibly more omega-6 than omega-3. For this reason, farmed fish are not a good source of usable omega-3s.

Plus, there are two other serious problems with relying on fish, even wild fish, for your EPA and DHA: bone-destructive mercury and environmental toxins called PCBs, both of which accumulate in fish. Mercury accumulates in a water-soluble form that is highly bioavailable (meaning easily absorbed by us). We absorb 7% to 15% of the mercury in the fish we eat. And mercury accumulates in us just like it does in fish. In humans, mercury deposits mainly in our kidneys, where it causes serious damage and disrupts essential kidney functions, including activation of vitamin D. (See Heavy Metals, Chapter 3.)

To minimize our consumption of mercury, we need to be careful which fish we eat, and it can be difficult to *safely* eat enough fish to provide optimal amounts of EPA and DHA. Some types of fish contain lower levels of mercury and can be eaten in moderate amounts without risk of harm to our kidneys and bones. Other types of fish contain high levels of mercury and are best avoided. The following table can help you choose the best seafood for your kidney and bone health. But, unless you really enjoy eating fish, you're not likely to consume enough EPA/DHA to keep your bones healthy.[566][567]

You'd have to eat at least 2 servings of fish every day to get the amount of EPA/DHA needed for healthy bones. Current research indicates *optimal* health benefits provided by omega-3s are associated with intakes of 2.6 to 4 grams of EPA and DHA per day. (And you want *optimal*, right?) As you can see from the table below, you'd need to consume *at least* two 3-ounce portions of low-mercury fish every day to provide enough EPA and DHA to beneficially impact the health of your bones. That's a lot of fish! Bottom line: you need an EPA/DHA supplement. What you need to know to choose the one that will serve you best and how you can determine how many grams of EPA/DHA you require daily is discussed next.

EPA/DHA Levels in Commonly Eaten Seafood vs. Mercury Contents	
Least Mercury (less than 0.09 parts per million) *Safe to enjoy these fish.*	**EPA + DHA** (grams in 3 ounces)
Anchovies (European, canned in oil)	1.7
Catfish	0.4
Clam	0.2
Crab (Alaska king)	0.4
Crayfish (Crawfish)	0.1
Flounder	0.2
Haddock (Atlantic)	0.2
Herring	1.2
Mackerel (N. Atlantic)	2.5
Mackerel (Chubb)	1.9
Oyster (Eastern, Farmed)	0.4
Perch (Ocean)	0.2
Pollock (Atlantic)	0.5
Salmon (Wild, Canned)	1.0
Salmon (Wild, Chinook)	1.4
Salmon (Wild, Sockeye)	1.2
Sardine (canned)	1.0

EPA/DHA Levels in Commonly Eaten Seafood vs. Mercury Contents	
Least Mercury (less than 0.09 parts per million) *Safe to enjoy these fish.*	**EPA + DHA** (grams in 3 ounces)
Scallop	0.3
Shrimp	0.3
Squid (Calamari)	0.2
Tilapia (farmed, so high in omega-6, also PCBs)	0.2
Trout (freshwater, wild)	3.0
Moderate Mercury (0.09 to 0.29 parts per million) *Eat no more than 6 servings per month.*	**EPA + DHA** (grams in 3 ounces)
Bass (Striped, Black, Freshwater)	0.8
Clam	0.2
Cod (Alaskan)	0.3
Halibut (Pacific)	0.4
Lobster	0.4
Mahi Mahi	0.1
Sablefish	1.4
Red Snapper	0.2
High Mercury (from 0.3 to 0.49 parts per million) *Eat no more than 3 servings per month*	**EPA + DHA** (grams in 3 ounces)
Tuna (Albacore, canned)	0.7
Tuna (Skipjack, also called Yellowfin)	0.2
Highest Mercury (more than .5 parts per million) *Don't eat these fish.*	
Mackerel (King)	
Marlin	
Orange roughy	
Shark	
Swordfish	
Tilefish	
Tuna (Bigeye, Ahi)	

Sources: NRDC Mercury Guide (www.nrdc.org/health/effects/mercury/guide.asp), Oregon State Omega-3 Fatty Acid Content in Fish (bit.ly/Oregon-OmegaFish)

What to Look for When Choosing your EPA/DHA Supplement

To choose the omega-3 supplement that will serve you best, you need to consider 3 factors. The rest of this chapter covers each fully.

- **Potency**: Your supplement must contain an amount of EPA/DHA that enables *you* to maintain an omega-6: omega-3 ratio of no more than 4:1. Current research indicates achieving this ratio and gaining the health benefits provided by omega-3s requires 2 to 4 grams per day of EPA/DHA.

- **Purity**: Your omega-3 supplement must be free of harmful contaminants, such as mercury and POPs (persistent organic pollutants) and must also be free of rancidity.

- **Palatability**: If your omega-3 supplement causes fishy-tasting burps, a common occurrence with many EPA/DHA supplements, you probably won't *remember* to take it every day. Obviously, if you don't take it, it won't help you.

Potency

The first thing you need to do is decode the supplement label. Some supplement manufacturers tell you clearly how much EPA/DHA their omega-3 supplement provides; others have made this a bit challenging. Here are the 3 things you need to look for and what it means in plain English.

1. **The *actual omega-3 content* per serving.** Don't rely on claims about the amount of *fish oil* a product contains. Fish oil contains *at least* six other fatty acids besides EPA and DHA, including myristic acid, palmitic acid, palmitoleic acid, oleic acid, gadoleic acid, and cetoleic acid.[568] Even if the front label touts 1,200 mg of fish oil, you have no idea the actual dose of omega-3s provided. To determine how much EPA/DHA you're getting in a serving, you have to read the Supplement Facts section of the label (often in small print on the back) and add up the amounts (listed in milligrams) for both EPA and DHA.

2. **The form of fish oil used, which affects bioavailability.** While you're reviewing your fish oil nutrition label, you may see listed the form of the EPA/DHA provided. However, manufacturers don't have to tell us which form is present in their products. Omega-3s

derived from fish oils are available in 3 forms, one of which offers far better bioavailability.

» **Natural triglycerides, as the name suggests, are the natural form**—the closest thing to eating omega-3-rich fish or other original food sources of EPA/DHA. Plus, these are far better absorbed and utilized than the other forms. The bioavailability of natural triglycerides is further enhanced if delivered in an emulsion—meaning they're suspended in another liquid (like oil in a vinegar-based salad dressing).[569]

» **Ethyl esters (EE) are processed to be more concentrated.** While ethyl esters begin as natural triglycerides, a chemical process called *transesterification* allows supplement manufacturers to double or triple the levels of EPA/DHA in a pill. While this sounds good on the surface, research has shown some major drawbacks. EE omega-3s are far less bioavailable, with 73% lower absorption than that from natural triglycerides. So, even if a supplement made from EE-type omega-3s offers more EPA/DHA, your body will absorb far less.[570]

What's more, the safety of the EE form has not been confirmed in humans. Pregnant women are advised not to take the EE form of omega-3s because they accumulate in major organs such as the heart, liver, pancreas, and potentially the placenta. Here's another big concern for pregnant women: When your body absorbs and then converts EEs back into their natural triglyceride form, alcohol is released. While only a tiny amount, it still has the potential to harm a developing fetus.[571]

» **Synthetic reverse triglyceride oils have the least bioavailability.** In this form, manufacturers first create ethyl esters and then go one step further to reconvert them to a synthetic form of triglycerides. Except they don't go back to being natural triglycerides. They're now a weird, new-to-nature *reverse* form of triglycerides (rTG). The molecule's overall structure is altered, which unhappily affects absorption of the oil, so it's even lower than that of EEs. Well, duh. How many billions of years has Mother Nature been working all this out for us? As they say, don't mess with Mother Nature![572]

The lesson is to choose an omega-3 supplement that contains natural triglycerides. If this information is not on the label, ask! For even better absorption, look for natural triglycerides that are emulsified. Emulsions definitely have Mother Nature's seal of approval. Milk is an emulsion of fat and water. In fact, the word *emulsion* comes from the Latin word for milk. Emulsions increase the physical stability of oil droplets in general and have been shown to increase the bioavailability of omega-3 fatty acids. [573] [574]

3. **Check that the serving size delivers a *full dose* of EPA/DHA.** Serving sizes vary dramatically between brands. Remember, you want to get at least 2 grams of EPA/DHA per day (likely 3 or 4 if your diet contains meat, eggs, or dairy products). Take a single pill or spoonful and you may get less than you need. And no one wants to have to swallow a bunch of fish oil capsules every day (which increases the chance of those nasty-tasting fish oil burps). Once again, look at the Nutrition Facts to decode the serving size and how much you'll need for a complete dose.

Comparison of Omega-3 Supplement Brands

Supplement	Serving Size	Omega Types	Form
Triple Power Omega 3 Fish Oil	1 tablespoon provides 1480 mg of omega-3s	750 mg EPA, 450 mg DHA, and 280 mg other omega-3s	Provides EPA/DHA in the form of emulsified natural triglycerides
Note:	Emulsification has been shown to to improve the bioavailability of omega-3 fatty acids. www.algaecal.com/product/triple-omega3-fish-oil		
Nordic Naturals® Ultimate Omega	Two soft gels provide 1,280 mg. The product actually contains 650 mg EPA and 450 mg.	650 mg EPA, 450 mg, and 180 mg other omega-3s	Not provided
Note:	The front label advertises 1,280 mg Omega-3. If you don't carefully read the label, you may not realize a serving is 2 soft gels. www.nordicnaturals.com/consumers/ultimate-omega		
NatureMade® Mini Omega-3	One softgel provides 540 mg of omega-3 (listed as serving size which implies this is all you need)	Provides 365 mg EPA, 135 mg DHA, and 40 mg other omega-3s	Ethyl esters (indicated in small print on box)
Note:	Ethyl esters form is significantly less bioavailable. www.naturemade.com/products/burp-less-mini-omega-3#		

Purity

How do you know if your fish oil contains the amount of omega-3s promised? Researchers out of New Zealand investigated some of the fish-oil-derived omega-3 supplements on the market in 2015 and discovered some shocking statistics. Only about 9% (3 out of 32) contained the full amount of EPA/DHA they claimed on their label. Over two-thirds contained less than 67% of the claimed EPA/DHA fatty acids.

Even worse, what the vast majority (92%) did contain were toxic contaminants at a level that exceeded international safety guidelines. Toxic compounds in a fish-oil supplement indicate that the oil has oxidized (i.e., become rancid).

- 83% of the products tested exceeded recommended levels of *peroxide*, the first toxic compound produced during oxidation.
- 25% exceeded *anisidine* thresholds. Anisidine is produced from peroxides and gives oil a rancid smell.
- 50% exceeded the recommended TOTOX value, an overall picture of an oil's overall oxidation based on the peroxide and anisidine levels.[575]

The Global Organization for EPA and DHA Omega-3s (GOED) found that peroxide values averaged 89% higher than its recommended level of 5 milliequivalents/kilogram (mEq/kg) in fish oils supplements sold in 13 countries. That included 80% of the fish oil supplements sold in the South African market and more than 93% of those sold in the Norwegian market. And the GOED requirement, frankly, is not low enough. FDA quality guidelines are more stringent, demanding a peroxide value of 2.5 mEq/kg or less.[576][577]

You don't want to consume oxidized, rancid oils of any kind! Rancid oils are highly pro-inflammatory and potentially carcinogenic. They promote free radical damage and increased osteoclast activation (and therefore bone loss) along with virtually everything we want to avoid, such as hardening of the arteries and increased blood clot formation, which increases heart attack and stroke risk.

Once oil has gone rancid, it will hurt rather than help you. And this is true of *all* oils, be it olive oil, flaxseed oil, or canola oil. Check your oils before using them. Any oil that tastes *off* or has even the slightest bitter aftertaste, has become oxidized. Throw it away! Keep your oils in opaque glass, ceramic, or stainless steel (not plastic) containers and out of direct light. Refrigerate flaxseed oil. Olive and canola oil can be stored out at room temperature though use within 2 to 3 weeks after you open the bottle.

| Fish Oil Purity Standards: U.S. Food & Drug Administration and Others ||
Chemical	Safe Limit
Polychlorinated biphenyls (PCBs) *toxic chemicals*	FDA: 20 parts per million EU: 75 parts per *billion*
Dioxins *toxic chemicals*	FDA: 0.7 picograms/kg body weight/day EU and WHO: 1 to 4 picograms per kg/bw/d
Peroxide *sign of oxidation*	FDA: less than 2.5 mEq/kg EFSA: less than 2.5 mEq/kg GOED: 5 mEq/kg or less
Anisidine Value *oxidation; gives oil a rancid smell*	FDA and EFSA: less than 20
TOTOX Value *overall measure of freshness*	FDA and EFSA: less than 25.0

EU: European Union; WHO: World Health Organization; EFSA: European Food Safety Authority; GOED: Global Organization for EPA and DHA Omega-3

Source: Fish and Fishery Products Hazards—FDA/EPA (bit.ly/FDA-EPA-FishJune2021), Food Politics Jan. 2012 (bit.ly/FPdioxins), European developments following incidents with dioxins and PCBs [578]

Avoid PCBs, a potential contaminant in omega-3 supplements. Polychlorinated biphenyls (PCBs) are highly toxic compounds that form as by-products of pesticide manufacture and other industrial processes. They are called *persistent* organic pollutants (POPs) because they don't degrade. Instead, they deposit in the water, soils, and plants grown in the soils, then bio-accumulate in the animals, fish, and humans who consume them. PCBs are endocrine disruptors which cause cancer and reproductive toxicity. In animal studies, PCBs have been shown to change some fetuses from male to female. PCBs are so harmful to our environment and human health that Congress banned their manufacture in 1979. Because they don't break down, they're still with us.

How can you avoid getting PCBs in your omega-3s? PCBs accumulate up the food chain, building up as predatory fish eat other fish (similar to mercury and other toxins). Choose an omega-3 supplement that's derived from wild-caught smaller, short-lived fish like sardines, anchovy, mackerel, and salmon. Check that the company also purifies the oil to remove PCBs and other toxins.

The companies offering omega-3 supplements worthy of your trust run independent lab analyses to confirm that their product (1) provides at least the amount of EPA/DHA claimed on the label and (2) meets the international standards for purity (see box above).[579 580 581 582]

Palatability

The number one complaint people have about fish oil supplements is that they come back as fishy burps. These unpleasant repeat performances may also be accompanied by gas, flatulence, bloating, and even diarrhea. This happens for two reasons touched on above:

- The unnatural forms of supplemental fish oils—ethyl esters and reverse triglycerides (rTGs)—are hard to digest. Natural triglycerides are digested and absorbed between 2.7- and 3.4-fold more effectively than the new-to-nature forms.
- The fish oil in capsules has frequently gone rancid.[583 584]

Protect your omega-3 supplement from oxidation. The more unsaturated a fat is, the more vulnerable it is to oxidation. EPA and DHA are the most unsaturated of all fats, so they are the most susceptible to becoming oxidized. You can take a couple of steps to ensure your omega-3 oils stay fresh and healthful:

- Store your omega-3 supplements in a dark, cool place. Or you can refrigerate them rather than putting them in a cupboard. After the bottle has been opened, definitely refrigerate!
- Make sure your fish oil passes the smell test. When you open a new supplement bottle, smell a spoonful of the oil. If it's encapsulated, break open a capsule. Do you detect a fishy odor or a bitter or fishy aftertaste? If so, it's oxidized. Don't take it!
- Check to see that antioxidants have been added, which can protect against oxidation. If you see only vitamin E, don't be satisfied. Many of the products tested in the New Zealand study cited above contained vitamin E but were still highly oxidized.[585] Recently published research shows two other antioxidants are far more effective than vitamin E: astaxanthin and curcumin. (See details below.)

People sometimes ask if freezing fish oil capsules can help. Once oil is oxidized, the best that freezing will do is prevent you from smelling the rancid oil (or tasting a foul fish burp) before it's delivered to your intestines, arteries, heart, bones, and throughout your body.

Here's the bad news: your fish oil may have gone bad before it has even reached you. Even smell and taste tests aren't enough to know for sure. After the initial onset of rancidity—when the spoiled fish odors and taste are most obvious—the oil continues to oxidize while the odors and flavors return to neutral. And the *best before date* printed on the packaging is not much help either. Researchers found that this had no relationship to the level of oxidation. You might think the cost of the supplement would be a good guide. Yet, the most expensive EPA/DHA supplements were the most oxidized! These products often use the unnatural EE and rTG forms to produce a more concentrated product.

So, what steps can you take to ensure your fish oil is fresh?

1. Check out an independent lab report examining end-stage rancidity. The manufacturer of your omega-3 supplement should have this run and be happy to make it available to you. Check the values against those on the Fish Oil Purity Standards box, especially confirming that the TOTOX value is below 25.

2. Choose a product that contains EPA/DHA as natural triglycerides.

3. Look for a product that protects against oxidation with antioxidants besides just vitamin E. You'll often see vitamin E on omega-3 product labels. However, the study we discussed above showed this antioxidant is not up to the task of protecting the highly vulnerable omega-3s, EPA and DHA, from oxidation. The most recently published research indicates two other antioxidants are far more effective: curcumin and astaxanthin.

Curcumin not only prevents the formation of compounds that indicate oxidation is occurring but significantly increases production of the most potent antioxidant that cells produce, glutathione.[586][587]

Curcumin has so many beneficial effects—in addition to preventing omega-3-rich oils from turning rancid—that a PubMed search on curcumin limited to human studies over the past 5 years returns 3,202 medical journal articles.[588] In relation to bones specifically, studies of curcumin in animal models have shown outstanding results:

- Curcumin lessens bone turnover, increases femur size, and greatly increases bone strength and resistance to fracture in animal models of postmenopausal osteoporosis.[589]

- In a study of mice, curcumin had resulted in constant increases in trabecular bone and improved bone mineral density after 12 months. Researchers think curcumin's bone-building effects are due to its very strong antioxidant effects. Curcumin greatly lowers production of chemical messengers including the cytokines, TNF-alpha, and IL-6, both of which play leading roles in osteoclast production.[590]

Astaxanthin, a red carotenoid (organic pigment) produced by marine algae, is responsible for the beautiful peach color of the flesh of wild salmon, which consume astaxanthin-rich algae. Astaxanthin is a potent antioxidant that neutralizes singlet oxygen (a highly reactive form of oxygen and one of the most destructive oxidizing agents) and scavenges (eliminates) free radicals. In numerous studies, astaxanthin has been shown to prevent the oxidation of lipids (including the fats EPA and DHA in fish oil) so effectively that in 1999 the FDA approved astaxanthin as a *nutraceutical,* a food providing a health benefit.

Astaxanthin also inhibits the activation of NF-kappa B, the signaling molecule that tells our genes to produce TNF-alpha and IL-6. In studies comparing astaxanthin to vitamin E and beta-carotene, astaxanthin's antioxidant abilities were far stronger than either of these well-known antioxidants. If this weren't enough, the effects of astaxanthin in combination with the omega-3s are synergistic. In other words, when you take astaxanthin along with EPA/DHA, far more beneficial effects occur than when either is taken by itself.[591 592]

What Supplemental Doses of EPA/DHA Have Proven Effective for Bone Health?

We'll share with you a couple of tools to determine your supplemental needs for EPA/DHA based on what your diet is providing and how much EPA/DHA is in your blood tissues. First, here's the latest research on what supplemental doses have been shown as effective for bone health:

- **1.2 grams EPA/DHA per day lessened bone turnover in postmenopausal women.** A double-blind study looked at the effects of EPA/ DHA supplementation on bone resorption in 126 postmenopausal women (age 68 to 82), who were also given 315 mg of calcium citrate and 1,000 IU of vitamin D3 each day. After 6 months, two key indicators of bone turnover (bone-specific alkaline phosphatase and osteocalcin) improved significantly in the women taking 1.2 grams of EPA/DHA daily. Their ratio of omega-3 to omega-6 increased by 42%. Neither of these bone-beneficial results was seen in the women given a placebo containing olive oil.[593]

- **4 grams/day of EPA/DHA significantly decreased bone turnover in postmenopausal breast cancer survivors on aromatase inhibitor therapy.** Aromatase inhibitors, often used to help prevent breast cancer recurrence, deplete estrogen levels, promote bone loss, and increase fracture risk. Omega-3s, known to prevent excessive bone turnover, were given in hopes of offsetting these harmful effects. Results were outstanding. This study only ran for 3 months, though even in this short time frame, 4 grams of EPA/DHA daily had significantly decreased bone turnover—without even a single adverse effect.[594] If you or someone you love have had breast cancer and are being treated with aromatase inhibitors, share the excellent results seen in this study with your doctor.

Genetic Variations Affect your Needs for Omega-3s

Apolipoprotein E (APOE) is a protein that binds to *lipoproteins* (fat-containing proteins), which include cholesterol and the fat-soluble vitamins (vitamins K, D, A, and E), so they can be carried throughout your body in the bloodstream. Fat and water don't mix well, so fat-containing compounds, like cholesterol and the fat-soluble vitamins, need help to move through our blood, which is primarily water. Moving them is the job of APOE. APOE comes in 3 flavors or SNP genetic variations: APOE2, 3, and 4. Most of us (78%) carry the APOE3 SNP. A few of us (7%) have inherited the APOE2 SNP, and 14% (1 in 7) of us, have inherited the APOE4 SNP. [595]

If you're among the 14% who have inherited the APOE4 SNP, you will need more vitamin K2 than *average* because this will be removed from your bloodstream more quickly. You will also require extra omega-3s to protect your bones, cardiovascular system (particularly EPA), and brain (particularly DHA).[596] Research findings on APOE4's effect on bone have been mixed, but APOE4 is the most pro-inflammatory of the three types of APOE, and some studies indicate lower bone mineral density in both hip and spine in APOE4 carriers.[597]

Carrying an APOE4 allele is also known to greatly increase the risk for Alzheimer's disease, for which EPA/DHA has been shown to lower risk—except in APOE4 carriers. Now we understand why this is the case. APOE4 carriers need more EPA/DHA than *average*. Unlike the rest of us, who carefully preserve EPA/DHA and put these essential fatty acids into our cell membranes, APOE4 carriers use most of the EPA/DHA they consume as fuel, burning it to produce ATP (the energy currency of the body).[598] The brain has your body's greatest need for omega-3 fatty acids, specifically DHA which plays a key role in many brain activities including neurotransmission (the process through which brain cells send signaling molecules called neurotransmitters to each other), neuron (brain cell) membrane repair and fluidity, and numerous brain-protective processes.

It's easy to find out your APOE type. Have your doctor run a blood test or you can order one yourself online as a lab offering the test, such as Quest Diagnostics (ADmark® ApoE Genotype Analysis and Interpretation).

What Amount of EPA/DHA is Right for YOUR Needs?

That answer varies by person, based on diet, metabolism, and genetics. However, we'll share some tools here to help determine the specific amount for your needs.

What ratio of omega-6: omega-3 should you be shooting for? Humans evolved on a diet with an omega-6: omega-3 ratio of about 1.5:1. Yet, the ratio in today's typical Western diet favors omega-6s by 20:1.

As we mentioned earlier, many experts suggest a ratio of no more than 4:1 for good health, though others suggest it should be even lower, 2:1 or even 1.5:1. And that's not just for healthy bones but also for cardiovascular and brain health.[599 600 601 602 603 604]

How to reach an omega-6: omega-3 ratio of at least 4:1. To determine how much supplemental EPA/DHA *you*'ll need depends upon a couple of factors, which you can identify with some helpful tools:

- **Your Omega-3 Index**, a measure of the amount of EPA and DHA in your red blood cell membranes. Now you can easily determine this with the OmegaQuant Kit, a simple finger-poke you do at home and send back for quick results (www.algaecal.com/product/omegatest).

  The kit provides an index that indicates what ratio of omega-6s: omega-3s you're currently getting. Your goal is an index of at least 8%, which translates to a ratio of omega-6: omega-3 of 4:1. An omega-3 index lower than 8% means your ratio is greater than our target of 4:1, and you'll need to increase your intake of omega-3s. *How much?* That's where the next tool comes in.

- **Calculating your current dietary ratio of omega-6 to omega-3 fatty acids.** You can figure this out in just minutes per day over 5 days by keeping a diet diary. In this chapter, we've provided a tracking chart, lists of omega-rich foods, and detailed instructions to make this easy.

We know this will take a small investment in time. You may be thinking, *why should I bother doing this?* First, you will see the real omega-6: omega-3 ratio that *your* current diet is actually providing for *you*. They say knowledge is power, and that truly applies here! Once you know where you are, you may choose to modify or tweak your diet for a healthier ratio.

Secondly, you will *know* (not just be guessing at) how much supplemental omega-3 (EPA/DHA) you need for your best health. If your goal is a ratio of omega-6: omega-3 of 4:1 (considered adequate), then you will need 1 gram of EPA/DHA for every 4 grams of AA your diet is giving you. If you shoot for an *optimal* ratio of omega-6: omega-3 of 2:1, then you will need 1 gram of omega-3 (EPA/DHA forms) for every 2 grams of omega-6 (AA form) that your diet is giving you.

We did this because, despite eating a healthy diet, Joe's Omega-3 Index results were far from optimal. And I (Lara) adore Joe and want to keep him! Plus, I tracked my own diet for two reasons: (1) my initial results were good—though not optimal—and I want optimal (not just *okay*) and (2) we're suggesting you do this, so we wanted to make the effort as well.

We kept our own diet diaries for 5 days. *What did we learn?* We discovered that despite eating a very healthy, organic, whole foods diet, both of us need supplemental EPA/DHA to reach even a 4:1 omega-6: omega-3 ratio. We are *pescatarians*, meaning we eat fish, dairy products, and eggs, but no meat. On the days we didn't eat fish, our EPA/DHA intake averaged less than 1 gram per day.

While our AA intake was low since we don't eat meat, we still averaged 8 grams AA per day (more on days homemade pizza or nachos were on the menu). That puts our average omega-6: omega-3 ratio at 8:1 (actually less than 1). Better than the 20:1 typical in America these days, but far from optimal. We knew we needed to increase our intake of EPA/DHA from less than 1 to 2 grams per day (for an omega-3: omega-6 ratio of 4:1) to 4 grams per day (for an optimal ratio of 2:1).

Joe and I made small changes to our diet AND started taking an omega-3 supplement daily. After several weeks, we ran our first Omega-3 Index test. Our results showed Joe's omega-6 (AA): omega-3 (EPA/DHA) ratio was 5.5:1, and mine was 4.1:1. I'm guessing my initial test ratio was a bit better because I eat far more ALA-rich vegetables and far fewer servings of Joe's homemade nachos. He's a guy after all. Plus, as mentioned above, women are much better at converting ALA into EPA than men.

Joe began taking 2 daily tablespoons of our omega-3 supplement (containing 2.4 grams of EPA/DHA). I took one tablespoon (1.2 grams daily). We also began to eat fish twice a week. We're both busy, so going out to buy fresh fish is not a good option, but eating more wild-caught, low-mercury varieties of canned and frozen fish is. After three more months, we ran a second Omega-3 Index test. Joe's omega-6: omega-3 ratio improved, dropping to 4.5:1. My omega-6: omega-3 ratio remained about the same: 4.4:1, a clear indication that I also need two tablespoons, so I've increased my dose.

Use this Diet Diary to Find Out Your Current Omega-6 to Omega-3 Ratio

Is your diet giving you enough healthy EPA/DHA fatty acids compared to inflammatory AA fatty acids? You can find out in less than a week, so you can make positive changes to your diet and determine your supplemental dosage needs. We've provided all the tools you need; just follow these easy steps:

STEP 1: Review the Omega-3 and Omega-6 Content of Commonly Eaten Foods chart. Familiarize yourself with this list, so you can see how many grams of EPA/DHA and/or AA each serving of common foods contains. Bookmark these pages, since you'll refer to them often to complete your diary. *Note: You don't need to record your intake of the parent form of the omega-3s (alpha-linolenic acid, ALA) or omega-6s (linoleic acid, LA), both of which are found in plant foods. As discussed earlier, humans are not good at converting either into their offspring omega fatty acids, so they are not likely to make a significant difference in your totals. However, we've included ALA content in the food lists and conversion instructions on the diary form for those who want the most accurate measure.*[605 606 607 608]

STEP 2: Use the Diet Diary to track your Omega-3 and Omega-6 foods for 5 days. Each day, record any food containing AA or EPA/DHA (and ALA if desired) on your Diet Diary (at the end of this chapter), along with the number of servings. At the end of each day, for each food you have listed, multiply the grams of omega-3 and the grams of omega-6 by the number of servings you have had for that food, and enter amounts consumed in the *Grams* omega-*3 ALA, Grams* omega-*3 EPA/DHA*, and *Grams* omega-*6 AA columns.* (The symbol for omega is ω, so we abbreviate ω-3 for omega-3 and ω-6 for omega-6 below.)

> **Example:** In the *Commonly Eaten Foods* list, in the Fats & Oils section, you'll see that one serving of butter = 1 teaspoon. Let's say you used a teaspoon of butter on some toast. That's 1 serving. Then, at dinner, you used a *tablespoon* of butter to season a baked potato; that's another 3 servings. So, during your day, you've had 4 servings. Each serving has given you 0.04 grams of ALA for a total of 0.16 grams ALA (4 x 0.04), and 0.31 grams of AA for a total of 1.24 grams of AA (4 x 0.31). So, in the Total ω-3 ALA column, you'll write 0.16, and in the Total ω-6 AA column, write 1.24.

STEP 3: Add up your totals for the day. You can simply get out your trusty calculator to add up the numbers in the Total ω-3, EPA/DHA, and Total ω-6, AA columns and see how much of each your diet provided that day. (Or you can create a table in an Excel, Google Sheets, or other spreadsheet and let it automatically tally them for you).

Remember, if you are tracking ALA, people don't convert efficiently. You'll need to multiply the day's total ALA by the conversion factors for men and women shown on the diary page. You can then add this derived amount of EPA and DHA to the amount you consumed directly.

STEP 4: After 5 days, get your average daily intake of EPA/DHA and AA. Add up the total grams of EPA/DHA (ω-3) your diet gave you and divide by 5 (the number of days you kept your diary). That's the average daily amount of EPA/DHA your typical diet is providing you. Do the same for your AA intake to get your average daily intake of omega-6.

> **Example:** If your total AA intake over the 5 days was 100 grams, you would divide 100 by 5 to get your average daily intake of ω-6, which would be 20 grams (which is the amount of AA most Americans consume). If your total EPA/DHA intake over the 5 days was 5 grams, you would divide 5 by 5 to get your average daily intake of ω-3, which would be 1 gram (which is the amount of EPA/DHA most Americans consume). This translates to an omega-6: omega-3 ratio of 20:1, the unhealthy ratio seen in people consuming the typical Western diet.[609]

STEP 5: Find out how many grams of EPA/DHA you need to maintain an omega-6: omega-3 ratio of 4:1. Now that you know your current omega-6: omega-3 ratio, you can go a step further to determine just how much additional EPA/DHA *you specifically* need to reach your goals. Say you want to maintain an omega-6: omega-3 ratio of 4:1. Simply divide your average daily ω-6/AA intake by 4. This will give you the number of grams of EPA/DHA that *you* require daily to achieve a 4:1 ratio.

> **Example:** If you are consuming an average of 20 grams of AA each day, for a ω-6: ω-3 ratio of 4:1, you would divide 20 by 4, which means *you* need 5 grams of EPA/DHA each day to achieve a 4:1 ratio of ω-6: ω-3.

In Step 4, you calculated how much EPA/DHA you already get daily. Subtract this amount from how much total you need to see how many additional grams of EPA/DHA you need. Knowing this amount, you can adjust your diet (eat more EPA/DHA-rich wild-caught fish and less meat, dairy, and eggs) or supplement with the proper amount of omega-3 (EPA/DHA). Or a combination of both, which is what Joe and I did after we kept and analyzed our own diet diaries.

Omega-3 and Omega-6 Content of Commonly Eaten Foods

Fish and Seafood	Serving Size	Omega-3 (EPA & DHA) grams	Omega-6 (AA) grams
Clams, canned	6.5 ounces	0.18	0.07
New England clam chowder	1 cup	0.70	4.94
Manhattan clam chowder	1 cup	0.16	1.10
Cod, Pacific	4 ounces	0.15	0.03
Crab, Alaskan King	1 leg	0.25	0.08
Halibut, Pacific or Atlantic	4 ounces	0.31	0.07
Mackerel, Pacific	4 ounces	2.53	0.29
*Pollock, Alaskan, raw	3 ounces	0.15	<0.01
Sablefish	4 ounces	2.58	0.39
**Salmon, wild Atlantic	4 ounces	3.05	0.64
**Salmon, farmed Atlantic	4 ounces	3.28	2.20
Salmon, wild sockeye, Pacific	4 ounces	1.18	0.45
Salmon, sockeye, canned	4 ounces	1.58	0.19
Sardines, canned in water	4 ounces	2.18	0.17
***Sardines, canned in oil	3.75 ounces	1.48	3.26 (LA)
Scallop	1 large	0.03	<0.01
Snapper, fillet	3-ounces fillet	0.29	0.02
Tuna, light, canned in water	4 ounces	0.26	0.02
Tuna, blue fin	4 ounces	1.94	0.14
Tuna, yellow fin	4 ounces	0.14	0.05
Tuna, albacore, canned in water	4 ounces	1.14	0.12
Tilapia, farmed, fillet	3.45 ounces	0.64	5.89
Catfish, farmed, fillet	5.23 ounces	0.28	1.46

*Pollock: Compared to pure, cooked fish fillets, breaded and pre-fried Alaska pollock fillet contains extraordinarily high fat and omega-6 levels. Pure fish fillet contained an average of 0.30% of weight as omega-3 and 0.17% of weight as omega-6. Breaded and fried pollock fish fingers contained an average of 0.30% of weight as omega-3 and 4.04% as omega-6! [610]

**Farmed versus wild salmon: Wild salmon is a significantly better source of usable omega-3s than farmed salmon. (See Omega Fatty Acids, Chapter 1.)

***contains LA, not AA

Source for all food tables: : Cronometer Nutrition Tracking App (cronometer.com)

A few practical tips to share: When reviewing the medial journals and nutrient databases to create these food charts, we learned that:

- Steak, surprisingly, has the lowest omega-6: omega-3 ratio (5.75:1) of all the meats. Pork has the highest: 21:1.

- Omega-3-rich free-range eggs are worth the extra money. Their omega-6: omega-3 (AA: EPA/DHA) ratio is 4.9:1, while that of eggs from conventionally caged and fed chickens is 16.8:1.

- Fishsticks and other breaded and fried fish products typically contain more omega-6 than omega-3.

- Farmed fish contains more than three times as much omega-6 (AA) as wild-caught fish. The omega-6: omega-3 ratio in farmed salmon is 0.7:1, while that of wild-caught salmon is 0.2:1.

- You are better off eating canned salmon (all of which is wild-caught) than farmed salmon.

- Avoid farmed tilapia and catfish. Tilapia is the worst, with an omega-6: omega-3 ratio of 9.2:1. You'd be better off eating a steak, which, as noted above, has an omega-6: omega-3 ratio of 5.75:1.[611]

Why Farmed Tilapia/Catfish are Not Good Omega-3 Choices

A recent study revealed that the average omega-6: omega-3 ratio (AA: EPA ratio) in farm-raised tilapia was 11:1. Two of the fish samples that had been harvested in central America contained greater than 20 times more AA than EPA! Farm-raised tilapia and catfish contained an average of 134 mg and 67 mg AA, respectively, and some tilapia samples from central America contained more than 300 mg of AA in a 3-ounce portion. To put this into perspective, a 3-ounce portion of hamburger (80% lean) contains 34 mg of AA, and a 4-ounce serving of steak tenderloin contains even less, just 23 mg. You'd be better off eating a Big Mac® or a Whopper® than farmed tilapia or catfish, which is what virtually all restaurants offering these fish will serve. [612]

Omega-3 and Omega-6 Content of Commonly Eaten Foods

Eggs and Dairy	Serving Size	Omega-3 (EPA & DHA) grams	Omega-6 (AA) grams
Egg, hard boiled	1 medium	0.3	0.59
Eggs, fried	2 medium	0.13	2.15
Eggs, cooked	2 medium	0.07	1.18
Eggs, omega-3-rich	2 medium	0.23	1.13
Cheese, Blue	1 ounce	0.07	0.15
Cheese, Cheddar	1 ounce	0.04	0.23
Cheese, Cottage 2%	4 ounces	0.01	0.06
Cheese, Feta	1 ounce	0.08	0.09
Cheese, Gruyere	1 ounce	0.12	0.37
Cheese, Swiss (Jarlsberg)	1 ounce	0.10	0.18
Cheese, Jarlsberg reduced fat	1 ounces	0.06	0.10
Cheese, Gouda	1 ounces	0.11	0.07
Cheese, Parmesan, hard	1 ounces	0.08	0.08
Cheese, Roquefort	1 ounces	0.20	0.17
Yogurt, 2%, Greek	1 cup	0.02	0.14
Milk whole	1 cup	0.18	0.29
Milk, 2%	1 cup	0.12	0.15
*Soy milk, unsweetened	1 cup	0.31	2.32

* contains LA, not AA

Omega-3 and Omega-6 Content of Commonly Eaten Foods

Meats	Serving Size	Omega-3 (EPA & DHA) grams	Omega-6 (AA) grams
Turkey, breast, roasted	4 ounces	0.03	0.31
Bacon, pork, pan fried	1 slice	0.03	0.63
Steak, sirloin, no visible fat	4 ounces	0.04	0.23
Steak, tenderloin, grass fed	4 ounces	0.13	0.28
Lamb chop	1 medium	0.03	0.34
Chicken breast	4 ounces	0.11	0.93

Omega-3 and Omega-6 Content of Commonly Eaten Foods

Fast Food	Serving Size	Omega-3 (EPA & DHA) grams	Omega-6 (AA) grams
Cheese pizza, medium	½ pizza	1.06	7.41
Pepperoni pizza, medium	½ pizza	0.93	7.23
Taco Bell, beef soft taco	1	0.07	0.62
Taco Bell, chicken soft taco	1	0.02	0.20
Taco Bell, bean burrito	1	0.63	3.39
McDonald's, chicken nuggets	1 nugget	0.16	1.17
Wendy's, chicken nuggets	1 nugget	0.07	1.37
Burger King, cheeseburger	1 burger	0.19	1.08
Domino's, chicken wings	1 wing	0.06	0.72

Omega-3 and Omega-6 Content of Commonly Eaten Foods

Fats & Oils	Serving Size	Omega-3 (ALA) grams	Omega-6 (LA) grams
*Butter	1 teaspoon	0.04	0.45
Coconut oil	1 tablespoon	0	0
Safflower oil	1 tablespoon	0	3.39
Soy oil	1 tablespoon	0.93	6.94
Corn oil	1 tablespoon	.05	2.43
Canola oil	1 tablespoon	1.28	2.61
Olive oil	1 tablespoon	0.10	1.32
Mayonnaise	1 tablespoon	0.65	5.18
Mayonnaise, made with tofu	1 tablespoon	0.31	2.18
Cottonseed oil	1 tablespoon	0.03	7.03
Margarine	1 tablespoon	0.24	1.02
Flaxseed oil	1 tablespoon	7.27	1.94
Salad Dressings			
French	1 tablespoon	0.44	2.93
Ranch	1 tablespoon	0.49	3.33
Thousand Island	1 tablespoon	0.34	2.57
Blue cheese	1 tablespoon	0.48	3.65
Sesame seed	1 tablespoon	0.30	3.48
Green Goddess	1 tablespoon	0.41	3.07

*contains AA not LA

Omega-3 and Omega-6 Content of Commonly Eaten Foods

Nuts and Seeds	Serving Size	Omega-3 (ALA) grams	Omega-6 (LA) grams
Walnuts	1 ounce	2.57	10.8
Sunflower seeds	1 ounce	<0.01	2.62
Pecans	1 ounce	0.28	5.85
Brazil nuts	1 nut	<0.01	0.97
Pistachios	1 ounce	0.07	3.74
Almonds	1 ounce	<0.01	3.68
Cashews	1 ounce	0.05	2.17
Mixed nuts	1 ounce	0.05	2.99
Macadamia nuts	1 ounce	0.06	0.37
Pine nuts	1 tablespoon	0.07	2.11
Pumpkin seeds	1 ounce	0.05	5.61
Sunflower seeds	1 ounce	0.02	6.53
Peanuts dry roast	1 ounces	0.01	2.75
Peanut butter	1 tablespoon	0.01	2.27
Tahini	1 tablespoon	0.06	3.47
Sunflower butter	1 tablespoon	<0.01	1.56
Chia seeds	1 tablespoon	2.90	1.00
Flax seeds	1 tablespoon	1.60	0.41

Omega-3 and Omega-6 Content of Commonly Eaten Foods

Snacks	Serving Size	Omega-3 (ALA) grams	Omega-6 (LA) grams
Popcorn microwave	1 cup	0.13	5.30
Popcorn air popped	1 cup	<0.01	0.2
Popcorn oil popped	1 cup	0.31	2.51
Potato chips	1 ounce	0.01	6.53
Potato chips, low fat	1 ounce	0.01	4.63
Corn puffs, twists	1 ounce	0.09	4.87
Corn chips, white corn	1 ounce	0.07	2.75
Corn chips, blue corn	1 ounce	0.01	2.64
Sweet potato fries	1 ounce	0.11	2.01
French fries, McDonald's	Medium order	1.09	7.80
Nachos with cheese	20 chips	0.66	8.41

Omega-3 and Omega-6 Content of Commonly Eaten Foods

Snacks	Serving Size	Omega-3 (ALA) grams	Omega-6 (LA) grams
Kind Fruit & Nut Bar	1 bar	0.12	2.16
Kind Bar Peanut/Dark Chocolate	1 bar	0.28	2.85
Rice crackers	1 ounce	0.01	0.76
Ritz crackers	1 ounce	0.38	3.79
Dark chocolate bar	1 ounce	<0.01	0.35

Omega-3 and Omega-6 Content of Commonly Eaten Foods

Cereal, Grains, Bread, Pasta	Serving Size	Omega-3 (ALA) grams	Omega-6 (LA) grams
Oatmeal, regular cooking	1 cup	0.04	0.92
Kashi Go Lean Crunch	1 cup	0.22	0.74
Arrowhead Mills 7 Grain	1 cup	0.03	0.45
Crispy brown rice cereal	1 cup	0.01	0.25
Granola Cascadian Farm	1 cup	0.06	1.16
Wheat bread	1 slice	0.03	0.29
Sourdough	1 slice	0.03	0.47
Rye bread	1 slice	0.02	0.24
Gluten-free bread	1 slice	0.03	0.41
Pasta, whole wheat, cooked	1 cup	0.01	0.28
Pasta, corn, cooked	1 cup	0.01	0.44
Pasta, brown rice, cooked	1 cup	0	0
Buckwheat soba noodles, cooked	1 cup	<0.01	0.03
Brown rice, steamed	1 cup	0.03	0.60
Millet, cooked	1 cup	0.05	0.84
Quinoa, cooked	1 cup	0.19	1.80
Buckwheat groats, cooked	1 cup	0.07	0.87

Omega-3 and Omega-6 Content of Commonly Eaten Foods

Vegetables	Serving Size	Omega-3 (ALA) grams	Omega-6 (LA) grams
Spinach	1 cup	0.04	<0.01
Romaine lettuce, shredded	1 cup	0.05	0.02
Kale, 1" pieces	1 cup	0.03	0.02
Swiss chard	1 cup	<0.01	0.02
Lettuce, mixed greens	1 cup	0.04	0.02
Collards	1 cup	0.04	0.03
Arugula	1 cup	0.03	0.03
Broccoli, chopped	1 cup	0.02	0.02
Cauliflower, chopped	1 cup	0.02	0.01
Brussels sprouts, cooked	1 sprout	0.04	0.02
Corn	1 cup	0.01	0.51
Olives, black, green	1 medium	0.01	0.035

Omega-3 and Omega-6 Content of Commonly Eaten Foods

Beans, legumes	Serving Size	Omega-3 (ALA) grams	Omega-6 (LA) grams
Garbanzos, canned, drained	1 cup	0.06	1.53
Hummus	1 tbls	0.01	0.54
Black beans, canned, drained	1 cup	0.30	0.23
Pinto beans, canned, drained	1 cup	0.27	0.20
Lentils, cooked from dried	1 cup	0.07	0.27
Split peas, canned, drained	1 cup	0.05	0.27
Split pea soup, no meat, canned	1 cup	0.11	0.78
Navy beans, canned, drained	1 cup	0.32	0.25
Tofu, firm	4 ounces	0.73	5.47
Natto	1 cup	1.28	9.58

Your Diet Diary for Omega Fatty Acids

Day: _____

Food	Servings	Derived EPA/DHA from ALA (optional)				Total Omega-3 EPA/DHA	Total Omega-6 AA
		ALA Calculate EPA/DHA in Next Columns	Men: 8% of ALA = EPA	Women: 21% of ALA = EPA	Women: 9% of ALA-derived EPA = DHA		
DAY 1 TOTALS		ALA =	Men's EPA from ALA =	Women's EPA from ALA =	Women's DHA from ALA-derived EPA =	EPA/DHA =	AA =

Step 1: Use the provided food charts to track your omegas.
Step 2: Record EPA/DHA and AA above. Optional: Record ALA and calculate derived EPA/DHA as indicated.
Step 3: Add your daily totals of EPA/DHA and AA.
Step 4: Repeat for 5 days and total for more accurate results.
Step 5: To get your omega-6: omega-3 ratio, divide your total AA by your total EPA/DHA and enter here: _____ :1

The result shows the grams AA you're getting for each gram of EPA/DHA. Your goal is a ratio no greater that 4:1, or at least 1 gram of EPA/DHA per 4 grams of AA.

BONE-HEALTHY ACTION ITEMS

- Aim for a ratio of omega-6: omega-3 of no more than 4:1 (and preferably 2:1) to lessen osteoclast production and encourage MSCs to become osteoblasts instead of fat cells.

- Get 2 to 4 grams of EPA/DHA per day (total from diet and supplements) to maximize omega-3s' beneficial effects on bone.

- To determine how much additional EPA/DHA you need to maintain a healthy 4:1 ratio, keep a 5-day food diary to compare your omega-3 and omega-6 dietary intakes.

- Use the Omega Quant finger prick test to measure your Omega-3 Index, another way to indicate your omega-6:omega-3 status.

- To reduce your intake of omega-6 (arachidonic acid) from diet, choose organic meats from pastured animals, free-range chickens, and wild-caught fish.

- Choose your omega-3 supplement based on three factors:

  » **Potency:** Make sure your supplement delivers 2 to 4 grams of EPA/DHA in just a few servings and is provided in a natural triglycerides form.

  » **Purity:** Check an independent lab analysis to confirm PCBs, dioxins, and oxidation markers (peroxide, anisidine, and TOTOX values) meet recognized international standards.

  » **Palatability:** Check for fishy smell or taste and look for products that contain curcumin and/or astaxanthin to prevent rancidity (not just vitamin E).

CASES FROM THE COMMUNITY

*The Community is a sponsored group of more than 17,000 men and women
supporting each other to build stronger bones naturally.
(www.algaecal.com/community)*

Jane's Story

Jane's doctor called her *the poster child for osteoporosis.* She's
petite, small-boned, and has a family history of bone loss (all
traits she shares with me, Lara). So, Jane wasn't surprised when
her DEXA scan showed she had bone loss. Jane's doctor recommended that Jane take conventional medication, which she did
for the next nine years.

Despite Jane's troubling DEXA scan, she was keen to continue her active lifestyle. She had already walked a couple of
half-marathons (over 13 miles each) to prepare for the 60-mile
Susan G. Komen® 3-Day. But while Jane was training, she
broke her femur. The advice Jane received? More conventional
bone medications.

Jane wanted to try something different, so started taking calcium citrate with vitamin D. Over the next few years, her DEXA
scans showed a slower rate of bone loss. But bone loss all the
same. So Jane started researching again. And she found Algae-
Cal Plus, a plant-based calcium that included over a dozen
bone-building nutrients, many she realized had been missing
from her diet. She also began supplementing with Strontium
Boost, which provides strontium, an element known to build
bone strength.

Just short of a year later, Jane sent this message to members of
The Community: "When the technician printed out my results,
she said 'Oh, wow!' and I knew I was going to hear good news.
My AP Spine went from -3.0 to -2.7, a 4.4% increase! I still
have osteoporosis, but I'm headed in the right direction!"

Lara's Take: Calcium alone can at best slow the rate of bone loss. Be sure you are benefiting, like Jane, from Team Calcium—which includes all of the vitamins, minerals, and healthy fats we discuss in Part Two.

See details on supplements for calcium on page 135 and strontium citrate on page 273. Statements regarding the products above have not been evaluated by the Food and Drug Administration. These products are not intended to diagnose, treat, cure, or prevent any disease.

CHAPTER 6

Minerals

Minerals are an essential component of the human body. All cells, tissues, and internal fluids contain minerals: teeth, muscle, blood, nerve cells, and, of course, our bones.

Yet, the body cannot produce a single mineral element and relies on those derived from the water, food, and supplements we consume. Whether the amount required of a specific mineral is large (such as calcium) or merely trace amounts (such as copper or zinc), you need to have sufficient levels of each available to fuel bodily processes occurring at the cellular level billions of times per second.

We already covered the important roles of calcium and magnesium in Chapter 5. Now, let's take a look at the other critical minerals your body needs to build strong bones.

Boron

BONE ESSENTIALS

- Boron boosts osteoblast production and activity.
- Boron cuts the amount of calcium lost in urine by almost half and helps put more calcium into your bones.
- Boron improves your body's ability to absorb and utilize magnesium.
- Boron helps men and women get the most bone-building benefit from their sex hormones and vitamin D.

For more than a century, boric acid (a compound containing boron) has been used as an astringent and to treat certain infections.[613] Over the past several decades, scientists have gained a new appreciation for boron's significance to human health. Boron can aid wound healing, improve short-term memory of older adults, and reduce the toxicity of heavy metals. Boron can even help you maintain the romance in your life (more on that later).[614]

This micronutrient plays diverse and vitally important roles in metabolism that render it necessary for plant, animal, and human health—and possibly for the evolution of life on Earth. Many of these roles are critical to the development and regeneration of your healthy bones.

Boron Boosts Osteoblast Activity

Boron serves as a key player in mineralization, the process by which osteoblasts lay down the bone matrix. Boron turns on the genes in osteoblasts that produce mineralization-related proteins. These include *bone morphogenetic proteins* (BMPs): *collagen type I* (COL I), *osteopontin* (OPN), *bone sialoprotein* (BSP), and *osteocalcin* (OCN). The combined boron-induced effects of these proteins make for robustly active osteoblasts—and plenty of them—at work increasing new bone formation.

In fact, BMPs are now offered as pricey bone supplements—you may have seen the ads. If you take one, make sure it has the right BMPs that impact bone (BMP-2, -4, -6 and -7). However, if you're getting enough boron, your body will produce all the key bone-building BMPs for you, naturally, at no extra charge.

Boron also increases your production of *bone-specific alkaline phosphatase* (BSAP), an enzyme secreted by osteoblasts. BSAP releases phosphate to build the bone matrix, by cleaving phosphate groups from many types of molecules. If you've had your bone turnover markers tested, you may have seen it on your lab reports because it's a marker of osteoblast bone-building activity.[615][616][617] (See Lab Tests, Chapter 10.)

Boron regulates your body's production of bone-building RunX2. *Runt-related transcription factor 2* (a.k.a. core-binding factor subunit alpha-1 [CBF-alpha-1]). *Who comes up with these wacky names?* Fortunately, you don't have to remember this. Just know that RunX2 is essential to osteoblast production and bone formation. Without boron, your body can't produce RunX2.

RunX2 works cooperatively with the above-mentioned BMPs to turn on the genes that direct your production of osteoblasts. RunX2 also helps convince your *mesenchymal stem cells* to develop into osteoblasts. Plus, RunX2 stays on the job in mature osteoblasts. When RunX2 levels drop, so does the activity of the genes that encode the BMPs. When boron's at work for you, so is RunX2.[618]

Boron Helps Us Maximize Other Bone-Building Nutrients and Hormones

Boron helps you keep more of the calcium you consume instead of peeing it away. We've known this healthy-bone effect of boron for many years. In 1985, the U.S. Department of Agriculture ran a study in which postmenopausal women, who took 3 mg of boron per day, lost 44% less calcium in their urine! The results were more dramatic in women eating a low-magnesium diet who reduced the amount of calcium they peed away by 52 mg per day. Even for women with adequate levels of magnesium (which also reduces calcium loss), boron resulted in the loss of 22 mg less of calcium per day.[619]

Boron maximizes your use of vitamin D as well as estrogen. Boron inhibits *24-hydroxylase*, an enzyme that breaks down both estradiol and vitamin D for elimination from the body.

- In a clinical trial, 15 middle-aged men and women were placed on a diet low in boron, and also low in magnesium and copper for 63 days. After study participants were given boron (3 mg/day) for an additional 49 days, their circulating 25(OH)D levels rose an average of 39%.[620][621]

• Similar results were seen in an open pilot study of 13 middle-aged subjects who were extremely vitamin D deficient (with average 25(OH)D blood levels less than 12 ng/ml). For 60 days, study participants were given a boron supplement (6 mg/day), and their blood levels of 25(OH)D rose an average of 20%. This study, which was conducted in Serbia, began in October and concluded in January; in other words, it took place during the fall transition to winter, a time when sunshine decreases and vitamin D levels are expected to drop. Yet, with boron supplementation, their 25(OH)D increased significantly.[622]

Boron boosts magnesium absorption. Because boron slows the rate at which estrogen is degraded and eliminated from the body, and estrogen boosts magnesium's absorption and deposition in bone, so does boron. This means that boron plays a supporting role in all of magnesium's many beneficial effects. That's a big deal because magnesium is the required co-factor for more than 350 enzymes whose activity is essential to your health. The opposite is also true: not having enough boron available lowers your ability to absorb and utilize magnesium, with widespread unhappy ramifications. (See Magnesium, Chapter 5.)

Boron helps you get the most bone-building benefit from your sex hormones. *Wouldn't it be great if we had a natural, safe way of getting back some of the beneficial effects of our sex hormones after menopause?* Well, we do: boron. Supplementation with boron maximizes the effect of estrogen to increase calcium and magnesium absorption into bone. Estrogen levels plummet during and after menopause, so getting the most bone-building benefit from the estrogen that remains becomes critical to maintain healthy bones as we age.[623][624][625]

In the study we mentioned earlier, where boron helped postmenopausal women lose less calcium in their urine, the researchers also found increases in blood levels of estrogen and testosterone. This was more pronounced in women eating a low-magnesium diet where estrogen nearly doubled and testosterone more than doubled! Even women eating a *magnesium-adequate* diet benefitted almost as much.[626] Remember, the RDA for magnesium is way too low, so *adequate* did not mean they were getting enough. (See Magnesium, Chapter 5.)

Could boron increase your estrogen or testosterone to unsafe levels? Don't worry. Despite their rise, levels of both hormones remained far lower than before menopause. Still, getting back a little more estrogen activity can make a big difference in a woman's ability to build bone. And in her sex life. When testosterone goes away, so does a woman's sex drive. Boron may help put a little romance back in your life.

And in your man's life as well. A study of boron's effects on healthy men found a significant increase in free testosterone, which rose an average of 22%, and a significant decrease in estrogen, which dropped an average of 39%. [627]

Personal note from Lara*: I recently wrote a review article entitled, Nothing Boring About Boron.*[628] *You can find it on PubMed (PMID:26770156) if you'd like to read more. By now, you can understand why I wrote this title. After writing this review, I added boron to Joe's daily vitamins. How can I put this? We're getting older, but no aspect of our life together is boring!*

How Much Boron Do You Need?

While we don't have an RDI for boron, research indicates 3 mg/day will meet our needs. Since 1987, the peer-reviewed medical literature has provided us with data from numerous studies, all of which indicate boron's beneficial effects on bone, sex hormones, and vitamin D do not appear until at least 3 mg of boron is consumed daily. So, the next question is: *Can your diet supply that 3 mg of boron your bones require daily?*

Unless you live in Turkey, where the soils are extra-rich in boron, you need a boron supplement. In boron-rich areas of the world, such as Turkey, daily boron intake averages 12.6 mg with no adverse effects, a good indication of how safe boron is for us. That's the good news.[629]

The bad news is that in the U.S., our soils are not boron-rich, and our food provides far less than the 3 mg we need to be healthy. Back in 1998, researchers estimated that the average daily intake of boron in the U.S. was 1.17 mg/d for men and 0.96 mg/d for women. And people were eating more fruits and vegetables back then. Today, the U.S. population is consuming fewer boron-rich plant foods, so it's a sure bet that our average intake of boron has also dropped.

Unfortunately, providing a full listing of the food sources of boron isn't possible, since the most widely relied upon source for this kind of data greatly overestimates the boron content of foods. You'll likely see these inaccurate results reported everywhere.

What we can provide for you is the *actual* boron content, derived from chemical analysis, of boron-rich foods. You can see from the table below that unless you eat multiple avocados or 15 ounces of peanut butter every day—neither of which is an option if you want to continue to fit into your skinny jeans—you'll need a boron supplement to get your daily 3 mg.[630] Check your bone health supplement. A day's dosage may provide 3 mg of boron. If not, look for a boron supplement delivering 3 mg per capsule.

Best Food Sources of Boron	
Food	Boron (milligrams per 3 ounces)
Raisins	1.80
Avocado	1.43
Peanut butter	0.59
Peanuts, dry	0.58
Prune juice	0.56
Chocolate powder	0.43
Red wine	0.36
Granola-raisin cereal	0.36
Grape juice	0.34
Pecans	0.26
Raisin Bran	0.26

Source: Meacham, S., et al. Boron in human health: evidence for dietary recommendations and public policies. Open Mineral Processing Journal 3.1 (2010): 36-53.

Boron Safety

Boron is considered safe at the dosages discussed here. Just don't exceed boron's Tolerable Upper Intake Level (UL) of 20 mg/d for adults 18 years or older.[631]

BONE-HEALTHY ACTION ITEMS

- Consume at least 3 mg of boron daily, though much of the research shows 6 mg produces better outcomes.
- Since most food sources provide small amounts, you will need a supplement.
- Don't exceed 20 mg of boron per day.

Manganese

BONE ESSENTIALS

- Manganese is required for our production of chondroitin sulfate, a compound required for bone formation.
- Insufficient manganese promotes lower bone mineral density.
- An antioxidant called mitochondrial superoxide dismutase (Mn-SOD) requires manganese as its cofactor. Without MnSOD, our cellular energy production would unleash an unstoppable cascade of free radicals.
- Low MnSOD activity increases the risk for osteoporosis, along with cancer, diabetes, cardiovascular disease, and Alzheimer's disease.
- Manganese is also required for our production of thyroid hormones and cholesterol, including estrogens, progesterone, and testosterone.

How important is manganese for building strong bones that resist fracture? The simplest illustration can be seen in deer antlers. After an exceptionally cold winter prevented deer from eating manganese-rich plants, researchers found breaking their antlers took 27% less impact energy. Antlers are considered an ideal experimental model for bone biology because they grow rapidly (and can be humanely obtained).

In another animal study, manganese deficiency inhibited both osteoblast and osteoclast activity in lab rats. In other words, without manganese, healthy bone remodeling was shut down.[632][633][634]

Manganese is Required for the First Steps in New Bone Formation

Bone mineralization cannot start without manganese. This trace mineral plays a critical role in our production of chondroitin sulfate. Chondroitin sulfate partners with an enzyme called osteocalcin (which is activated by vitamin K2) to form the *extracellular matrix*—the ground substance to which collagen adheres. This material helps you to maintain healthy bone, ligaments, and cartilage.[635]

Manganese is required for *chondrogenesis,* the process through which *chondrocytes,* the cells that secrete cartilage, are produced. It used to be thought that *chondrogenesis* was a separate process from *osteogenesis,* the production of new mineralized bone. Now we know it's one continuous process: chondrocytes secrete not only cartilage but also cells that become osteoblasts and eventually *osteocytes*—the key regulators of bone homeostasis that osteoblasts become as they are embedded in the bone matrix. Manganese is required for the initial steps in this entire process.[636]

Osteoblasts build bone using enzymes that require manganese. In addition, our osteoblasts produce several enzymes used to build bone which require manganese as their cofactor. (For those interested in the details, these manganese-dependent enzymes include polymerase and glycosyltransferase.)[637]

Human Studies Show Manganese's Importance for Bones

While manganese doesn't have the same wealth of research as more prominent nutrients, several studies demonstrate its relation to healthy bones:[638]

- In research conducted in Belgium, women with osteoporosis were found to have significantly lower blood levels of manganese compared to healthy controls (0.02 vs. 0.04 mg/L, respectively). Those with osteoporosis also had lower trabecular bone volume and lower BMD. (Trabecular bone is the interior, more metabolically active portion of our bones.)

- Another study found that men fed a diet lacking in manganese became manganese deficient in just 39 days, and their blood levels of calcium increased significantly. This indicates that manganese deficiency hindered calcium deposition into and/or increased calcium withdrawal from their bones.

- A 2.5-year study examined the effect of several trace minerals on 225 healthy postmenopausal women from the San Diego metro area (of whom 137 completed the study). The women were given either 1,000 mg of supplemental calcium (calcium-citrate-malate split into 4 doses); a trace mineral supplement containing copper (5 mg), manganese (2.5 mg), and zinc (15 mg); both the calcium and trace mineral supplements; or a placebo. Results: Spine BMD dropped in those given the placebo (-2.23%), calcium alone (-0.50%), *or* trace minerals alone (-1.66%). However, for those given *both* calcium and trace minerals, spine BMD increased by 1.28%.

Besides manganese's involvement in building bone, this trace mineral is critical for our production of many hormones and even our survival as we'll see shortly.

Manganese is required for thyroid and sex hormone production. Manganese is required for normal thyroid function and is involved in the formation of the primary hormone produced by the thyroid gland, thyroxine (T4). Low manganese levels are frequently found in hypothyroid patients. Hypothyroidism slows down all metabolic processes, including our ability to build new bone, which promotes osteoporosis.

Manganese is also involved in cholesterol synthesis. We need cholesterol to produce hormones, including estrogen, progesterone, DHEA, and testosterone. A manganese deficiency can impair normal hormone production, adversely affecting our ability to build bone.[639]

Manganese Prevents Our Own Production of Energy from Killing Us by Activating MnSOD

While this sounds a bit dramatic, manganese really is critical for keeping us safe (and alive) during our body's production of *adenosine triphosphate* (ATP). We produce ATP in our mitochondria, tiny organelles that act as the powerhouse of our cells. Think of ATP as the body's energy currency, which we spend to fuel all our metabolic activities. Generating ATP uses about 90% of the oxygen we breathe in.

During this process, 2% to 5% of the oxygen escapes in the form of a highly reactive oxygen free radical called superoxide anion (O_2-). Superoxide anion is so unstable and reactive that it will attack any other molecules it contacts, turning them into free radicals, too. It's a deadly pachinko game whose end result is a tsunami of free radical production and cellular damage.

Fortunately, our bodies come equipped with a number of specific enzymes that neutralize these free radicals. The most important one may be manganese-dependent superoxide dismutase (MnSOD), which lives within our mitochondria, the primary site of superoxide (O_2-) production. (As they say in real estate, location, location, location!) That makes MnSOD our first line of defense in the entire antioxidant enzyme repertoire. It initiates superoxide anion's breakdown into oxygen (O_2) and peroxide (H_2O_2), which the selenium-containing glutathione peroxidases are then able to dismantle. If no manganese is available, then all hell breaks loose.

MnSOD is a major big deal for your bones and many other body activities:

- You're probably aware that smoking causes bone loss. You might even know that nicotine kills our bone-building cells, the osteoblasts. What you probably don't know is that the way nicotine destroys osteoblasts is by shutting down their MnSOD.[640]
- Inhibition of MnSOD activity is also a hallmark of breast cancer. It's easy to understand why: a decrease in MnSOD activity increases damage to cell DNA, and abnormal DNA is much more likely to not replicate normally, promoting cancer.[641]

The importance of MnSOD cannot be overstated. This enzyme is essential for the survival of all oxygen-breathing life forms. Mice bred to lack functioning MnSOD die shortly after birth. The lifespan of those bred to produce MnSOD that is only 50% active is very short and unpleasant.[642] To put it bluntly, your survival, not just that of your bones, depends on manganese.

How Much Manganese Do You Need?

While no RDA has been set for manganese, the Institute of Medicine recommends an *Adequate Intake* (AI) of 2.3 mg/d per day for men and 1.8 mg/d for women (increasing to 2.0 mg/d for women are pregnant or 2.6 mg/d for those who are breastfeeding). These amounts are *not enough* to promote optimal health.

Remember the study cited above in which postmenopausal women taking calcium with trace minerals experienced an increase in BMD? The trace mineral supplement used in this study provided the women with 2.5 mg/day of bioavailable manganese, significantly higher than the AI level.[643]

Other human studies have found that even dietary intakes of 3 mg/d were not enough to maintain a positive balance (i.e., prevent a decline in the body's manganese levels). In one study, slightly more than 5 mg/d was needed. In sum, the research indicates that daily intake of 3 to 5 mg of manganese should be recommended—a level that should be quite safe. The Upper Tolerable Limit (UL) has been set at more than twice that, 11 mg/d, and no adverse effects have been reported at this level.[644]

Your Genetics May Impact Needs for Manganese

Might you have inherited genes that make your MnSOD enzymes less active than *normal*? More than 190 gene variations—single nucleotide polymorphisms (SNPs)—are known to affect the activity level of the MnSOD we produce.

The most important so far is a SNP called Ala16Val, containing amino acids alanine (represented by a C) and valine (represented by a T). Variations on which amino acid appears in each part (alleles) of the SNP affect your level of MnSOD activity.

- If both alleles produce an enzyme that contains valine at this position (a SNP called TT), MnSOD produced is far less active (meaning far less antioxidant protection).

- If one allele produces an enzyme that contains alanine at this position, the other an allele that contains valine (a SNP called CT), MnSOD produced will be lessened, though not as severely.

- If you are fortunate enough to have inherited a SNP called CC (both alleles produce an enzyme that contains alanine at this position), you are producing a highly active MnSOD.

These variations are not uncommon, as worldwide the slower TT

SNP appears in approximately 45% of individuals and the slightly less active CT SNP in 40%. Only about 15% of us are among those fortunate enough to have inherited the CC SNP, which produces a highly active MnSOD.[645]

If you've had your DNA tested by 23andMe®, you can find out what SNP you have. Click on your name in the upper right corner and select *Browse Raw Data*. In the resulting search box, enter rs4880 to reveal what Ala16Val SNP you have. It's a bit confusing because 23andMe® reports the "T" allele as "A" and the "C" allele as "G." So if rs4880 appears as AA or AG, this means you have inherited the TT or CT SNP.

What can you do about this? You can maximize the activity of your MnSOD by ensuring that you consume an optimal amount of manganese—somewhere between 3 to 5 mg per day.[646]

Dietary Sources of Manganese

Fifty years ago, your diet would have likely been rich in manganese. Back then, people typically ate abundant amounts and varieties of *whole* grains and cereal foods that were grown without the *assistance* of chemical herbicides.

Unfortunately, the U.S. and other developed countries have shifted from eating whole foods prepared at home to consuming a majority of highly-processed *Frankenfoods*. Our 21st-century diet is high in refined grains, processed meats, and energy-dense but nutrient-poor *foods*—all of which provide little if any manganese.[647]

- According to data collected from 2007 to 2012 by the FDA's Total Diet Study program, 27.6% of food samples tested had manganese concentrations below the limit of detection. In other words, *no* manganese was present.[648]

- Other studies have shown that the trace mineral content of the food supply in developed countries—particularly the content of manganese—has dropped greatly over the last 30+ years.[649 650 651]

So why has this happened?

Refining grains removes 90% of the manganese present. Conventionally grown grains are already lacking in manganese, as described below. However, even refined flours made from organically grown whole grains are missing 90% of their manganese content.[652]

Exposure to glyphosate severely depletes manganese in plants and animals. America gets the award for most glyphosate used worldwide as 72% of the chemical is applied on U.S. soil. Sadly, glyphosate doesn't just sit on the soil or stay on or inside plants. It gets into the water and air and migrates to untreated crops. We're breathing, drinking, and eating glyphosate. (See diagram below.) [653] [654]

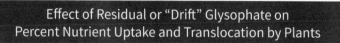

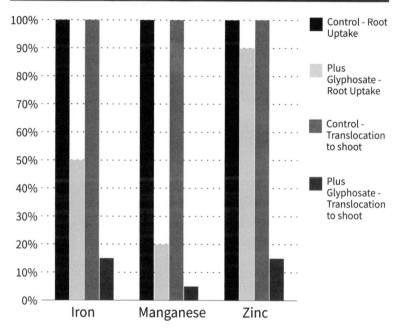

Source: Samsel A, Seneff S. Glyphosate, pathways to modern diseases III: Manganese, neurological diseases, and associated pathologies. Surg Neurol Int. 2015 March. PMID: 25883837

Why might this be a problem? See the box at the end of this section for details on the far-reaching effects of glyphosate on our food supply and ability to get essential nutrients from our diet. Know that unless you regularly eat organic whole grains, you will likely need a supplement to ensure you get 3 to 5 mg of manganese daily.

Food Sources of Manganese

Take a look at your diet and the chart below to estimate how much manganese you're getting. If you're eating organically grown foods, your diet is probably providing you with 3 to 5 mg of manganese daily. If your diet contains mostly chemically grown foods, which provide little to no manganese, you'll need to rely on supplements to get the manganese you need.

Best Food Sources of Manganese		
Food	**Serving Size**	**Manganese (mg)**
Cloves	1 teaspoon	1.27
*Oats, cooked	½ cup	3.84
*Brown rice, cooked	1 cup	1.76
*Garbanzo beans, cooked	1 cup	1.69
Spinach	1 cup	1.68
Pineapple	1 cup	1.53
Pumpkin seeds	¼ cup	1.47
Tempeh	4 ounces	1.46
Tofu	4 ounces	1.34
*Quinoa	0.75 cup	1.17
Walnuts	¼ cup	1.02
Sweet potato	1 cup	0.99
*Lentils, cooked	1 cup	0.98
*Lima beans, cooked	1 cup	0.97
Collard greens	1 cup	0.97
*Navy beans, cooked	1 cup	0.96
*Tea (green)	1 cup (8 ounces)	0.41–1.58
*Tea (black)	1 cup (8 ounces)	0.18-0.77

*Absorption is limited for these foods.

Source: World's Healthiest Foods (bit.ly/WHF-Manganese), Oregon State Univ. Micronutrient Information Center (bit.ly/Oregon-Manganese).

When you look at the food sources of manganese, remember that it's not just how *much* manganese is present in a food, but *how much is available* for absorption. Tea is a perfect example. While tea contains lots of manganese, it also contains lots of tannins, which bind to manganese and prevent its absorption from the gastrointestinal tract.[655]

Similarly, cereal grains and beans are rich in manganese but are also well endowed with phytates and fiber that may bind manganese, limiting its absorption. Fortunately, simple food preparation techniques can greatly improve manganese's availability. (See Zinc and Copper, page 288.)

Glyphosate Depletes Minerals from Food and Harms our Healthy Gut Bacteria

Glyphosate works by poisoning the shikimate pathway in plants. The shikimate pathway is a metabolic pathway used by plants (plus bacteria, fungi, and algae) to produce the B vitamin, folate, and several amino acids essential for plants' survival, including phenylalanine, tryptophan, and tyrosine. Phenylalanine and tryptophan are essential amino acids for humans, too.

Glyphosate is assumed non-toxic since humans don't possess the shikimate pathway, but our healthy gut bacteria do, depending on it for essential amino acids. Our gut bacteria are harmed by glyphosate, as underscored by the fact that glyphosate has been patented as an antimicrobial agent. This also overlooks the more far-reaching toxic effects, which are not corrected by genetically modifying plants. Glyphosate's actions go beyond poisoning the shikimate pathway to cripple a plant's nutritional pathways and immune system.[656]

Glyphosate blocks a plant's absorption of manganese from soil. Glyphosate oxidizes the manganese present in the soil changing it into a form that plants can no longer absorb. Plus, glyphosate is a very efficient mineral chelator—it binds easily to manganese and other critical trace minerals in the soil, preventing the already small amounts in conventional soil from being absorbed and used inside plants. Along with weakening plants by depriving them of trace minerals, glyphosate also promotes the growth of soil-borne pathogens—effectively killing all the pathogen-inhibiting beneficial microbes in the soil. The soil-borne pathogens then attack the weakened plant, killing it.[657] [658]

Let's connect the dots here. Glyphosate poisons both the shikimate pathway in plants along with the soil, while preventing plants from absorbing trace minerals. This is supposed to be fine for us because humans don't use the shikimate pathway, but we sure do use trace minerals! And we rely on plants—or animals that eat plants—to supply them. Oops! Guess the scientists who created this chemical and companies that market it didn't think about that!

If your diet relies on conventionally grown foods, you'd better also rely on a supplement for your manganese—as well iron, magnesium, zinc, and other nutrients.[659]

What to Look for in a Manganese Supplement

First, check the supplements you are taking. Manganese is often included in multi-vitamins and in products for osteoarthritis along with chondroitin sulfate and glucosamine hydrochloride. You don't want to exceed 11 mg of manganese per day.

If you find you need a separate manganese supplement to maintain a daily intake of 3 to 5 mg, manganese is available in a number of forms: manganese aspartate, manganese citrate, manganese gluconate, and manganese amino acid chelate. To date, no peer-reviewed published research indicates one form is preferable, but since citrate is known to easily disassociate from its stabilizing partner even in the absence of stomach acid, this form might be a better option.[660]

Manganese Safety

At a dietary and/or supplemental intake level of 3 to 5 mg/d, manganese is safe and beneficial. No adverse effects have ever been reported for up to 11 mg manganese per day, its Tolerable Upper Intake Level (UL).

Industrial exposure to airborne manganese at very high levels can be toxic. Reports of manganese toxicity due to oral intake are quite rare. Manganese toxicity is usually caused by chronic airborne exposure of workers in iron and steel factories, manganese ore mining, welding, chemical plants, dry cell battery production, and the fuel-oil industry.

Such workers may develop nervous system disorders including behavioral changes and slow, clumsy movements. When sufficiently severe, this combination of symptoms, called *manganism*, resembles Parkinson's disease and may be misdiagnosed as such. Geographical studies in the U.S. have found a higher incidence of Parkinson's disease in urban areas with higher industrial release of manganese and fuel oil consumption.

However, the manganese concentrations causing such adverse effects are about *20,000-times higher* than normal environmental concentrations and about *a million times higher* in workers with developed manganism.[661][662] For the general population, environmental exposures to unsafe levels of manganese can occur in populations living near industrial manganese emissions, from manganese-containing pesticides, and from the consumption of water with elevated manganese levels.[663]

Variations in an individual's genetic inheritance that result in that person producing a slow or less effective version of the SLC30A10 gene can increase the risk for toxic accumulation of manganese in the brain (i.e., manganism). Fortunately, this can be easily and safely treated with chelation therapy.

BONE-HEALTHY ACTION ITEMS

- Get 3 to 5 mg/d of manganese to prevent insufficiency, ideally from organically grown foods.
- If you eat conventionally grown foods, you will likely need a supplement. Both the use of glyphosate and the refining process of wheat and other grains deplete manganese (along with many other nutrients).
- Note that multivitamins often include manganese, as do supplements for osteoarthritis (along with chondroitin sulfate and glucosamine hydrochloride). Don't consume more than 11 mg/d of manganese from all sources.

Selenium

BONE ESSENTIALS

- Selenium is the cofactor for selenoenzymes and deiodinase enzymes, both of which are essential for bone health.
- The selenoenzymes include the glutathione peroxidases, which neutralize free radicals and restore used antioxidants, such as vitamins C and E.
- The glutathione peroxidases help eliminate bone-damaging toxic metals, such as lead, arsenic, cadmium, and mercury.
- The deiodinase enzymes support healthy thyroid function, preventing conditions that can cause bone loss.
- Adequate selenium intake significantly lowers the risk of hip fracture—even in smokers!
- Vegetarians, especially vegans, are more likely to get insufficient selenium from their diets.

Our osteoblasts, like all of our cells, generate energy from within to run their metabolic machinery. This process produces highly damaging free radicals. When not quickly neutralized, free radicals cause damage that results in the production of more free radicals, which promote bone loss in many ways. For example, free radicals prevent the mesenchymal stem cells (MSCs) in our bone marrow from developing into new osteoblasts.

Here's where selenium helps save the day. Selenium is a cofactor for some of the body's most important antioxidant enzymes. In other words, this trace mineral must activate these enzymes to neutralize the free radicals before they cause rampant damage. Selenium is the required cofactor for a family of 25 antioxidant enzymes called the *selenoenzymes*, including at least 9 produced by osteoblasts.

In fact, MSCs produce antioxidant selenoenzymes to protect themselves, allowing their development into osteoblasts. But MSCs can only produce these selenoenzymes when adequate selenium is available.

Selenium protects bones in other ways, including reducing osteoclast development, promoting healthy thyroid function, and clearing the body of toxic metals. You'll soon see how getting the right amount of selenium could be the difference between bone loss and bone gain.[664][665]

Selenium Activates the Powerful Glutathione Peroxidases to Protect Bones

One of the selenium-dependent enzymes that MSCs produce is the powerful *glutathione peroxidases*. These enzymes both neutralize free radicals directly and also restore other already used antioxidants, such as vitamins C and E, back to their reduced form in which they're ready to disarm more oxidizers.

One of the most bone-harmful free radicals is *hydroxyl radical*, which has the dubious honor of being considered *the* major culprit in triggering osteoclast generation. Glutathione peroxidases are our primary defense against hydroxyl radicals. They protect us by preventing hydroxyl radical's release from hydrogen peroxide, a compound secreted by defensive cells in our immune system (macrophages and microglia). Selenium is required to activate our glutathione peroxidase enzymes, so they can neutralize hydrogen peroxide before it releases hydroxyl radical.

After menopause, women's production of glutathione drops, while needs increase. We know the loss of estrogen during menopause is harmful to women's bones. A main reason is that estrogen increases our production of the glutathione peroxidase enzyme (GPx1). When we lose estrogen, our production of GPx1 plummets, greatly increasing our risk for excessive osteoclast production and bone loss.[666][667]

Along with producing less glutathione, postmenopausal women use up their remaining glutathione far more quickly. *Why?* Because when estrogen production drops off, the number of free radicals we need our glutathione peroxidase enzymes to neutralize increases. And more free radicals trigger an increase in the production of osteoclasts and bone resorption. Having enough selenium available to activate our glutathione peroxidase enzymes becomes especially important after menopause.[668]

When adequate selenium is available, mesenchymal stem cells produce more glutathione. When blood levels of selenium are low, our MSCs produce far less glutathione and antioxidant selenoenzymes and show increased free radical damage as a result. When selenium is provided, levels of key compounds involved in bone-building activity (type I collagen and bone alkaline phosphatase) increase—and so does the ability for osteoblasts to deposit calcium in our bones.[669][670]

How Selenium Supports Bone Building

Similar as with menopausal women, research shows selenium is also essential for the bone health of aging men. Research evaluating a group of 387 healthy European men (average age 77) found BMD in those with the lowest blood levels of selenium (quartile 1) was quite a bit lower than those with the highest blood levels (quartile 4):

- BMD in the femoral neck averaged 846.6 mg/cm^2 (quartile 1) compared to 924.5 mg/cm^2 (quartile 4).

- BMD in the femoral trochanter averaged 813.9 mg/cm^2 (quartile 1) vs. 903.6 mg/cm^2 (quartile 4).

- BMD in Ward's triangle averaged 678.4 mg/cm^2 (quartile 1) vs. 760.3 mg/cm^2 (quartile 4).

The differences clearly demonstrate that having low levels of selenium negatively impacts BMD. *Love your man?* Make sure he gets his selenium! One or two (but not more!) Brazil nuts eaten daily will do the job.[671]

Selenium enables osteoblasts to control *thioredoxin reductase* (TrxR)—a selenoenzyme with a Dr. Jekyll and Mr. Hyde split personality. When selenium is available, TrxR acts as an antioxidant that protects osteoblasts. In selenium-deficient osteoblasts, TrxR activates a signaling agent called *nuclear factor-kappa B* (NFκB). NFκB initiates a series of events that result in osteoclast production and bone resorption. (Curcumin also inhibits the Dr. Jekyll version of TrxR to inhibit osteoclast production. This is one of the key ways curcumin, the main compound in the spice turmeric, supports bone health.)[672][673]

Selenium lessens osteoclast development from its precursor cells. Osteoclasts are produced in our bone marrow from hematopoietic stem cells, the same precursor cells that give rise to our blood cells. The activation of the signaling agent NFκB (mentioned above) regulates whether these hematopoietic stem cells will develop into blood cells or into osteoclasts. NFκB activation occurs when RANKL (receptor-activator of nuclear factor κB ligand) attaches to NFκB, beginning cellular signaling that causes free radical production and stimulates the production and maturation of osteoclasts. Selenium suppresses the binding of RANKL to NFκB, preventing free radical generation and inhibiting the signaling that causes osteoclast production and development.

Selenium Supports Healthy Thyroid Function

Our thyroid glands affect our bone health by producing the thyroid hormones *thyroxine* (T4) and *triiodothyronine* (T3), which play a vital role in orchestrating our metabolic rate, including the rate at which bone maintenance occurs. Our thyroid glands primarily produce T4—we typically have 14 to 20 times more T4 than T3 in our bloodstream. T4 is much less active than T3 (3 to 4 times less potent). In fact, T4 is considered a *prohormone*, an inactive form of a hormone that serves as a ready-to-activate version. (You may recognize this scenario as 25(OH)D, the form in which vitamin D circulates in your bloodstream, works similarly.)

So how do we get our active (T3) thyroid hormone? Almost all our T3 is made from T4 inside our cells by the action of enzymes called *deiodinases*, which convert T4 to T3 by removing one of T4's iodine molecules. Except for some special deiodinase enzymes in the brain, the deiodinase enzymes in all of our body's other cells (including in our bones) require selenium. For this reason, poor conversion of T4 to T3 due to low selenium status has been proposed as one important reason for the age-associated increase in *underactive* thyroid (a condition called hypothyroidism, see Chapter 4).[674][675]

Hypothyroidism, from insufficient selenium, leads to bone loss. Thyroid hormones regulate the rate of all our metabolic machinery, including the rates at which osteoclasts demolish old bone, and osteoblasts work to build new bone. However, osteoclasts' bone removal takes just a few weeks, while osteoblasts need several months to rebuild new bone. So, not producing enough T3 tips the bone remodeling process in favor of osteoclasts and results in delayed or impaired bone formation and bone loss. Our bones need T3, which we cannot produce from T4 without the help of the deiodinase enzymes. And these enzymes won't work without selenium.[676]

Selenium deficiency also contributes to hyperthyroidism. A *hyperactive* thyroid (a condition called hyperthyroidism, see Chapter 4) is also well known to cause bone loss, regardless of sex or age. When thyroid hormone levels (particularly T3) are too high, the body goes into over-drive, accelerating all metabolic activities, including the rate at which bones are remodeled.

During a normal bone remodeling cycle, our osteoclasts spend 3 to 5 *weeks* breaking down bone, while our osteoblasts take about 3 *months* to replace this with new bone. In other words, it's much faster to break down old bone than it is to build new bone. Therefore, high T3 levels fast forward the bone remodeling process, resulting in bone loss, around 10% of bone mass per remodeling cycle. Not surprisingly, this quickly results in lowered bone mineral density and increased risk of fracture. The deiodinase enzymes work together to regulate how much T3 is cir-culating in the bloodstream and is in our tissues—not too much or too little. But none of these enzymes work without selenium.[677 678 679]

The good news here is that restoring normal thyroid function (in med-speak, healthy thyroid function is called *euthyroidism*) can restore bones' BMD in as little as 24 months.[680]

Selenium Helps Your Body Clear Toxic Metals That Cause Bone Loss

You saw in Part One how damaging toxic metals—like lead, arsenic, cadmium, and mercury—can be to your bones. Selenium not only helps reduce the free radical damage caused by toxic metals but also helps us eliminate these toxins from our bodies.

Higher selenium levels are associated with lower lead levels in high-risk workers. A study examined 324 men whose work chronically ex-posed them to lead. Researchers divided the men into two groups, based on their blood level of selenium, and checked their lead every 3 months. Those in the high-selenium group averaged 6% less lead floating around in their bloodstreams over a 5-year period.

In addition, the high-selenium group had far more protective antioxi-dants working for them: 9% more glutathione, 23% more glutathione peroxidase activity, and 3% more *catalase*. Catalase is another enzyme that, like the glutathione peroxidases, breaks down hydrogen peroxide into safe components: hydrogen and water, before it can release the free radical terrorist, hydroxyl radical. By increasing the production and activity of the glutathione peroxidases, selenium also spares catalase, increasing its availability to clear hydrogen peroxide.[681]

Selenoenzymes combine with arsenic and cadmium to change them into biologically inert compounds. In both humans and animals, if selenium is present in adequate amounts, it:

- reduces arsenic accumulation and combats its free-radical generating and DNA-damaging effects, according to human studies
- protects against free radical production caused by cadmium, as shown by animal studies[682]

You may think you're not exposed to arsenic or cadmium. Think again! More than 10% of the water supplies in the U.S. contain levels of arsenic known to cause disease. And if you eat rice or chicken, both deliver arsenic. Rice plants are especially good at absorbing arsenic from the soil. Chickens may be fed that rice, and arsenic may be added to chicken feed, a practice used to improve the color of the meat—a practice still not officially prohibited in the U.S.[683]

If you consume chemically grown foods, smoke, or are exposed to secondhand smoke, you are loading up on cadmium. Most people know that smoking is toxic, but you probably didn't know that the phosphate fertilizers used in conventional agriculture contain cadmium—and therefore so do the plants grown using phosphate fertilizers.[684]

Our vulnerability to methylmercury toxicity depends on selenium status. Mercury exposures that are neurotoxic and lethal to animals fed a diet low in selenium are far less serious in those whose diets provide normal selenium intakes. In animals with selenium-enriched diets, those same exposures had no observable consequences. Until recently, we didn't understand why. Now we know that mercury binds to selenium and prevents it from activating the selenoenzymes. That's now considered the reason behind mercury's pathological effects and explains several interesting findings:

- Studies of mothers in populations consuming foods that contain more mercury than selenium (shark or pilot whale meats) have found adverse effects from mercury toxicity on their children's IQs, while studies of populations exposed to mercury by eating selenium-rich ocean fish find improved IQs in the children instead of harm.[685]

- Speaking of fish, a new selenium-containing compound called *selenoneine* has recently been identified in the bloodstream of tuna. That may help explain why fish that contain more selenium than mercury are good for us. Selenoneine increases the rate at which mercury is detoxified and excreted by the fish—and thus the healthful effects of these fish on us, when we eat them.[686][687]

Selenium lowers the risk of hip fracture—even in smokers! The Osteoporosis and Ultrasound Study (OPUS), a 6-year prospective study of 2,374 healthy postmenopausal women from five European cities, confirmed that selenium status significantly impacts bone turnover, BMD, and susceptibility to fracture. Higher blood levels of selenium were associated with higher hip BMD when the study began and after the 6-year follow-up. Conversely, lower selenium levels were associated with higher bone turnover rates and lower hip BMD. The researchers concluded that the data collected clearly showed adequate selenium intake is required to maintain bone.[688]

Selenium's importance for your bones is vividly illustrated by a recent case-control study that investigated the link between antioxidants and the risk of osteoporotic hip fracture. They also looked at whether cigarette smoking, which is well known to greatly increase hip fracture risk, affected this link. Smokers (including those who had smoked in the past) were divided into five groups according to their intake of selenium. Those with the highest intake of selenium had a 73% lower risk of hip fracture compared to those with the lowest selenium intake. We're certainly not suggesting you smoke, but if you or someone you love does, make those two daily Brazil nuts a habit.[689]

How Much Selenium Do You Need?

For healthy men and women 19 years and older, the Recommended Dietary Allowance for selenium is 55 mcg daily. Keep in mind, the Institute of Medicine set this back in 2000 to prevent deficiency, not promote optimal health.

The dosage we recommend for optimal health is 200 mcg/d. This is the typical dose used in human clinical trials with no adverse effects and the dose provided by many nutritional supplements containing selenium.

Can you get 200 mcg/d from food or do you need to take a supplement? This depends upon a couple factors:

1. **Where you live:** Since selenium is present in soil, the amount present in food depends on where it was grown. Although daily intake of selenium in the U.S. and Canada is estimated to range from 60 to 224 mcg/d, dietary surveys have shown that as many as 25% of people in the Pacific Northwest and Northeast (low selenium regions) consume less than 50 mcg/d (even less than the non-optimal RDA). However, people living in selenium-rich areas of South Dakota consume an average of 209 mcg/d without adverse effects.

   While the extensive transport of foods should enable even those living in low-selenium areas to get a minimum RDA amount from diet, a surprising number of Americans don't. And even fewer get an optimal amount. If you live in a low-selenium area, you may want to get a lab test to check your glutathione peroxidase activity. (See Lab Tests, Chapter 10.)

2. **Your dietary preferences:** Vegetarians have far lower blood levels of selenium than omnivores. And vegans are at even greater risk for insufficient dietary selenium consumption compared to vegetarians who eat eggs and/or dairy products. One reason is that vegan diets are low in the amino acid methionine, which our bodies require for optimal utilization of selenium. Foods high in methionine tend to be animal products, including beef, lamb, cheese, turkey, pork, fish, shellfish, eggs, and dairy. However, some non-animal options for methionine include soy, nuts, and beans, so vegans should incorporate these as staples in their diet.

   For that same reason, omnivores may already be consuming 200 mcg/d of selenium or more. Knowing how much selenium your typical diet is providing is important because too much selenium can be toxic. Before taking supplemental selenium, omnivores and pescatarians should keep a diet diary for 5 to 7 days and use the table below to estimate typical daily intake.[690]

Best Food Sources of Selenium	
Food	Selenium (micrograms)
Brazil nuts, 1 nut	140
Tuna, yellowfin, cooked dry heat, 3 ounces	92
Halibut, cooked dry heat, 3 ounces	47
Sardines, canned in oil, drained, 3 ounces	45
Ham, roasted, 3 ounces	42
Shrimp, canned, 3 ounces	40
Beef steak, bottom round, roasted, 3 ounces	33
Turkey, roasted, 3 ounces	31
Chicken, light meat, roasted, 3 ounces	22
Cottage cheese, 4% milkfat, 1 cup	20
Rice, brown, long-grain, cooked, 1 cup	19
Beef, ground, 25% fat, broiled, 3 ounces	18
Bread, whole-wheat, 1 slice	13
Baked beans, canned, vegetarian, 1 cup	13
Oatmeal, regular or quick, cooked with water, 1 cup	13

Source: NIH Fact sheet, Selenium (ods.od.nih.gov/factsheets/Selenium-HealthProfessional)

Slow Version of Selenoenzyme (GPx1) Can Affect Your Selenium Needs

If your genetic inheritance includes a SNP that results in the production of a slow version of the selenoenzyme glutathione peroxidase 1 (GPx1), you could have increased levels of bone turnover markers and are at increased risk for low BMD. SNPs that result in an individual producing slower versions of other selenoenzymes are also associated with increased inflammatory signaling and risk of osteoarthritis.[691]

Ensuring an adequate supply of selenium is even more important for those producing slower versions of the selenoenzymes. Providing optimal amounts of their cofactor, selenium, will maximize the potential level of activity of these enzymes. The reason for this is a complicated principle in biochemistry called Michaelis–Menten kinetics, which shows that supplying more of an enzyme's cofactor helps increase its activity.

What to Look for in a Selenium Supplement

Selenium exists in two forms: inorganic (selenate and selenite) and organic (selenomethionine and selenocysteine). As mentioned earlier, researchers recently discovered an unusual organic form called sele-noneine, found in tuna.

Soils contain the inorganic forms, which plants accumulate and convert to organic forms, mostly selenocysteine and selenomethionine.[692] High-selenium yeast contains a mixture of organic selenium compounds, including both selenomethionine and selenocysteine. If a supplement is needed, this may be the best option since high-selenium yeast was found to increase glutathione peroxidase activity much more than inorganic selenium (sodium selenite).[693]

Selenium Safety

Selenium is a *Goldilocks* nutrient—either too little or too much is not good for you. The Institute of Medicine established a *no observed adverse effect level* (NOAEL) for selenium of 800 mcg/d for adults. To account for sensitive individuals, the NOAEL was reduced by 50% to set the Tolerable Upper Intake Level (UL), which is 400 mcg/d for adults.

If regularly consumed in *excessive* amounts (greater than the UL of 400 mcg/d), selenium can be toxic. On days when you eat selenium-rich foods, do not take additional selenium. This holds true especially for Brazil nuts, which may contain 140 mcg of selenium in each nut! (Eat no more than 2 Brazil nuts per day.)

If consumed in amounts no greater than 200 mcg/d selenium is safe and beneficial, as long as your calcium intake is at least 800 mg/d. A study conducted in Cáceres, Spain, involving 335 postmenopausal women (average age 60.9), found selenium, accompanied by at least 800 mg/d of calcium, showed a protective effect on bone mass. However, for those consuming less than 800 mg/d of calcium, higher selenium intake correlated with lower BMD.[694]

Therefore, as long as you're getting the 1,200 mg/d RDA for calcium (food and supplements combined), selenium should not negatively affect bone mass and instead do quite the opposite.

BONE-HEALTHY ACTION ITEMS

- Consume 200 mcg/d of selenium to match the dosage used in clinical trials, provided by most supplements containing selenium, and what we recommend for optimal health.
- For a rich food source of selenium, eat a couple of Brazil nuts, which contain about 140 mcg each.
- Don't exceed 2 Brazil nuts per day as frequent consumption of too much selenium can be toxic.
- Your best supplement option may be high-selenium yeast providing no more than 200 mcg per daily dose.
- Avoid exceeding selenium's Tolerable Upper Intake Level of 400 mcg/d.

Silicon

BONE ESSENTIALS

- Silicon plays a key role in bone formation by stimulating the production of bone-building osteoblasts and the synthesis of type 1 collagen, and by increasing calcium's incorporation into bone.
- Silicon's beneficial effects are boosted by estrogen, another reason to consider BHRT (bioidentical hormone replacement).
- The form of silicon used as a food additive and present in plants is not bioavailable. Only liquids contain orthosilicic acid, the bioavailable form of silica.
- The richest sources of bioavailable orthosilicic acid are mineral waters and (men rejoice) beer, which is the most concentrated dietary source of silicon.

Although silicon (Si) is not yet considered an essential trace mineral, the more we learn about it, the more likely this trace mineral will be awarded *essential* status. Silicon is the second most abundant element in the Earth's crust—bested only by oxygen. You can find *silicon dioxide* (SiO_2, silicone bound with oxygen) in silica or silicate compounds as a major component of sand, granite, quartz, and other types of rocks, clays, and gems. Silica is also used as a common additive in processed foods and beverages, and in many drugs.

In our blood, silicon makes up similar concentrations as iron, copper, and zinc—all elements that play essential roles in human physiology. Plus, the element has a significant beneficial impact on bone formation and quality.

What Silicon Does to Keep Our Bones Healthy

Silicon plays a host of roles for our bodies and is present in all of our tissues. However, its highest concentrations are found in our bones. Most importantly, it both reduces bone breakdown and stimulates new bone formation—a rare combination most nutrients don't offer.

Silicon plays an essential role in the synthesis of collagen, a critical protein for our bones, connective tissues, skin, hair, arteries, and nails. For proteins to do their work, they need to *fold* properly into distinct shapes. A process called *glycosylation* combines proteins with a carbohydrate through the help of enzymes, creating *proteoglycans*, which allow proteins to function properly. Silicon is required to form cross-links between *proteoglycans* and collagen (type I).

Silicon stimulates osteoblasts' production and their bone-building actions. *In vitro* (cell culture and tissue) studies have confirmed that silicon increases:

- osteoblasts proliferation and activity
- *bone-specific alkaline phosphatase*, an enzyme involved in osteoblasts' bone-forming activity
- *osteocalcin*, the vitamin K-dependent protein that escorts calcium into bone
- synthesis of the extracellular matrix, a collection of molecules secreted by cells to provide structural and biochemical support to surrounding cells.[695][696]

Silicon improves calcium's incorporation into bone. Silicon makes the bone matrix more receptive to calcium deposits. Silicon concentrations are 25 times greater in *osteoid*—the not yet mineralized, organic portion of the bone matrix that forms before bone mineralization occurs—than in surrounding areas, and the silicon content in osteoid gradually declines as calcification occurs.

Silicon helps maintain a healthful calcium: magnesium balance. In animal models of menopause, silicon lessens the typically seen imbalances in calcium and magnesium. Typically, blood levels of calcium increase, a sign that calcium is being withdrawn from bone, while those of magnesium decrease, increasing the risk of high blood pressure. Bioavailable silicon lowers blood levels of calcium and increases those of magnesium.[697]

Silicon improves how bone implants bond to bone. *In vitro* (cell) and *in vivo* (animal and human) studies of silicon-containing implants and ceramics show that these implants bond far more effectively to bone than their non-silicon-containing counterparts because silicon:

• causes the formation of a biologically active layer on the implant's surface

• increases the production of *calcium apatite*, a combination of phosphate and calcium that serves as the scaffold upon which bone is built

• increases osteoblast proliferation and differentiation

• increases type I collagen synthesis[698]

How does silicon trigger all this bone-building magic? It's a player in what Walt Whitman might poetically term the *Body Electric*. As the nickname *Silicon Valley* attests, silicon is a well-known conductor of electrical charges. Without silicon, your laptop and iPhone would not exist. Piezoelectricity—the technical term for silicon's semiconducting actions—is the negative electric charge that accumulates in certain solid materials (such as crystals and certain ceramics) and biological matter (such as bone, DNA, and various proteins) in response to applied mechanical stress.

How does this apply to bone, specifically? Bone mineralization takes place in the electronegative areas generated by compression. Silicon crystals accumulate piezoelectricity when subjected to stress, and the collagen matrix of immature bone uses piezoelectricity in the electrochemical process of bone mineralization. Silicon literally *turns your bones on.*[699]

Silicon Shown to Improve Bone Quality

As you can see, silicon plays several critical roles in bone health. A variety of animal and human studies illustrate the real-life benefits of getting enough of this trace mineral.

Silicon improves bone quality in animal studies. Studies of dietary silicon supplementation in growing animals (quail, chicks, horses) and fish (rainbow trout) have consistently reported improved bone strength and density.

Let's look at horses, the largest, longest-lived of the animals studied. In a randomized study, racing quarter horses supplemented with silicon at an age of six months old through 18 months were found to have significantly faster race times and greater training distances before any bone problems developed. The horses getting the highest level of silicon supplementation also had increased bone mineral density in the third metacarpal (cannon bone). Fracture of the cannon bone is the most common major long bone fracture in horses.

A convincing research model if you're equine, slightly less cogent if you're human. Studies designed to examine dietary silicon on bone metabolism on postmenopausal women often use female rats whose ovaries have been removed. A series of reports using this model found that the rate of mineral deposition and bone formation was an average of 30% greater in the mice supplemented with silicon. They also experienced less bone resorption.[700]

Silicon improves bone mineral density in human studies. Two large U.S. population studies, one involving participants in the original Framingham study and a second study of their children (the Framingham Offspring Study), have reported that the risk of osteoporosis was lower in those whose dietary intake of silicon was higher. Consumption of *at least* 40 mg of bioavailable silicon daily was the amount associated with increased BMD. And we're talking large differences in BMD here— up to 10% more BMD between those individuals with the highest (above 40 mg/d) and lowest (below 14 mg/d) intakes of silicon.[701]

Silicon boosts trabecular bone formation in postmenopausal women. Trabecular bone is the inner, more metabolically active part of our bones and the predominant form of bone in the spine. Study participants, all postmenopausal women with osteoporosis, were divided into three groups: a control group, a group given an injection containing 16.5 mg of silicon each week for four months, and a third group receiving an oral silicon supplement providing 27.5 mg per week for three months. The women consumed their normal diets, with no supplemental calcium or vitamin D. Both groups receiving supplemental silicon had significant increases in trabecular bone volume compared to the control group.[702] [703]

Silicon helps maintain bone density in women with osteopenia. Osteopenic women were divided into four groups and given daily silicon doses of either 3 mg, 6 mg, 12 mg, or none (the control group). All four groups received calcium and vitamin D supplementation. After one year, the control group showed a decrease in femoral bone density, while the groups given silicon maintained but did not further improve bone density. However, since *at least 40 mg/d is* the amount found to improve BMD in the Framingham studies, the doses of silicon provided here were far too low, even for the group receiving the highest dose.[704]

Estrogen Boosts Silicon's Beneficial Effects

In the Framingham studies discussed above, higher silicon intake correlated with increased bone mineral density for men and premenopausal women, though not postmenopausal women, except for those on hormone replacement therapy (HRT). Researchers suggest that estrogen, already known to improve our absorption of calcium, may also boost silicon's absorption as well. Or perhaps silicon and estrogen interact synergistically in women.

If this is the case, supplemental estrogen would boost silicon's beneficial effects, a big help when consuming low amounts of silicon daily, as were the women in these studies. As mentioned, these women's *average* intake of silicon was just 24 to 25 mg/day, while 40 mg/day is the amount clearly associated with increased BMD.

The potential importance of estrogen for women's utilization of silicon was noted again in a later study conducted in Aberdeen, Scotland. This study involved 3,198 women (aged 50 to 62) of whom 1,010 were premenopausal, 1,170 were using HRT, and 1,018 had never used HRT. Higher silicon intake had a very beneficial effect on femoral BMD, but only in the women who were *estrogen replete* (had adequate estrogen as they were premenopausal or postmenopausal on HRT). Among these women, femoral BMD was an average 2% higher in those consuming the most silicon (an average of 31.5 mg/d) compared to those consuming the least (an average of 16.5 mg/d).[705]

So, what does this research mean for you? If you are postmenopausal and not on hormone replacement therapy, please consider bioidentical hormone replacement (BHRT). In addition to its numerous other beneficial effects on your bones, cardiovascular system, and brain function, supplementing with bioidentical estrogen may significantly improve silicon's bone-building effects in postmenopausal women. (We strongly urge you to use *only* bioidentical hormone replacement, not conventional HRT. (See Lab Tests, Chapter 10.)

How Much Silicon Do You Need and In What Form?

Only one form of silicon, orthosilicic acid, is bioavailable. Silicate additives are not useful dietary sources of silicon because they are insoluble in water and thus have very low biological availability. Water-soluble, biologically available forms of silicon are derived from the gradual release of silica from volcanic and sedimentary rocks into the soil, where further exposure to water results in the formation of soluble forms of silicon in mineral waters.

Orthosilicic acid (OSA, $SiOH_4$), the major bioavailable form of silicon formed this way, is present only in liquids. Its two richest sources are mineral waters and beer, the latter being the most concentrated dietary source of silicon. At least 50% of the OSA present in mineral waters or the beer we drink is absorbed. The silica present in plant foods is also largely insoluble and was thought to be unavailable, until recent research revealed that an average 41% of the silica compounds in plant foods are broken down into much smaller soluble species such as orthosilicic acid, which is absorbed. Several supplements, discussed below, contain plant-derived bioavailable silicon.[706][707][708]

Are you getting at least 40 mg/d of silicon? Not likely, based on the Framingham and Framingham Offspring studies that examined this. However, the average U.S. silicon intake for men (30 mg/d and 33 mg/d, per each study) is significantly higher than that in women (24 mg/d and 25 mg/d). *Why?* Men drink more beer, a rich dietary source of bioavailable silicon. Women tend to get their silicon from bananas and string beans, sources of silicon that are poorly absorbed.[709] [710]

In India and China, countries in which far more plant foods are consumed, the typical diet provides far more silicon: 143 to 204 mg/d in India, and 139 mg/d in China. These higher silicon amounts have never been associated with any adverse effects. However, it's important to repeat that not all dietary silicon consumed is absorbed: only about 49% of the silicon in cereals and grains, and about 21% of the silicon in vegetables and fruits (and just 2% in bananas) is bioavailable. Apply these facts to the average dietary intake of silicon in Western countries (i.e., the U.S., Canada, and Europe), and you can see that our consumption of silicon is way below adequate.[711] [712]

In addition, several factors lessen our ability to absorb silicon:

- **Phytates and Fiber:** A diet that contains lots of legumes, whole grains, fruits, and vegetables is good for us, but the phytates and fiber it provides can reduce our absorption of minerals, including silicon. Fortunately, simple cooking techniques can greatly boost mineral availability. (See Zinc/Copper, Chapter 6.)

- **Aging:** Our ability to produce stomach acid typically decreases as we age. The lack of adequate stomach acid compromises our ability to liberate silicon from food. The use of acid-blocking drugs further exacerbates this problem. And if this weren't trouble enough, population studies have found that dietary intake of silicon drops with aging.

- **Hypothyroidism:** Insufficient thyroid hormone production and/or activity decreases our ability to metabolize silica and absorb silicon.[713] (See Hypothyroidism, Chapter 4.)

If any of these factors apply to you, increase your intake of silicon to compensate and make sure you are getting 40 mg of highly bioavailable silicon each day. You can drink mineral waters, enjoy a beer (see below) or take one of the supplements mentioned later that provides *bioavailable* silicon.

Best Food and Beverage Sources of Silicon

Mineral waters and beer are, by far, the richest dietary sources of bioavailable silicon. Following these, the silicon in whole grains and grain products (breakfast cereals, breads, rice, and pasta) is moderately well absorbed, while even less is absorbed from green beans and fruits. The reason bananas provide virtually no usable silicon, despite their relatively high silicon content, is that the silicon is a highly polymerized form that is not soluble. (This is similar to colloidal silica supplements, as we'll explain below.) This means you can't just look at the amount of silicon contained within foods to determine how much may reach your bones. A food that contains fewer milligrams of silicon may deliver more. (See table on the next page.)

To get the most silicon from beer, drink India pale ales (IPAs). The silicon contained in all beers is highly soluble (50% to 80% bioavailable), but IPAs retain more because they are exposed to less heat during the malting process. The beers produced from darker malts—such as chocolate, roasted barley, and black malt—all undergo substantial roasting and thus have far lower silicon content. Also, look for beers with the highest amounts of hops. Hops contain surprisingly high levels of silicon—as much as four times more than is found in malt. However, hops are used in much smaller quantities than grains in beer production.[714]

Best Silicon Supplements

Remember that silica, where silicon dioxide is commonly found in nature, is insoluble in water and therefore not bioavailable. The human body is unable to convert it into a soluble form we can absorb. Fortunately, companies have developed supplements, some from natural plants or ocean algae that can do the job.

- **AlgaeCal**: The marine algae species from which it is derived, *Lithothamnion superpositum*, naturally contains bioavailable silicon. Independent laboratory analysis of AlgaeCal powder indicates that 1 gram contains 10.81 mg of silicon. The daily 4-capsule serving of AlgaeCal Plus provides 24.9 mg of orthosilicic acid.
- **Other plant-based formulas:** Some plants (*horsetail, nettle, and bamboo*) can also convert silica into orthosilicic acid and various companies have incorporated this bioavailable form of silicon into supplements. Be sure to check any supplement's label carefully. The amount of OSA provided per serving varies greatly and is sometimes not specified at all.

Best Food and Beverage Sources of Silicon		
Beverages	**Serving Size**	**Silicon (mg)**
Beer (IPA)	1 liter (2 beers)	41.2
Beer (ale)	1 liter (2 beers)	32.8
Beer (lager), 1 liter	1 liter (2 beers)	23.8
Beer (light lager), 1 liter	1 liter (2 beers)	17.2
Beer (nonalcoholic) 1 liter	1 liter (2 beers)	16.3
Mineral water (Volvic)	0.5 liter (16.9 ounces)	7.23
Mineral water (Evian)	0.5 liter (16.9 ounces)	3.44
Wine, rose	4.4 ounces	2.89
Cider	1 pint (20.4 ounces)	2.3
Wine (red)	4.4 ounces	0.85*
Foods	**Serving Size**	**Silicon (mg)**
High-bran cereal,	3 ounces	10.17
Raisins	3 ounces	8.25
Green beans, fresh, boiled	3 ounces	7.86
Dates, dried	3 pieces (1.58 ounces)	7.47
Granola	2 ounces	7.35
Banana	1 medium, no skin	4.77**
Mango, fresh, smooth	1 medium (5.29 ounces)	4.73
Beans, runner, fresh, boiled	3 ounces	4.73
Brown rice, boiled, with husks	3 heaping tablespoons (4.23 ounces)	4.51
Whole grain bread	6 ounces	4.5
Spinach, fresh, boiled	2.8 ounces	4.1
Oats, porridge	2 tablespoons dry, 1 ounce	3.42
Pineapple, raw, sliced	2.8 ounces	3.14
Tofu	2.1 ounces	1.78
Lentils, red, boiled	1 tablespoon (1.4 ounces)	1.77
Currants	1 heaping tablespoon	1.52
Cucumber	raw 1-inch piece	1.52

*Red wine ranged 0.2 to 2.35. **Silicon in bananas is very poorly absorbed

Source: Casey TR, Bamforth CW. Silicon in beer and brewing. J Sci Food Agric. 2010 Apr 15;90(5):784-8. doi: 10.1002/jsfa.3884. PMID: 20355113

Jugdaohsingh R, Anderson SH, Tucker KL, et al. Dietary silicon intake and absorption. Am J Clin Nutr. 2002 May;75(5):887-93. PMID: 11976163

Powell JJ, McNaughton SA, Jugdaohsingh R, et al. A provisional database for the silicon content of foods in the United Kingdom. Br J Nutr. 2005 Nov;94(5):804-12. PMID: 16277785

Sripanyakorn S, Jugdaohsingh R, Dissayabutr W, et al. The comparative absorption of silicon from different foods and food supplements. Br J Nutr. 2009 Sep;102(6):825-34. doi: 10.1017/S0007114509311757. Epub 2009 Apr 9. PMID: 19356271

- **BioSil®** is OSA concentrated from liquids and then combined with choline to stabilize. One capsule of BioSil provides 5 mg of OSA and 100 mg of choline. The recommended dose is 2 capsules per day.[715]

Silicon Supplements to Avoid

You may come across *monomethyl silanetriol* (MMST), which is synthesized in the lab from petrochemicals. MMST has also been shown to increase the body's pool of silicon but only in one very small study in which 22 healthy premenopausal women (aged 22 to 38) were given the maximum daily recommended dose (providing 10.5 mg/d of silicon) for 4 weeks in a double-blind, randomized, placebo-controlled study. Although the study ran for 8 weeks in total; the women getting MMST only received it for 4 weeks.[716]

This research has been criticized as insufficient evidence to demonstrate safety, and we do not recommend MMST for the following reasons:[717]

- Four weeks is far too short a time to evaluate potential toxicity, and the standard battery of toxicity studies has not been run on MMST. (Such testing typically includes acute, subchronic, and chronic toxicity, genotoxicity, and reproductive and developmental toxicity studies.)

- Study participants were not representative of the general public. Excluded were men, older premenopausal women, and most importantly, postmenopausal women.

- Participant diets were not checked, so we don't know if they frequently consumed mineral waters or beer, the two best dietary sources of bioavailable silicon.

- Orthosilicic acid was not measured in serum and urine samples, only MMST. Researchers simply assumed that when less MMST appeared in blood and urine, this was due to MMST's conversion to OSA. However, MMST can deposit in tissues and organs, which would also result in a drop in its levels in blood and urine.

Colloidal silica products are also not recommended because this form of silicon is very poorly absorbed. Colloidal silica products contain large, negatively charged polymeric silica species. These larger silica compounds will either interact strongly with the mucus layer of the digestive tract, making them less able to migrate through it to the bloodstream, or will be too large to even penetrate the mucus layer. In either case, colloidal silica species will simply be excreted in stools. Colloidal silica has a rate of absorption of *less* than 2%—even lower than that of bananas![718]

You may notice that silicon is present in some *antacids,* such as *magnesium trisilicate.* Unfortunately, the silicon in antacids is present in the form of silicate, a highly polymerized form that is very poorly absorbed.[719]

Silicon Safety

Daily consumption of 40 mg/day of silicon—the amount shown to improve bone quality—is very safe. Oral toxicity has not been seen in animals or humans from elemental silicon (SiO_2) or organic silicon (orthosilicic acid), even when rats and mice have been fed up to 1,000 times the normal dietary intake. The only exception is one study in which rats were given absurdly high doses and experienced a loss of bone strength. (See details below.)

Because no evidence of toxicity has been seen in animals or humans (except for the rat study mentioned), silicon's safe upper level for humans has been set as a range of 700 mg/d to 1,750 mg/d. You only need 40 mg/d, so play it safe. Don't ingest more dietary bioavailable silicon than you would consume in a liter of mineral water plus a 12-ounce beer (for women) or perhaps a couple beers for men.[720]

Individuals with CKD who are on dialysis may accumulate silicon. Renal failure could impair the excretion of water-soluble forms of silicon, which are absorbed in the intestinal tract and eliminated by the kidneys within 4 to 8 hours. However, even in patients with renal failure who reported blood levels of silicon up to 10 times normal, no adverse effects were seen. There have been rare cases of silica kidney stones in patients with renal failure who were also consuming large quantities of magnesium in the form of antacids. But no adverse effects from oral silicon have been observed in healthy individuals.

Can Silicon Reduce Bone Strength?
Only in Ridiculously High Doses

Two experimental studies in rats reported small reductions in bone strength when excessively high and prolonged levels of dietary silicon were added to the animals' diet. However, we're talking ridiculously high doses of silicon here—500 parts per million (ppm), which translates to 500 mg/liter per day. The average human weighs in at 70,000 grams (about 154 pounds) and the typical lab rat weighs 300 grams. That means 500 ppm for these little furry critters would equal 116,667 mg of silicon per day— nearly 3,000 times more than the 40 mg/d a typical Westerner would get drinking mineral waters and beer. *Why do they run these nonsensical studies?*

Researchers evaluating the silicon content of 100 commercial beers found the average ranged from 6.4 mg/L to 56.5 mg/L. To experience the small loss of bone strength of the lab rats, humans would have to consume between 2,065 and 18,229 beers. Some men may consider this as a personal challenge; we honor your devotion to scientific experiment but don't recommend this one.

On a serious note, light alcohol consumption has been found to actually improve bone mineral density and bone mass, particularly in postmenopausal women and men over age 50. For women, this means about one 4- to 6-ounce glass of wine or an 8-ounce glass of beer, and for men, two equivalent drinks per day. Consume more alcohol than this and even the silicon in beer won't save you. The excess alcohol will decrease your bone mass via a number of mechanisms. (See Alcohol, Chapter 1.)

BONE-HEALTHY ACTION ITEMS

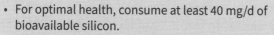

- For optimal health, consume at least 40 mg/d of bioavailable silicon.
- To get bioavailable silicon from your diet, you can drink mineral water and enjoy a beer. Look for India pale ales (IPAs), which retain more silicon than darker ales, and beers with a high hops content.

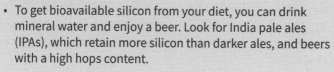

- For silicon supplementation, consider the bioavailable silicon in AlgaeCal Plus (25.94 mg per daily dose) and BioSil (10 mg per daily dose).

Strontium

BONE ESSENTIALS

- Strontium lowers the rate of bone resorption *and* promotes the rate at which new bone is built.
- Strontium's beneficial effects are not due to its replacing calcium in your bones. Less than 1 calcium ion out of 10 is replaced by a strontium ion.
- Strontium builds bone because of its beneficial effects on a wide range of processes, including calcium absorption into bone; promoting osteoblasts' production, activity, and mineralization; and lessening osteoclasts' production and activity.
- Confusion on the safety of strontium persists because of two unsafe forms—strontium ranelate (an unnatural salt) and radioactive (unstable) strontium.
- The safety of natural stable strontium salts (e.g., strontium citrate) has been shown in more than 100 years of research, as long as the amount of calcium consumed is at least twice that of strontium.
- Strontium molecules are twice as large as calcium's, which can impact DEXA readings—though only by a small amount. This can account for up to 10% of BMD increases, meaning 90% of the increase is accurate.

When it comes to healthy bones, think of strontium as calcium's best friend. They get along famously, like Lucy & Ethel or Laverne & Shirley. Both minerals have so much in common: they're absorbed in your gut, eliminated from your body through your kidneys, and incorporated into bone the same way. In fact, 99% of the total amount of strontium in the body is localized in bone, just like calcium. And years of research—going back as early as 1910—show this mineral has incredible bone-strengthening properties. Yes, in our bones, strontium always has calcium's back.[721] [722]

However, many of us don't get enough of this trace mineral. We mainly get dietary strontium from seafood, as the mineral occurs naturally in oceans and rivers. While plants can be a source of strontium, the amount varies greatly based on how much of the mineral the local soil contains. Making matters worse, commercially produced food grown on fields using synthetic fertilizers, pesticides, and herbicides has far lower levels of strontium than their organic counterparts.

That means those eating conventionally grown foods—or who don't eat much bran, vegetables, or beans at all—are at higher risk of strontium deficiency. In the U.S., Canada, and Europe, the typical diet contains only 2 to 4 mg of strontium per day, far below the amounts shown to improve bone health.[723]

Further complicating things, many myths continue to persist about strontium. Undoubtedly, you've heard a lot of conflicting information online, from friends or even from medical professionals. Before we detail the many ways this mineral supports your bones, let's first sort out fact from fiction.

Natural Strontium Salts are Safe and Beneficial

Misinformation about strontium is often due to confusion over 3 different types of strontium salts, each of which act very differently: 1) natural strontium salts, 2) radioactive strontium, and 3) strontium ranelate. First, let's look at the type of strontium you're most likely to encounter:

Natural strontium salts contain the element strontium combined with another compound to form a salt. The most common are:

- *strontium sulfate* and *strontium carbonate*, which are found in soils
- *strontium citrate*, which is used for nutritional supplements

These stable forms of strontium themselves have never been found to cause any harmful effects—with one caveat. To maintain a proper balance between calcium and strontium, you must consume more calcium than strontium.

Unsafe Forms of Strontium Cause Confusion

Much of the confusion results from news about 2 unnatural forms:

Radioactive strontium is formed in nuclear reactors or during the explosion of nuclear weapons. This unstable form of strontium can damage bone marrow and act as a potential carcinogen at high enough doses. However, radioactive strontium is used to treat metastatic cancer, and some strontium isotopes (85Sr and 89Sr) are also used as delivery agents for chemotherapy drugs and for research purposes.[724]

However, you certainly wouldn't want to use radioactive strontium (or any radioactive nutrient) as a supplement for bone health. Another form of strontium you may have heard about is not radioactive, though it has its own dangers.

Strontium ranelate is an *unnatural* strontium salt. *Strontium ranelate* is stable strontium taken over by a *Darth Vader* compound called ranelic acid. It's strontium whose beneficent *Force* has been co-opted and corrupted by the *Dark Side*. In order to create a synthetic form of strontium which it could patent, a French company combined the mineral with ranelic acid to create a new-to-nature compound—one that is potentially toxic. Ranelic acid is called an *aromatic hydrocarbon* (like benzene, toluene, and polycyclic aromatic hydrocarbons present in coal, gasoline and car exhaust). Such compounds are known to adversely affect the skin, liver, and immune system.[725]

You won't be surprised that these body areas match the sites where side effects of strontium ranelate treatment occur, including skin irritation and nausea. Serious, though less common, effects include venous thromboembolism (blood clot formation in the deep veins) and autoimmune reactions such as the potentially deadly DRESS (a severe drug reaction with an extensive skin rash, rapid facial swelling; a spike in white blood cells; and lymph, liver, kidney, and cardiac involvement).

The use of strontium ranelate has never been approved in the U.S. and is now significantly restricted in Europe, while strontium citrate is safe and freely available.[726][727]

Here's the takeaway: In more than 100 years of research on strontium, including a number of recent human studies, no adverse effects have been reported for any natural stable strontium salt, as long as more calcium than strontium is consumed. Natural strontium salts are safe (at reasonable dosages, of course) and highly beneficial as we'll share shortly.

Strontium and Calcium: Similarities and Differences

Strontium often mimics the actions of calcium in ways that support your bones. Both strontium and calcium promote insulin secretion which helps maintain healthy blood sugar (though strontium does so to a lesser extent). That helps to avoid the activation of osteoclasts, which can promote bone loss.

Similarly, strontium, like calcium, inhibits the release of parathyroid hormone (PTH), which activates osteoclasts when blood levels of calcium are low.

Strontium competes with calcium for absorption—and loses every time. Strontium and calcium share a common carrier system in the intestinal wall. These carriers always choose to ferry calcium, rather than strontium, from the digestive tract into our bloodstream. Therefore, strontium does not prevent calcium from being absorbed. Strontium's typical absorption rate is about 25% to 30%, but if taken when calcium is present, virtually no strontium will be absorbed. Calcium will monopolize all absorption pathways.[728]

Strontium and calcium both require vitamin D for absorption, and our absorption ability decreases as we age. Ensuring your vitamin D levels are in the optimal range (a blood level of 25(OH)D of 60 to 80 ng/mL) is essential for your ability to absorb either mineral.

Strontium, like calcium, is incorporated into both trabecular and cortical bone. However, strontium deposits almost entirely into new trabecular bone. Trabecular bone is the soft, spongy, more metabolically active inner portion of your bones. Cortical bone is their hard, outer layer. If your bones were M&M's® candies, cortical bone would be the hard, outer candy shell and trabecular bone, the soft chocolate center. Newly forming apatite crystals in trabecular bone incorporate more strontium ions than the larger crystals in cortical bone, which grow far more slowly. Plus, in either type of bone, strontium substitutes for *less than 1 calcium ion in 10* in apatite crystals. Claims that strontium causes cortical bone to become thicker, reducing tensile strength and increasing risk of fractures, have no scientific basis.[729]

Strontium impacts DEXA readings—though only slightly. At the atomic level, strontium (atomic number of 38) is almost twice as large as calcium (atomic number of 20). Strontium's larger size affects X-ray penetration during DEXA scans, causing a slight overestimation of bone mineral density. However, this effect is relatively small, from 6% to 10% depending upon the type of DEXA scanner. *What does a 10% overestimation really mean?*

> **EXAMPLE:** Let's say your DEXA score shows a BMD improvement of 3%. Taking strontium means 10% of that 3% (just 0.3%) of that improvement may be overestimated. In other words, 2.7% of that 3% was real improvement. Not too shabby, especially when you consider that we typically lose at least 1% to 2% of our BMD every year. That overall gain of 2.7% plus the 2% you normally would have lost adds up to a real-life gain of 4.7%.[730] [731]

When strontium supplementation is stopped, its concentration in bone drops rapidly. Strontium's larger size makes its reabsorption in the kidneys more difficult than calcium, so we eliminate strontium far more quickly. Three times as much strontium is lost in urine compared to calcium. In humans, strontium elimination from the skeleton occurs in 2 phases: an initial rapid clearance—where 50% will be eliminated within 41 days—followed by a slower phase of elimination during which the remaining half is lost over the following 3 years.[732] [733]

What Strontium Does for Your Bones

Strontium's beneficial effects are not due to it replacing calcium in your bones. They are the result of strontium's bone-building effects on key molecules involved in bone remodeling. If your bones were contestants on *The Dating Game*, interviewing potential trace minerals with an exhaustive list of all the qualities they wanted in their prospective mate, strontium would blow away the competition. The research reveals that strontium:

- **Increases our ability to absorb and deposit calcium in our bones.** Yes, calcium!

- **Boosts our ability to absorb calcium by activating calcium-sensing receptors (CaSR),** which sense extracellular calcium and increase its absorption. In the kidneys, CaSRs increase reabsorption of calcium when blood levels drop too low. In our bones, CaSRs are found on osteoblasts, the cells that build new bone. While strontium was previously known to activate osteoblasts (though not as strongly as calcium), researchers have identified a new CaSR version in osteoblasts that is activated *only* by strontium.[734]

- **Regulates RANKL and OPG, the key molecules that control our rate of bone breakdown.** Strontium inhibits RANKL, which activates osteoclasts and increases bone resorption, and increases osteoprotegerin (OPG), which serves as a decoy for RANKL to slow bone resorption. This becomes even more important as we reach menopause, and our drop-in estrogen production does 3 things that are very bad news for our bones: 1) increases RANKL production, 2) decreases OPG production, and 3) generates more pro-inflammatory messenger molecules (the cytokines, IL6, TNFα, and IL-17). The result is too much osteoclast activity and bone loss. Strontium shuts down this entire bone-breaking cycle.

- **Boosts the rate at which new bone-building osteoblasts are formed from *mesenchymal stem cells* (MSC) and increases their survival.** Strontium turns on genes that help MSCs become osteoblasts (instead of fat cells, i.e. adipocytes), grow up more quickly, and stay alive longer.

Strontium plays other important roles in gene expression, both reducing those that encourage adipocytes while also promoting those that support the production and activity of 3 critical proteins:

1. RunX2 is a protein required for osteoblastic differentiation.

2. Bone sialoprotein (BSP) constitutes approximately 8% of all non-collagen containing proteins found in bone and directs the formation of the first apatite crystals produced as new bone is developed. Apatite crystals are the inorganic (mineral) component of bone tissue and give our bones the ability to withstand compression without breaking. Apatite constitutes as much as 50% by volume and 70% by weight of human bone.

3. Osteocalcin, once activated by vitamin K2, brings calcium into bones.

- **Increases the number of *osteoid surfaces* (bone-forming sites).** Osteoblasts begin the process of forming bone tissue by secreting osteoid, the not-yet-mineralized, organic portion of the bone matrix. When osteoid has been mineralized, it and the adjacent bone cells have graduated *summa cum laude*—they are now fully developed new bone tissue. Strontium increases the rate at which we produce osteoid.

- **Improves healthy bone mineralization and formation of *hydroxyapatite* (healthy bone crystal).** Strontium not only helps produce more apatite crystals, but it also produces crystals that are more stable and resistant to compression damage (i.e., from heavy weight loading). Furthermore, the tiny amount of strontium ions that incorporate into cortical bone lowers its porosity, improving bone microstructure and resistance to fracture. Strontium is the *only* trace mineral present in human bone whose level in bone correlates with bone compression strength (i.e., resistance to fracture).[735]

- **Activates *Wnt signaling*, a cellular pathway that plays a crucial role in osteoblast production and bone formation.** When strontium binds to the calcium-sensing receptor, it triggers the translocation into the nucleus of an important player in the Wnt signaling pathway, *Catenin beta-1* (β-catenin). β-catenin sets off a whole chain of osteoblast-boosting activities, including inhibiting the production of *sclerostin*, another protein in the Wnt signaling pathway. Strontium inhibits sclerostin's *make-no-more-new-bone* signaling.[736] [737]

- **Inhibits osteoclast production and activity.** Strontium inhibits osteoclasts' ability to mature, reduces their ability to adhere to bone and start the bone removal process, and increases the rate at which osteoclasts commit apoptosis (a suicide program cells initiate as they become old or dysfunctional).[738] [739]

As you can see, strontium is a bone-health rock star!

Note from Lara: When my DEXA report in 2016 showed bones as healthy as those of a 30-year-old woman, I stopped taking strontium. However, after reading the current research on how many ways strontium helps us maintain healthy bones, I started taking strontium citrate again.

Now, I take a prophylactic (preventive) dose of 340 mg/d, which I also recommended to Joe to help keep his knees, hips, and spine healthy. We will continue to take strontium, since we want our bones to stay in great shape for the next 50 or so years. (I'm now 72, Joe is 73, and maximal life expectancy is said to be 120 years.)

Getting the Most from your Strontium Supplement and Deciding on Dosage

If you have either osteopenia or osteoporosis, you will receive the most benefit from a 680 mg/d dose of strontium citrate, the amount used in almost all the human research conducted on stable strontium salts. A half dose of 340 mg/d will also be supportive of healthy bone renewal, although benefits will occur more slowly. If your bones are now in great shape, you may still wish to consider supplementing with strontium citrate at a dose of 340 mg/d. This dose will help protect and maintain the long-term health of your bones. Regardless of which dosage you use, follow these tips to help you get the most benefit:[740] [741]

Adjust your supplemental intake of certain nutrients: Strontium affects our absorption of certain minerals and increases our need for others. Be sure you are getting optimal amounts of:

- **Calcium**: Make sure you maintain a higher intake of calcium (diet and supplemental) than strontium. (See Strontium Safety below.)

- **Magnesium**: Because strontium increases our calcium absorption, our needs for magnesium may also increase slightly for us to maintain a proper 2:1 balance between calcium and magnesium. (See Calcium and Magnesium, Chapter 5.)

- **Vitamin D3**: We depend on D3 for our active intestinal absorption of strontium, and this decreases with age. While aging is non-negotiable (consider the alternative), you can age very well and further optimize your strontium absorption by consuming enough vitamin D3 to bring your blood level of 25(OH)D into the 60 to 80 ng/mL range. (See Vitamin D, Chapter 5.)

Take strontium at night, and consider splitting doses to improve absorption. If you're taking 680 mg of strontium citrate per day, your absorption may be best if you can take one 340 mg capsule twice daily rather than both at once. But take at least part of your daily dose at night to help optimize its beneficial effects. Bone renewal is a housekeeping function that ramps up when we're sleeping and the body is not otherwise occupied.

Avoid eating processed foods. Phosphate significantly lowers strontium absorption. Phosphates are used as preservatives in most processed foods. Read labels![742] [743] (See Phosphate Additives, Chapter 2.)

Avoid consuming calcium for at least 2 hours before or after taking strontium. Calcium will be preferentially absorbed over strontium. Humans absorb about 25% to 30% of the dose of elemental strontium consumed when it is administered alone. Our absorption of strontium is reduced by 60% to 70% if it's taken with calcium. For at least 2 hours before and after taking your strontium citrate supplement, avoid consuming supplements containing calcium; foods naturally rich in calcium; calcium-fortified nut-milks, tofu, or juice; and medications that contain calcium, such as certain antacids and oral tetracyclines.[744]

Here are other items you should stagger from your strontium doses:

- **Kelp**. Alginate, which is found in kelp, reduces strontium absorption so greatly that it's used to prevent strontium toxicity in cases of poisoning caused by exposure to radioactive strontium.

- **Quinolone antibiotics**. Like calcium, strontium is likely to form complexes with quinolones in the gastrointestinal tract, preventing absorption of the antibiotic and strontium. Broad-spectrum antibiotics, the quinolones include ciprofloxacin, levofloxacin, ofloxacin, moxifloxacin, gatifloxacin, and others.

- **Antacids** that contain aluminum hydroxide or magnesium hydroxide

- **Chelating agents**. If you have been prescribed an oral chelating agent, such as DMSA, take strontium citrate 3 to 4 hours before or after consuming your medication.

Strontium Safety

As mentioned earlier, the *unnatural* forms (strontium ranelate and radioactive strontium) have caused much confusion, even among medical professionals. However, *natural*, stable forms of strontium (strontium citrate) have an excellent safety record over more than a century of research, including in a number of recent human studies. A couple of caveats:

Consume twice as much calcium as strontium. The only potential concern with strontium citrate supplementation would be *if both calcium intake were low and strontium intake was high*. Only one human study has ever reported an adverse effect from natural stable strontium. A paper published in 1996 reported an increased incidence of rickets in children in the Sivas province of Turkey due to high levels of strontium in the soil *and* a low intake of calcium there. The recommendation made to prevent this: calcium supplements.[745]

Certain patients with chronic kidney disease should avoid strontium. Since strontium is eliminated by our kidneys, it may accumulate in CKD patients whose blood-filtering capabilities are compromised. In patients with chronic renal failure, blood levels of strontium are increased 4-fold when creatinine clearance (eGFR) is less than 50 mL/minute, so avoid supplementation. If your eGFR is between 50 mL/minute and 60 mL/minute, discuss your use of strontium with your doctor.

BONE-HEALTHY ACTION ITEMS

- For maximum benefit, take 680 mg/d of strontium citrate. A half dose, 340 mg/d, will also provide support, although gains may occur more slowly. Once your bones are in great shape, a maintenance dose of 340 mg/d will support long-term bone health.

- Avoid consuming calcium-rich foods, medications that contain calcium, and calcium supplements for at least 2 hours before or after taking strontium.

- Adjust your supplemental intake of certain nutrients: calcium (twice as much as strontium), magnesium (needs could slightly increase with higher calcium absorption), and adequate amounts of vitamin D.

- Take your strontium at night to optimize its beneficial effects.

- Avoid processed foods since they contain phosphate additives, which interfere with strontium absorption.

Zinc and Copper

BONE ESSENTIALS

- Zinc and copper intake must be in a 15:1 balance due to the special relationship between the two minerals.

- An imbalance in the zinc/copper ratio promotes inflammation and increases the risk for and progression of all chronic degenerative diseases, including osteoporosis.

- About 300 enzymes and 2,500 transcription factors—about 8% of the human genome—require zinc.
- Zinc both increases the production of bone-building osteoblasts and inhibits that of bone-clearing osteoclasts.
- Zinc is required for the creation of the bone matrix and its calcification, and for our production of 1,25-D, the hormonal form of vitamin D that helps us actively absorb calcium.
- Not having enough zinc around disrupts healthy bone remodeling, as well as immune, thyroid, reproductive, and brain-sensory (e.g., taste and smell) functions.
- Regularly consuming more than 40 mg of zinc per day can cause a copper deficiency, which promotes poor bone quality, periodontal disease, and osteoporosis.
- Copper is required for healthy collagen and bone matrix formation.

Zinc is perhaps most well-known for its role in immune system health. And for good reason! If you search for "zinc and the immune system" in the PubMed database of scientific studies, you'll return more than 6,000 scientific studies, over 35% of which were published within the past decade![746]

As important as zinc is to our immune system, zinc is also the *cofactor* for about 300 enzymes involved in cellular metabolism, including many processes critical to our bones. Without zinc, these enzymes don't work. In addition, about 2,500 *transcription factors*—proteins that bind to our DNA and turn our genes on or off as needed—require zinc. That's about 8% of the human genome! Zinc is an essential trace mineral, not just for humans, but for all animals, plants, and even microorganisms.

So, it's no surprise that having too little zinc damages health in many ways, including impairing physical growth (like bone renewal) and disrupting the balance necessary for healthy bone remodeling, immune function, thyroid function, reproductive function, and brain-sensory functions (like taste and smell).[747 748 749 750]

We'll discuss this essential trace mineral's role in fighting pathogens along with its important relationship with copper. First, let's explore how critical zinc is for our healthy bones.

Zinc Plays Structural and Formative Roles for Healthy Bones

Zinc plays a combination of roles in the health of our bones:

- **Structural**: Bone mineral is composed of hydroxyapatite crystals, a compound that gives bones their rigid structure and contains several different elements, including zinc.

- **Formative**: Zinc is the cofactor for bone alkaline phosphatase (B-ALP), a key enzyme involved in bone building. The bone-specific version of ALP found on the surface of osteoblasts plays a role in bone mineralization and is often used as a marker of bone formation.[751][752][753]

Zinc is critical for bone development and maintenance. In growing animals, zinc deficiency causes greater impairment of bone development than protein or calorie restriction. Even when zinc is finally provided, bone recovery is hampered until zinc status is fully restored. In young adult lab rats, zinc deficiency causes a loss of bone mineral density (BMD) in the spine.[754][755][756][757]

Zinc boosts osteoblast activity and the formation of collagen and trabecular bone. Zinc increases the production, development, and activity of our bone-building osteoblasts, and their formation of bone's extracellular matrix, a collection of molecules that provides structural and biochemical support for surrounding cells. Think of this as the scaffolding for your bones, one primarily made of type I collagen. Zinc encourages the formation of that collagen along with the development of our trabecular bone, the spongy, highly active interior portion of our bones.[758]

Zinc inhibits the bone-resorbing activity of osteoclasts. Zinc inhibits the two major signaling pathways that encourage these bone-resorbing cells to develop: the RANKL and Tumor Necrosis Factor differentiation pathways. (See Magnesium, Chapter 5.)[759][760]

Zinc helps protect against our absorption of toxic heavy metals that destroy our bones. Zinc reduces the accumulation of lead in bone, disrupts cadmium's inhibition of osteoblast activity, and protects our kidneys from heavy metals. Healthy kidneys are essential for healthy bones because our kidneys are the primary place where we convert vitamin D into 1,25-D, the form in which it helps us absorb calcium. When zinc levels are marginal, growing animals accumulate more lead and produce less bone.[761][762][763]

Zinc Defends Our Immune System

Zinc's reputation as a defender of healthy immune function is well deserved. Without adequate zinc, your immune system is far less effective. The immune system consists of two parts, both of which require zinc to function at their best:

- The *innate immune system* is our first line of defense against bacteria, viruses, and other invaders. It includes our skin, mucus membranes, and white blood cells, which are programmed to just kill anything that looks potentially *pathogenic* (capable of causing disease). These immune cell types include mast cells, macrophages, neutrophils, basophils, eosinophils, and natural killer cells. (You may recognize these cells—and the resulting sneezing, coughing, and mucous responses—from their role in hay fever and asthma.)

- Our *acquired immune system* remembers all the pathogens we've encountered, so its T and B cells can quickly target and eliminate known invaders.

Zinc signaling orchestrates our immune cell communication and activity. Plus, the mineral is essential for the growth and development of all of our immune cells, which are hamstrung by not having enough. A less effective immune system takes longer to clear infections and pathogen-related damage and can trigger key signaling molecules, such as NF-kappa B, which turns on RANKL, which in turn activates osteoclasts.[764][765]

However, inadequate zinc promotes bone loss in another way, as the body attempts to conserve this critical trace mineral. After first decreasing excretion, the body then breaks down tissues where our tiny pool of zinc is stored. Bone contains about 30% of total body zinc. While this amount is only about 700 mg, it represents 3 times the zinc present in all our other tissues combined. Bone becomes our last-ditch, back-up source for zinc when other tissues have a vital need. When this happens, zinc is no longer available for collagen formation, osteoblast proliferation, or the creation of the bone matrix and its calcification—resulting in loss of bone mass and deterioration in trabecular bone architecture and quality.[766][767][768]

Zinc supplementation is shown to have positive effects on elders (those over age 65), all of which support healthy bones:

- a decrease in oxidative stress (when more free radicals are present than a cell can neutralize)
- fewer infections
- an increase in *zinc finger proteins*, which have antioxidant effects
- a decrease in blood levels of cytokines, which are signaling molecules that promote osteoclast activation and bone loss.

Surprisingly, nearly 30% of elders in the developed countries (e.g., America, Great Britain, Europe, and Canada) are zinc deficient and a significant proportion of all adults get far too little for positive effects on their bone mineral density.[769]

Can You Get Enough Zinc from Food?

The human body contains just 2 to 3 grams (2,000 to 3,000 mg) of zinc—a tiny amount compared to the 1,200 grams (*1,200,000 mg*) to 1,400 grams (*1,400,000 mg*) of calcium typically residing in the bodies of young women and men respectively.[770] And we lose only 20 to 30 mcg/day (just 0.1%). Maintaining this level should be easily accomplished by consuming foods containing zinc. (See table.) Yet, a surprisingly high percentage of the U.S. population is zinc deficient.[771][772]

Best Food Sources of Zinc		
Food	Serving Size	Zinc (milligrams)
Oysters, cooked, breaded, fried	3 ounces	74.0
Beef, chuck roast, braised	3 ounces	7.0
Crab, Alaska king, cooked	3 ounces	6.5
Beef patty, broiled	3 ounces	5.3
Breakfast cereal, zinc fortified	¾ cup	3.8
Lobster, cooked	3 ounces	3.4
Pork chop, loin, cooked	3 ounces	2.9
Baked beans, canned, vegetarian	½ cup	2.9
Sesame seeds	¼ cup	2.8
Lentils	1 cup	2.5
Pumpkin seeds	¼ cup	2.5
Chicken, dark meat, cooked	3 ounces	2.4
Cashews, dry roasted	¼ cup	2.3

Best Food Sources of Zinc		
Food	Serving Size	Zinc (milligrams)
Turkey	4 ounces	2.0
Quinoa, cooked	¾ cup	2.0

Source: NIH Fact Sheet, Zinc (ods.od.nih.gov/factsheets/Zinc-HealthProfessional),
World's Healthiest Foods, Zinc (bit.ly/WHF-Zinc)

The Recommended Dietary Intake (RDI) for zinc is inadequate to support bone health or health overall. The RDI is set at 11 mg/d for men and 8 mg/d for women (who are not pregnant or breastfeeding). Research shows that 15 mg/d is necessary to increase bone density. For an estimated 17.3% of the global population, dietary consumption of zinc is less than the already inadequate RDI—low enough to result in frank zinc deficiency.

In the United States, more than 6% to 7% of Americans risk zinc deficiency according to the 2006 NHANES-III. Even more concerning is that among older women (50+) and men (60+)—adults with the greatest age-related risk of osteoporosis—almost *none* were consuming even the inadequate RDI for zinc. Across most age and gender groups, Black and Hispanic people were lower in their zinc intake than white people. (See table below.)[773][774]

Average U.S. Zinc Intake and Difference by Population						
Age	Men			Women		
	White	Hispanic	Black	White	Hispanic	Black
50 to 59	12.27	9.73	8.4	7.94	8.13	7.01
60 to 69	11.52	8.71	8.77	7.71	6.80	6.93
70 to 79	10.34	8.13	7.84	7.18	6.42	6.37
80+	9.06	7.74	7.04	6.59	5.26	5.92

Source: NHANES III, Zinc requirements...[775], BOND-Zinc Review...[776], Dietary phytate...[777]

Since zinc's UL is 40 mg/d, it's safe to consume at least 15 to 20 mg daily. However, some people might need more, as much as 30 or 35 mg/d.[778][779][780]

Vegetarians and vegans are more likely to be zinc deficient. Meat, dairy, and crustaceans—especially oysters—are among the richest food sources of zinc. (See previous Best Food Sources table.) While a number of plant foods provide zinc, it's not nearly as well absorbed as from animal-derived foods.

Many plant foods—particularly cereals, nuts, and legumes (beans)—contain compounds called *phytates*, which bind to minerals during digestion, including zinc, forming an insoluble complex that prevents the mineral's absorption. Phytate levels vary from crop to crop, but you can get an estimate from the following table. Researchers have found that increasing the phytate content of the diet from 300 to 1200 mg/d *doubles* the amount of dietary zinc a person requires.[781]

Phytate Content of High Phytate Foods	
Food	**Phytate (mg/3 oz. dry weight)**
Brazil nuts	1,719
Cocoa powder	1,684 to 1,796
Brown rice	650
Oat flakes	1,174
Almond	1,138 to 1,400
Walnut	982
Peanuts, roasted	952
Lentils	779
Hazelnuts	648 to 1,000
Refried beans	622
Corn tortillas	448
Corn	367
Coconut	357
Wheat (refined) flour	258
Wheat (refined) flour tortillas	123

What can vegetarians and vegans do to get more zinc from plant foods? Vegetarians have been found to require as much as 50% more zinc than the already insufficient RDA. While similar research has not been conducted on vegans—whose diet does not even include dairy products—they'd likely require *at least* 50% more zinc than the RDA.

Here's the good news: special preparation and cooking techniques can reduce the phytate content of plant foods and significantly increase the availability and absorption of the minerals they contain.[782] For those of you who are vegans and vegetarians, we've provided instructions on several centuries-old—and scientifically proven—prep methods, so you can absorb more zinc (and other nutrients) from phytate-rich foods and safeguard the health of your bones.[783] (See box)

How to Get the Most Minerals from Plant Foods

Many plant foods, such as cereals, nuts, and legumes, contain compounds called phytates, which bind to minerals, including zinc, during digestion, forming an insoluble complex that prevents mineral absorption.

Fortunately, you can improve the bioavailability of zinc (and other minerals) in plant foods by preparing them using the methods below. Along with significantly reducing the phytic acid content in these foods, you render them far more digestible. As an extra benefit, you'll be able to say goodbye to gas after eating beans![784]

- **Soaking**: Cereals and legumes can be soaked in water overnight, then drained and rinsed with fresh water before cooking, to reduce their phytate content. If oatmeal or porridge is a favorite breakfast, try soaking your cereal overnight before cooking. You'll not only remove most of its phytate content, your breakfast will cook in half the time.

  Soaking uncooked beans, peas or lentils overnight as described above removes at least 50% of their phytic acid content. One report with peas and lentils found that almost 80% of their phytic acid was removed by soaking, rinsing, adding fresh water, and boiling.

  Note from Lara: I prefer using our Instant Pot, an electronic pressure and slow cooker. Set the cooking time desired and walk away. It automatically stops cooking your food and keeps it warm until you're ready—even hours later.[785]

- **Sprouting**: The sprouting of seeds, grains, and legumes, also called germination, degrades phytates. In one study, fava and adzuki beans were soaked for 12 hours and then allowed to sprout for 1, 3, or 5 days. This germination process greatly increased the phytase enzyme activity within the fava beans (up to 210%) and adzuki beans (up to 596%) and reduced their phytate content by up to 81% in the fava beans and 63% in the adzuki beans.[786]

- **Fermentation**: Organic acids, which form during fermentation, promote phytate breakdown. A preferred method uses lactic acid, which is used to make sourdough bread (and is available in vegan varieties). Even slight acidification of dough (to a pH of 5.5) with the addition of either lactic acid or sourdough starter results in significant phytate breakdown (70% of the initial phytate content of the dough disappears).

  Plus, it imparts a tangy sourdough flavor to your bread. For preparing beans, you can add lactic acid to the water. Presoak your beans overnight, then drain, and add fresh water before cooking.[787]

You can find Lara's favorite bone-building recipes online, including this one for creating your own gluten-free sourdough starter (www.algaecal.com/expert-insights/gluten-free-sourdough).

Factors that Increase Your Needs for Zinc

The human body contains only 2 to 3 grams of zinc. Therefore, we have virtually no reserve available and a regular, *adequate* supply of zinc is essential. Other factors can *greatly* increase our needs for zinc, including growth or repair (think bone remodeling) and infection because of zinc's key role in immune function. In addition, many factors increase what's *adequate* for each of us.

1. **How well you digest your food and absorb its nutrients.** As mentioned, deficiency can arise from poor absorption of zinc from foods. If you're not producing enough stomach acid or pancreatic enzymes, you'll be unable to break down food components into smaller zinc-containing peptides. This is often the case in inflammatory bowel disease, ulcerative colitis, Crohn's disease, and gastric bypass surgery. However, everyone's ability to release zinc from food often decreases as we age.[788] [789] [790]

2. **Your level of inflammation, from infection or chronic disease.** Your needs for zinc increase sharply when you're fighting an infection,

such as a cold or flu. The same holds for gastric bypass surgery or any condition that chronically increases your level of inflammation, such as obesity, type 2 diabetes, asthma, any inflammatory bowel disease, or cardiovascular, kidney, or liver disease. Remember, chronic inflammation is the driving force behind excessive activation of osteoclasts. If you deal with such chronic conditions, your needs will be 30 mg of zinc daily rather than 15 mg (for *healthy* individuals) to support increased bone density.

3. **Liver or kidney disease**. These diseases impair our conversion of vitamin D into its active hormonal form of 1,25-D. In this form, vitamin D not only increases our absorption of calcium, but also increases the expression of key genes involved in the transport and maintenance of stable levels of zinc (plus manganese and iron).[791]

4. **Chronic diarrhea.** This causes increased losses of zinc.

5. **A high calcium diet, particularly for lacto-ovo vegetarians and vegans.** When both calcium and zinc combine with phytate, the resulting calcium-zinc-phytate complex is even more insoluble than the compound formed with phytate and either element. While this can inhibit zinc's absorption, animal studies showing the formation of this insoluble complex have used dietary calcium levels *much* higher than those typical of human meat-containing diets.

   Those at increased risk of zinc insufficiency here are lacto-ovo vegetarians and vegans, whose diets are relatively high in both phytate and calcium, and low in sources of readily available zinc. This is particularly true when foods containing zinc are eaten at the same time as calcium sources. Vegetarians and vegans whose diet provides less than 25 mg of zinc daily should consider taking a zinc supplement. Make your goal a daily total intake of 25 to 30 mg/d from diet and supplements.[792]

6. **Pregnancy and lactation.** Needs for zinc are increased during pregnancy and breastfeeding. Remember, you're providing essential nutrients for a rapidly developing baby as well as yourself.

7. **Anemia or other hemoglobin disorders.** New evidence suggests that much iron deficiency anemia is due to an underlying zinc deficiency. Zinc controls iron's availability for hemoglobin production because one of the zinc finger proteins (myeloid zinc-finger 1) regulates the production of ferroportin, the only known transporter of iron out of

cells. Ferroportin's availability determines whether iron will accumulate inside cells or move into the bloodstream.[793 794 795 796 797]

A high prevalence of zinc deficiency has also been seen in patients with *thalassemia*, an inherited blood disorder in which the body produces an abnormal form of hemoglobin. Studies of individuals with thalassemia reveal a blood level of zinc below normal in 70% to 100% of patients. In one recent study, zinc deficiency was found in all 333 thalassemia patients, and 98.5% had severe deficiency. Fortunately, taking supplemental zinc has been shown to improve total body bone mass in individuals with thalassemia.[798 799 800]

Studies have linked low hemoglobin levels to low bone density and osteoporosis.

» Low hemoglobin levels, a key characteristic of anemia, correlate with low bone density in individuals with sickle-cell anemia, chronic inflammatory conditions (e.g., chronic obstructive pulmonary disease [COPD], and kidney failure.) Significant associations between bone mineral density and hemoglobin levels have also been found in *healthy* older men and women in studies conducted in the Chianti area of Italy and in Tuscany.

» Low hemoglobin results in low oxygen concentration in the blood (the medical jargon for this is *hypoxemia*), which studies have determined is a risk factor for osteoporosis. In one study involving 289 subjects with normal hemoglobin values and 82 anemic subjects, hemoglobin cutoff levels less than 12 grams/decaliter predicted low spinal bone mass with 100% accuracy.

If you are anemic or have inherited any form of thalassemia, you'll want to ensure you're getting *at least* 15 mg (at least 25 mg if also vegetarian or vegan) but no more than 40 mg of zinc daily.

Supplemental Forms of Zinc: Which One is Best?

As you can see, getting the zinc we need from food can be tricky, depending on our individual needs. Given how this mineral promotes healthy bone rebuilding, supplementation can be a good insurance policy to make sure we're getting enough. Zinc supplements come in several forms, each with different levels of elemental zinc. (See table below.) *So, which supplemental form of zinc might be best?*

Zinc picolinate was found better absorbed than zinc gluconate or zinc citrate in research conducted in 1987. According to Joe, one of the authors of this paper, the reason for zinc picolinate's greater absorption is that our bodies secrete picolinate (which we produce from the essential amino acid, tryptophan) specifically for its use in enhancing zinc's absorption from foods. And not just into the bloodstream, but into our cells. Zinc picolinate is the form in which our bodies preferentially absorb and utilize zinc.[801]

- A recent study compared the bioavailability of 3 other forms of supplemental zinc in healthy adults. Fractional absorption of zinc from zinc citrate averaged 61.3%, essentially the same as zinc gluconate, which averaged 60.9%. Absorption from zinc oxide was lower at 49.9% with 3 study participants absorbing little or no zinc from this form. However, note that the supplements were taken *without food.* Zinc oxide is not soluble in water alone but is well absorbed when stomach acid is present. That occurs when zinc oxide is taken with a meal, and as the table below shows, zinc oxide provides far more elemental zinc than other common supplemental forms.[802]

Overall, we'd say zinc picolinate is your best option, followed by zinc oxide if consumed with food, and then zinc citrate or zinc gluconate.

Zinc Oxide Provides Most Elemental Zinc		
Zinc Supplement	**% Elemental Zinc**	**Elemental Zinc (mg/25 mg)**
Zinc acetate	30%	7.5
Zinc citrate	31%	7.75
Zinc gluconate	14.3%	3.5
Zinc oxide	80%	20
Zinc picolinate	20%	5
Zinc sulfate	23%	5.75

Source: Zinc: An Essential Micronutrient...[803], Comparative Absorption of Zinc... [804]

How to take zinc for best absorption. Since phytate-rich foods and calcium can bind zinc and prevent its absorption, taking supplemental zinc apart from food with a glass of water is often recommended. However, taking zinc (or other mineral supplements) without food can result in stomach upset, nausea, and impaired absorption. *Why?*

Because food stimulates the production of stomach acid, which is needed *both* to release minerals from the food matrix (though not for supplements) *and* also to release the mineral ions from their stabilizing partners. Therefore, stomach acid production is required for optimal mineral absorption, especially that of zinc oxide.

Joe typically just tells people to do what works best: if you don't get an upset stomach taking zinc without food, fine. If you do, take it with a meal or snack. Ideally choose foods low in phytate and calcium, such as fruits, vegetables, or meats. Beans, seeds, nuts, and grains contain phytates, and dairy foods are rich in calcium, so don't take your zinc supplement with a meal or snack containing these foods.

Zinc Safety

The Food and Nutrition Board set zinc's Tolerable Upper Intake Level (UL) at 40 mg/day for adults, based on data showing that daily long-term intakes greater than 50 mg/day reduced the activity of an important antioxidant enzyme called *copper-zinc superoxide dismutase*. As its name indicates, this enzyme requires both copper and zinc. The 40 mg/day limit, from both food and supplements, establishes an additional margin of safety. Zinc is sometimes prescribed at higher amounts for medical treatment, but individuals receiving daily doses of zinc greater than the UL should be under the care of a physician who is carefully monitoring them for any adverse health effects.[805] [806]

Do not take more than 30 mg of *supplemental* zinc daily—unless you are ill, in which case up to 75 mg/d can be used for about 10 days. Excessive long-term zinc consumption can cause a copper deficiency, and copper plays a number of essential roles, including being required for our manufacture of collagen. Copper deficiency causes a loss of tissue integrity, particularly in our bones and blood vessels. See below on the importance of maintaining a balanced intake of zinc to copper.

Drug interactions: Zinc and certain drugs can affect each other's absorption:

- Antibiotics: both quinolone antibiotics (such as ciprofloxacin) and tetracycline antibiotics interact with zinc in the gastrointestinal tract, lessening the absorption of both zinc and the antibiotics. If you must take an antibiotic, ask your pharmacist if it impairs the absorption of zinc and vice versa.

- Penicillamine: the absorption of this drug used for treatment of both Wilson's disease (genetically caused copper excess) and rheumatoid arthritis, is reduced by zinc supplements.
- Diuretics increase urinary zinc excretion and decrease plasma zinc concentrations.

Zinc and Copper: a Special Relationship

It's important to check your intake of both zinc *and* copper. Because of how zinc and copper affect each other, you must compare your intake of both minerals. Make sure you are *not* consuming—from both your diet and supplements—more than 40 mg of zinc daily and that your intake of copper provides a balanced ratio of zinc to copper of 15:1. This translates to zinc intake of 15 to 30 mg/d balanced by copper intake of 1 to 2 mg/d.[807]

This is important for not just your bones but your overall health, for two reasons:

1. Long-term consumption of zinc in amounts greater than 40 mg/d can cause a copper deficiency, which can adversely affect your *lipid profile* (increase your total cholesterol and decrease your level of protective HDL cholesterol) and trigger *arrhythmia* (an erratic heartbeat).

2. Excessive copper intake in relation to zinc, however, can greatly increase *oxidative stress*, which is medical jargon for the production of more free radicals than the body can quickly neutralize. By increasing oxidative stress, an imbalance in the zinc/copper ratio increases the risk for and progression of *all* chronic degenerative diseases including osteoporosis and the rate of aging overall.[808 809]

Elders with chronic degenerative disease were found to have higher blood levels of copper and *ceruloplasmin* (the major copper-carrying protein in the blood). The study examined the *lipid peroxides* (fat-containing molecules damaged by oxidative stress) in 81 healthy elders and 62 elders who had a chronic degenerative disease. Both groups had too much copper in relation to zinc as compared to younger healthy adults. However, the unhealthy elders not only had elevated copper but low zinc concentrations as well—a double whammy for both bone and overall health.

In their conclusions, the researchers strongly suggest that the increase in chronic degenerative diseases, rather than being an inescapable result of aging, is due, in part, to an insufficiency of zinc. Recent studies have provided further evidence to support this:

- An elevated ratio of copper to zinc predicts death from all causes in elders, particularly if we have any type of chronic degenerative disease—including osteoporosis. An imbalanced zinc/copper ratio exacerbates the damage by increasing oxidative stress especially as we get older. Researchers have hypothesized that subclinical zinc and/or copper deficiency is a significant factor contributing to bone loss in the elderly.[810 811 812 813]

This provides yet another reason to check your zinc/copper status, as well as that for *all* of the vitamins and minerals discussed in this section. (See Lab Tests, Chapter 10.)

Taking too much zinc can cause adverse effects. The take-away to remember here is that *optimal is good. More than optimal is NOT good!* Do not overdose on any nutrient. Determine what your body requires and supply it. More is not only *not better,* but potentially harmful. Safe intakes of bioavailable zinc are dependent upon a balanced intake of copper. Disproportionately high dietary and/or supplemental intake of zinc increases the risk of copper deficiency.

What Copper Does for Your Bones

Like zinc, copper is a cofactor required by a wide array of enzymes. Enzymes that cannot function without copper are involved in energy production, cholesterol metabolism, blood sugar regulation, hemoglobin synthesis, the production of red blood cells and immune cells, wound healing, the ability of the heart muscle to contract, the formation of collagen and connective tissue, and tooth and bone mineralization.

Copper is also employed as the cofactor for two powerful antioxidant enzymes, *ceruloplasmin* and *superoxide dismutase.* Normally, 90% to 95% of the copper in the blood is bound to ceruloplasmin, and only a tiny amount of copper is present in a free (unbound) state. This is important because free copper ions can act as pro-oxidants and increase the production of free radicals and oxidative stress.

Copper deficiency promotes poor bone quality, periodontal disease, and osteoporosis. In animal studies, copper deficiency results in reduced bone strength and deterioration of bone quality leading to *osteoporotic lesions* (damaged areas of bone). Similar results have been seen in research involving humans.

- A study on postmenopausal women found those with osteoporosis had significantly lower blood levels of copper compared to controls with healthy bones.

- Other research has reported an important and common coincidence among periodontal disease, copper insufficiency, and osteoporosis in both men and women. Low copper content in tooth enamel is a common finding in adult dental patients with severe tooth wear accompanied by markedly reduced bone mineral density (BMD) in the lumbar spine. And this phenomenon—low spine BMD accompanying severe tooth wear—has been found to occur even when blood levels of vitamin D (25(OH)D), parathyroid hormone (PTH), and osteocalcin are within normal range.

Vitamin D enables us to actively absorb calcium; PTH causes calcium's removal from bone when blood levels of calcium dip too low; and osteocalcin is the vitamin K2-dependent protein that ushers calcium into our bones. The fact that copper insufficiency causes bone loss—even when these 3 key players in maintaining healthy bone mass are at normal levels—should tell you how important copper is for your bones (and teeth).[814 815 816 817]

More reasons why you don't want to become deficient in copper. The main adverse effect caused by copper deficiency is that *lysyl oxidase*, an enzyme whose activity is essential for crosslinking between collagen and elastin, stops working. This quickly results in greatly reduced strength in the bone matrix. Plus, copper deficiency results in decreased activity of copper-dependent enzymes, including the potent antioxidant enzyme, superoxide dismutase. That can lead to unhappy changes in your immune function and lipid profile (more cholesterol, but less protective HDL cholesterol), along with inhibition of osteoblast activity (because these bone-building cells are sensitive to the increase in free radicals that occurs when superoxide dismutase is not working.)[818]

How Much Copper Do You Need?

The Recommended Dietary Intake (RDI) of copper for adequate bone quality in adults is 0.9 mg/day. Even the usually very conservative authorities say this may be too low. Plus, an age-related drop in the digestive tract's ability to absorb copper increases the risk for copper deficiency in elders.

As discussed above, you should peg your copper intake to that of zinc, at the recommended ratio of 1 mg of copper for every 15 mg of zinc consumed per day. Experts in nutritional medicine, including Joe, recommend an intake of zinc of 15 to 30 mg/d balanced by copper intake of 1 to 2 mg/d. According to national surveys, the average dietary intake of copper for U.S. adults is 1.0 to 1.1 mg/day for women and 1.2 to 1.6 mg per day for men. So, depending upon your zinc intake, your diet may be providing all the copper you require. Check the following table to be sure.[819 820 821 822]

Best Food Sources of Copper		
Food	Serving Size	Copper (mg)
Liver (beef), cooked, braised or pan-fried	3 ounces	15
Lamb, cooked	3 ounces	10
Shiitake mushrooms, dried	3 ounces	5
Mollusks, oysters, eastern, canned	3 ounces	4.4
Tahini (sesame seed paste)	3 ounces	4.2
Cashews, roasted	3 ounces	2.0
Peanuts, dry roasted	3 ounces	1.3
Pistachios, dry roasted	3 ounces	1.3
Pumpkin seeds	3 ounces	1.3
Flaxseed	3 ounces	1.2
Pecans	3 ounces	1.2
Kidney beans	3 ounces	1.1
Buckwheat	3 ounces	1.1
Almonds	3 ounces	1.1
Crab meat, Alaskan king, cooked	3 ounces	1.0
Soybeans, roasted	3 ounces	1.0
Adzuki beans	3 ounces	1.0
Crab meat, blue, cooked, moist heat	3 ounces	0.7

Best Food Sources of Copper		
Food	**Serving Size**	**Copper (mg)**
Mollusks, clams, mixed species, cooked, moist heat	3 ounces	0.6
Sunflower seed kernels, dry roasted	1 ounce	0.5
Hazelnuts, dry roasted	1 ounce	0.5
Almonds	1 ounce	0.3
Peanut butter, chunk style, without salt	2 tablespoons	0.2
Lentils, mature seeds, cooked, boiled, without salt	1 cup	0.5
Mushrooms, white, raw	1 cup (sliced)	0.2
Shredded wheat cereal	2 biscuits	0.2
Chocolate (dark or semisweet)	1 ounce	0.2

Source: NIH Fact Sheet, Copper (ods.od.nih.gov/factsheets/Copper-HealthProfessional)

Copper Safety

Set your copper intake to maintain a zinc to copper 15:1 ratio. Note that regularly consuming more than 40 mg/d of zinc can cause a copper deficiency.

BONE-HEALTHY ACTION ITEMS

- Maintain a balance of zinc to copper of 15:1, ideally 15 to 30 mg/d of zinc balanced by 1 to 2 mg/d of copper.
- If you are a vegetarian or vegan, you may need up to 50% more zinc. The phytates in plant foods bind to zinc in the digestive tract and prevent its absorption.
- Improve the bioavailability of zinc in plant foods through soaking, sprouting, or fermentation.
- Your best option for supplemental zinc is zinc picolinate because it's absorbed and utilized more effectively.
- If your overall intake of zinc is less than 25 mg/d, calcium can affect zinc's bioavailability. Take your calcium supplement at least 2 hours before or after consuming zinc.
- You may already be getting enough copper from your diet since the U.S. dietary intake of copper for adults averages 1.0 to 1.1 mg/d for women and 1.2 to 1.6 mg/d for men. Use the *Best Food Sources of Copper* chart to find out.

CASES FROM THE COMMUNITY

*The Community is a sponsored group of more than 17,000 men and women
supporting each other to build stronger bones naturally.
(www.algaecal.com/community)*

Virginia's Story

"You are walking!" exclaimed Virginia's doctor, who was surprised to see her walk into his office given that she usually uses a mobility scooter.

Virginia had struggled with health problems since her twenties. Add to that age-related bone loss continuing into her 80s, and you can see why it was often painful for Virginia to move freely.

But Virginia has always adapted to her challenges. She's adopted a high-protein, low-carbohydrate diet and uses a special machine to help her blood circulate. Plus, Virginia has incorporated supplements into her diet for much of her life. But it was a particular plant-based calcium supplement that had Virginia's doctor so amazed. She'd been taking AlgaeCal Plus for a few months by the time she went for an appointment, but Virginia felt an impact within just 6 weeks, *"I was able to stand and walk and do things that I was not able to do before because of the pain."*

Fast forward a year and Virginia continues to thrive. At 87 years old!

Lara's Take: Good for Virginia for not accepting her mobility struggles as part of getting older. Here's proof positive that you truly can address bone issues at any age!

See details on supplements for calcium on page 135. Statements regarding the products above have not been evaluated by the Food and Drug Administration. These products are not intended to diagnose, treat, cure, or prevent any disease.

CHAPTER 7

Vitamins

In contrast to minerals, vitamins are organic substances (made by plants or animals). The Recommended Dietary Intake is set to avoid deficiencies, where the long-term lack of a particular vitamin is associated with disease. However, vitamins interact with each other and minerals to serve a variety of functions, including those that support bone building. Getting just enough of a particular vitamin to prevent deficiency will not provide you with the amount needed to produce optimal effects in the body.

Vitamins fall into two categories: fat-soluble and water-soluble. Since the fat-soluble vitamins (A, D, E, and K) dissolve in fat, your body can store them. However, water-soluble vitamins (C and the B vitamins) need to dissolve in water before your body can absorb them. Your body can't store these vitamins, so you need a fresh supply every day.

We already discussed the vital roles of vitamins D and K in Chapter 5. Here we explore how the other vitamins impact your ability to build strong bones.

Vitamin A

BONE ESSENTIALS

- When in balance with vitamins D and K2, vitamin A does not promote bone loss as has been reported and, in contrast, is highly beneficial for our bones.
- Vitamin A protects against vitamin D's potentially toxic effects: hypercalcemia and calcification of soft tissues.
- Vitamin A improves calcium's delivery to bone and increases urinary excretion of *excess* calcium, protecting against calcium oxalate kidney stone formation.
- Vitamin A is required for immune tolerance (preventing a hyperactive immune system from attacking the body's own cells, tissues, and organs).
- Beta-carotene (pro-vitamin A) from plant foods or supplements will not reliably allow us to meet our vitamin A needs.

Before we get into the many ways vitamin A helps your bones, know that some of what you've heard about this nutrient is likely incorrect. Vitamin A does *not* promote bone loss despite some reports. In fact, vitamin A, when balanced with vitamin D and K2, provides many benefits for your bones.

Vitamin A Must be Balanced with Vitamin D to Help Bones

Nutrients interact with one another, so you need to look at them together rather than in isolation. What the latest papers show is that *high* vitamin A intake—combined with *low* vitamin D intake—is what may contribute to decreased bone mineral density (BMD) and increased fracture risk. In contrast, human clinical studies consistently show that vitamin A, *in balance with vitamin D*—provides many protective benefits to your bones.

- **Vitamin A improves BMD when vitamin D status is adequate.** One good example looked at 6,481 subjects (2,907 men and 3,574 women) age 50 or older. When blood levels of vitamin D (25[OH]D) were at least 20 ng/mL, *higher* dietary vitamin A intake was associated with *increased* total hip and femoral neck bone mineral density in men and lumbar spine BMD in women. Vitamin A intake was negatively associated with BMD *only* in individuals who were vitamin D deficient (i.e., blood levels less than 20 ng/mL). Note that this level is even lower than the 30 ng/mL a rapidly diminishing number of authorities still say is adequate.[823]

- **High blood levels of vitamin A may increase bone resorption *only* when they coexist with a shortage of vitamin D**. That's the very situation known to affect at least half of subjects in Scandinavia, the area of the world where the majority of the research has been done suggesting vitamin A promotes fracture.[824] [825] [826] [827] [828]

Vitamin A and vitamin D balance each other's effects. Just as vitamin D protects us against the undesirable effects of unmitigated vitamin A on bone, vitamin A protects us against the toxic effects of unmitigated vitamin D, such as hypercalcemia (excessively high blood levels of calcium) and the calcification of soft tissues (e.g., our blood vessels and kidneys). (See details in the box.)

How Bonds Between Vitamin A and Vitamin D3 Help Us Use Vitamin K2

For vitamin A and D3 to team up in your body, 3 things must happen:

1. Vitamin A (as retinoic acid, its active, hormonal form) binds to the retinoic acid receptor (RAR) in your cells' DNA.
2. Vitamin D (as 1,25-D, its active, hormonal form) binds to the vitamin D receptor (VDR).
3. Together, vitamin D and vitamin A combine to form a *heterodimer*, a compound that binds to the retinoid X receptor (RXR).

This final binding is what fully triggers your genes to initiate the production of a very large number of enzymes and other proteins. Without vitamin A around, vitamin D (even bound to its VDR) only binds weakly to DNA and produces only a small effect on gene expression. However, when vitamin A is present, the resulting heterodimer partnership binds to DNA at the RXR very strongly, enabling vitamin D to achieve its full effect.

In other words, vitamin A *optimizes* the body's use of vitamin D inside our cells, including its effects on increasing the production of osteocalcin, matrix Gla protein, and other proteins needed to build healthy bones. Plus, since both vitamin D and vitamin A are needed to complete the above series of events, 1,25-D and retinoic acid naturally prevent one another's uncontrolled effects.

If you're lacking either vitamin A or vitamin D, the heterodimer cannot be made. Whichever vitamin is around will bind to your cells' DNA, but only half the message will be sent. Even if you are taking vitamin K2, its ability to help you build bone will be significantly lessened because far fewer of the vitamin K-dependent proteins will be produced, so fewer will be available to ensure your healthful use of calcium.

Even a defective vitamin D receptor (VDR) works much better when vitamin A is present. The genetic inheritance of somewhere between 34% to 44% of Caucasians (including Lara) and 24% to 36% of African Americans includes a faulty vitamin D receptor that does not bind vitamin D well. For anyone in this group of individuals, the importance of vitamin A for the health of their bones cannot be overstated.[829 830 831 832]

Why Vitamin A is Called the Anti-infective Vitamin

We'll dive further into how vitamins A and D work together, along with vitamin K2 in a moment. First, let's look briefly at how critical vitamin A is to our immune system and how that helps safeguard our bones.

Vitamin A promotes *immune tolerance* that would otherwise cause bone loss. Immune tolerance allows our bodies to recognize safe substances in our environment—food, pollen, pets, even our own body tissues—and not attack them. Vitamin A inhibits the production of *helper T cells* of the Th17 lineage, which produce IL-17 cytokines that marshal the immune system's most powerful battle troops. Vitamin A also promotes the production of *regulatory T cells* that secrete *IL-10*, which balances the effects of other cytokines.[833 834 835 836]

Vitamin A modulates our immune response by lessening our production of *naive B cells*. These cells are prone to overreact, activate osteoclasts and destroy healthy tissue (including bone tissue). When vitamin A stores become depleted, our regulatory T cells die off and free radical damage increases in our mitochondria (the energy production factories in our cells). Our mitochondria die, and our energy plummets. We need the energy our mitochondria produce for all the physiological processes that maintain a healthy body, including our constant rebuilding of healthy bones.[837 838 839]

Vitamin A protects against infection/infectious diseases. Vitamin A is required to produce healthy skin and mucous membranes (the lining of the respiratory tract, digestive tract, genitourinary tract), which are the barriers that protect us against infection. When healthy, these *epithelial* tissues have tight junctions between their cells to block viruses and pathogenic bacteria from penetrating. Vitamin A's role helps explain why its insufficiency predisposes an individual to infection.

If we do get infected, vitamin A is critical in mounting an effective immune defense, which is known to further deplete vitamin A as stores are used to increase immune cell production (such as *memory B cells*, which protect us from known threats we've encountered).[840 841 842]

How Vitamins A, D, and K2 Work Together for Your Bones

By now, we hope you're convinced that you need adequate supplies of vitamin A to protect and promote your overall health and that of your bones. As we've seen, balancing your intake of vitamin A with vitamin D3 is critical, and now we'll look at the important role vitamin K2 plays here as well. The key point here is that vitamin A is a *team player!*

Vitamin A improves calcium's delivery into bone. Vitamin A works with vitamin D to boost the production of osteocalcin, a protein vitamin K2 activates to deliver calcium into bone. Vitamin A also lowers the production of vitamin K-dependent matrix Gla protein, freeing up more vitamin K2 to activate osteocalcin. The result is that more calcium gets delivered to your bones rather than being deposited in your arteries, kidneys, brain, or breasts.[843 844 845 846]

While vitamin D boosts the production of matrix Gla protein, vitamin A does so only in certain types of cells. In other cell types, vitamin A *decreases* it. That's important because both matrix Gla protein and osteocalcin compete for the available K2 to turn them on. If you produce too much matrix Gla protein, thanks to the *help* of vitamin D, you can run out of the vitamin K2 you need to activate osteocalcin and deliver calcium to your bones. Plus, research shows that when vitamin K2 is unavailable, high amounts of *inactive* matrix Gla protein accumulate in the arteries, which calcify. Vitamin A restores balance by maintaining production of matrix Gla protein where we need it most.[847 848 849 850 851 852]

Vitamin A protects against vitamin D toxicity (*hypercalcemia* or above-normal blood calcium). Numerous animal studies have confirmed this since 1937. Even when massive doses of vitamin D were administered, vitamin A at just half of that dosage prevented bone demineralization and soft-tissue calcification. Vitamin A balances the calcium-absorbing actions of vitamin D by increasing our urinary excretion of calcium. That allows us to eliminate the *excess* calcium floating in our bloodstream that matrix Gla protein (activated by vitamin K2) has liberated from our soft tissues (e.g., blood vessels and kidneys) and the calcium released from worn-out bone by osteoclasts.[853]

Vitamin A deficiency is associated with kidney stone formation. Vitamin A's essential role in the balancing act required for our healthful use of calcium is illustrated by the fact that lack of vitamin A promotes kidney stone formation. In human studies published in the *Journal of Urology* in the 1930s and 1940s, over 90% of patients with kidney stones were found to be vitamin A deficient. More recent studies in animals have confirmed that vitamin A prevents the formation of calcium oxalate kidney stones.[854 855 856 857 858]

Vitamin A also prevents vitamin D toxicity by balancing blood levels of phosphorus. These 2 vitamins cooperate to maintain blood levels of calcium and phosphorus by stimulating their absorption in the intestine. Vitamin D increases calcium levels and decreases phosphorus levels, while vitamin A does the exact opposite. This balancing act is extremely important for your body's healthful use of calcium because hypercalciuria occurs not only when calcium levels are too high, but also when phosphorus levels are too low.[859]

Vitamin D increases your body's need for vitamin A. Animal research has revealed that vitamin D3 decreases liver stores of vitamin A. As explained in the previous box, vitamin D requires vitamin A to effectively bind to the DNA in our cells. High doses of vitamin D, without vitamin A, result in a functional vitamin A deficiency.[860 861]

Together, vitamin A and vitamin D optimize our production of osteocalcin, then vitamin K2 activates it. Osteocalcin is produced exclusively by osteoblasts, when they are signaled to do so by the active (hormonal) forms of both vitamins A and D. When osteoblasts are incubated with either vitamin A or vitamin D alone, their production of osteocalcin increases only minimally. When osteoblasts are incubated with activated vitamin A and vitamin D together, osteocalcin production increases dramatically.

However, the osteocalcin produced cannot become active without the help of vitamin K2, and blood levels of unactivated osteocalcin are strongly associated with an increased risk of fracture. People with the highest levels of inactive osteocalcin have 3 times the risk of fracture as those with normal levels. In other words, no one of these 3 nutrients can deliver healthy bones without the assistance of the other two.

So, now that you know your bones need not just vitamin D3 and vitamin K2, but vitamin A as well, what you need to know is: *How much vitamin A do you require and where can you get it?* Let's look at the sources of vitamin A first and then discuss how you can determine how much *you* specifically need.[862 863 864 865 866 867]

Dietary Sources of Vitamin A

Vitamin A deficiency is quite widespread both because it's lacking in the standard American diet (liver being the only good food source, though certain cheeses, eggs, and milk provide some) and because many people (including some medical professionals) have the mistaken belief that everyone can convert *beta-carotene* (pro-vitamin A) into vitamin A. We can't.

Beta-carotene is NOT vitamin A. You cannot rely upon plant foods or a supplement containing beta-carotene to meet your needs for vitamin A. The majority of humans do a very poor job of converting beta-carotene into vitamin A, which we've known since 2009 based on genetic research. (See details in the box below.)

While beta-carotene has some antioxidant effects, we want to underscore that beta-carotene is *not* vitamin A. Therefore, it does *not* protect you against possible vitamin D toxicity or optimize vitamin D's beneficial effects. Only the animal-derived foods listed in the Best Food Sources of Vitamin A table below contain actual vitamin A.

Best Food Sources of Vitamin A		
Food	**Serving Size**	**Vitamin A (IU**)**
Liver, beef*	4 ounces	3,207
Cod liver oil	1 tablespoon	1,440
Liver, chicken*	4 ounces	1,353
Milk, whole	1 cup	33
Cream cheese	1 ounce	31
Eggs, free range*	1 large	25
Cheddar cheese	1 ounce	22
Swiss cheese (Emmental)	1 ounce	18
Butter*	1 teaspoon	10

*Liver from pasture-raised animals, butter from grass-fed cows, and eggs from hens foraging in pasture will have an approximately 20% higher content of vitamin A. [868 869]

**Tool for converting UI to micrograms (www.thecalculatorsite.com/articles/units/convert-ui-to-mcg.php)

Source for both tables: cronometer.com

Foods high in beta-carotene are listed in the table below. However, the majority of us are unable to convert beta-carotene to real vitamin A (retinol).

Best Food Sources of Pro-vitamin A (Beta-carotene)		
Food (1 cup)	**Vitamin A (RAE*)**	**Vitamin A (IU*)**
Carrots, sliced	1,019	50
Sweet potatoes	1,922	96
Spinach	943	48
Kale	885	44
Winter squash, cubed, cooked	535	27
Broccoli	121	6
Cantaloupe, cubed	121	6
Mango, cubed**	63	3

*Retinol Activity Equivalents (RAE) are used to account for the different bioactivities of retinol and provitamin A carotenoids. For beta-carotene from food, 1 IU = 0.05 mcg RAE; approximate conversions are shown in the IU column.

**In the case of mangoes, up to 64% of the total beta-carotene is present as the cis-isomer, which is not taken up or transported as efficiently as the trans-isomer.

Genetic Variations Impair Conversion of Beta-carotene into Vitamin A

In 2009, Dr. Georg Lietz and his team published research showing that a very high percentage of women in the UK were likely to be vitamin A deficient. The reason: two SNPs (genetic variations) in at least 45% of the population greatly lessen the body's ability to convert beta-carotene to vitamin A.

- The SNPs (rs12934922 and rs7501331) found in the enzyme that converts beta-carotene into vitamin A (15,15'-monooxygenase (BCMO1), cause it to not work properly.[870]

- Further research in 2012 by Lietz and his team identified four more common SNPs. Three of these (rs6420424, rs11645428, and rs6564851) reduced the enzyme activity of BCMO1 in female volunteers by 59%, 51%, and 48%, respectively.[871]

Lietz's 2012 paper looked at the presence of these SNPs not just in the UK, but in people all over the world: people of African ancestry in Southwest U.S.; Utah residents with Northern and Western European ancestry; Han Chinese in Beijing; Chinese in Metropolitan Denver; Gujarati Indians in Houston; Japanese in Tokyo; Luhya in Webuye, Kenya; individuals with Mexican ancestry in Los Angeles; Maasai in Kinyawa, Kenya; Tuscan in Italy; Yoruban in Ibadan, Nigeria. The SNPs that hamper our ability to convert beta-carotene to vitamin A were found in frequencies varying from 43% to 84% (rs6420424), 52% to 100% (rs11645428), and 19% to 67% (rs6564851).[872 873]

Virtually everyone carries at least one, typically more than one of these SNPs. Therefore, your ability to convert beta-carotene to vitamin A almost certainly ranges from not great to lousy. Yet, authorities continue to equate beta-carotene with vitamin A and incorrectly tell you that various plant foods, such as sweet potatoes, carrots, or mangoes, can help you meet your needs for vitamin A. In reality, you need to get vitamin A from animal-derived food sources or through supplements containing retinoic acid.

Reasons You're Likely Not Getting Adequate Vitamin A

While many of us are now taking higher doses of vitamin D for our bones, the need for additional vitamin A to balance out our calcium is not as widely recognized. In the next section, we'll share how to determine your vitamin A needs based on your current vitamin D dosage. Several other items contribute to our needs:

Vitamin A stores are depleted by at least 5% each day. Despite being a fat-soluble nutrient, we lose 5% of vitamin A stores daily under normal conditions and even more if inflammation is present.

Normal absorption of carotenoids is minimal. About 70% to 90% of the vitamin A we consume is absorbed. However, even under optimal circumstances, we absorb only 3% or less of beta-carotene and other carotenoids. Plus, other factors, such as the processing and/or cooking of food, can affect their absorption as well:

- the type and amount of fat a meal contains (fat helps us absorb carotenoids)
- the amount and type of fiber, which inhibits carotenoid absorption (especially pectin)
- interactions among the different types of carotenoids (For example, lutein and beta-carotene inhibit one another's absorption.)
- availability of bile acids and minerals: The conversion of beta-carotene to vitamin A (through the enzyme beta-carotene 15,15'-monooxygenase or BMC01) occurs in a series of steps that require bile acids, iron, riboflavin, niacin, and zinc. Bile flow is compromised by liver diseases, including non-alcoholic fatty liver disease, now estimated to be present in at least 46% of the U.S. population.

Exposure to liver toxins. Numerous chemicals toxic to the liver (e.g., carbon tetrachloride, which has *supposedly* been banned since 1970) reduce retinol storage and or alter the metabolism of vitamin A compounds. Carbon tetrachloride continues to be present in many cleaning products as a result of manufacturers' mixing surfactants or soap with sodium hypochlorite (i.e., chlorine bleach).

Excess alcohol consumption promotes vitamin A deficiency via two mechanisms. Not only is bile flow compromised, but *alcohol dehydrogenase*—an enzyme that catalyzes the conversion of retinal to retinaldehyde, which is then oxidized to produce vitamin A (retinol)—is more attracted to ethanol than retinal. Rather than producing retinol (vitamin A), it gets used up metabolizing alcohol.

Drugs that deplete vitamin A, include:

- Antacids containing aluminum hydroxide can impair vitamin A absorption.

- Bile acid sequestrants, used to reduce cholesterol reduce fat absorption, also reduce the absorption of vitamin A and other fat-soluble nutrients, including vitamin D and vitamin K.

- Colchicine, used to treat gout, impairs vitamin A absorption by blocking the release of the protein (*retinol-binding protein*) that carries vitamin A into the body.

- Neomycin (e.g., in some topical antibiotics) if used in high doses over an extended period, may impair vitamin A absorption.

- Sucralfate, used to treat duodenal ulcers and GERD, decreases the absorption of all the fat-soluble nutrients (i.e., vitamins D, K, and E as well as vitamin A).

Finally, impaired digestion also increases the chances we're not getting enough vitamin A. In sum, the majority of us need supplemental vitamin A.[874 875 876 877 878 879 880 881]

Could You Have Vitamin A Insufficiency?

With few dietary sources of actual vitamin A (not beta-carotene) and several factors that can deplete it, you may not be getting adequate amounts, especially if you're supplementing with vitamin D. Check the below symptoms of vitamin A insufficiency, and tell your doctor about those you're experiencing. (See Lab Tests, Chapter 10.)

- Bone loss

- Impaired vision, initially most evident in reduced light (e.g., night blindness, due to lack of vitamin A at the back of the eye, the retina)

- Dry skin, itchy skin, dry hair

- Easily broken or ridged fingernails

- Skin lesions—actinic keratosis, increased susceptibility to basal and squamous skin cancers

- Epithelial cancers—lung, colon, breast, prostate cancers
- Viral infections (e.g., measles, chicken pox, pneumonia, and COVID)
- Infections of the respiratory, GI, and urinary tracts; the vagina; and possibly the inner ear
- Fungal infections (nail fungal infections, athlete's foot)
- Environmental and food allergies
- Inflammatory bowel disease
- Autoimmune disease

Choosing Your Vitamin A Supplement and Dosage

Make sure your supplement provides actual vitamin A (retinoic acid), not beta-carotene. The RDA for those age 14 and above is 3,000 IU for men and 2,333 IU for women (who are not pregnant or lactating).[882] However, you should set your needs for vitamin A based on what you need to maintain balance with your daily intake from total vitamin D intake.

Balance Intakes of vitamins A, D, and K2: Remember, your dosage requirement for vitamin D depends on several specific factors, which we previously detailed. That vitamin D amount not only affects your vitamin A needs but your vitamin K2 needs as well. (See Vitamin D, page 164; Vitamin K, page 182.)

If You Require Daily	Maintain Balance by Taking:	
Vitamin D	Vitamin A	Vitamin K2 (MK-7)
1,000 to 2,000 IU	1,000 to 2,000 IU	100 to 180 mcg
3,000 to 4,000 IU	3,000 to 4,000 IU	200 to 300 mcg
5,000 IU or more	5,000 IU or more	360 mcg*

*This is the K2 dosage being used in the current research involving postmenopausal women with osteoporosis and both men and women with coronary artery disease and chronic kidney disease. No adverse events have been reported in any of the studies.[883 884 885 886 887]

Vitamin A Safety

Vitamin A's Tolerable Upper Intake Level (UL) has been set at 10,000 IU for adults 19 and over, which includes total intake from food and supplements.[888] As long as you don't exceed this amount *and* take it in balance with vitamin D3, vitamin A is safe, exerts many beneficial effects on our bones, and promotes immune tolerance.

However, if not balanced by comparable intake of vitamin D3, vitamin A intake greater than 3,000 IU/day may increase the loss of BMD and risk of fracture in older people.

Pregnant or breastfeeding women should not consume more than 5,000 IU of vitamin A daily. At *high* levels, vitamin A has the potential to contribute to fetal development anomalies (teratogenic activity). *Adequate* supply of vitamin A, however, is *especially important* in pregnant women for normal fetal development, and for women who are breastfeeding to ensure adequate vitamin A is present in breast milk for healthy development after birth. The adverse effects of vitamin A deficiency during pregnancy cannot be compensated for by postnatal supplementation. Although the UL for pregnant women is 10,000 IU/d, we recommend a maximum of 5,000 IU/d of vitamin A (*total*, from both food and supplements). Any supplemental vitamin A taken during pregnancy or breastfeeding should be administered with your obstetrician's oversight.

Hypervitaminosis A. Taking *very large* amounts of vitamin A, that exceed the limited storage capacity of the liver, can supersaturate the body and produce toxic effects. Toxic effects appear when the ability of retinol-binding protein (the carrier for vitamin A in blood) to bind retinol, and to eliminate excess retinol in urine via a liver detoxification process called glucuronidation, is exceeded. Therefore, patients with liver and kidney diseases and children are more susceptible to developing hypervitaminosis A. So are individuals whose genetic inheritance has given them a slower, less effective UDP-glucuronyltransferase, the Phase II liver enzyme responsible for glucuronidation.

You are unlikely to develop hypervitaminosis A because very large amounts of vitamin A must be consumed. The most famous case of excessive vitamin A consumption was the fatal poisoning of polar explorers after they ate polar bear liver—in which vitamin A content is approximately 10 mg/gram. If these men consumed just a 4-ounce serving of polar bear liver (and they likely ate more than 4 ounces, which is a serving the size of a deck of cards), this would have delivered almost *4 million IU* of vitamin A! Since you are unlikely to be eating polar bear liver, especially as polar bears are a protected, endangered species, this is an interesting historical tidbit, but not of practical concern. However, hypervitaminosis A can result from an acute overdose of far less: 500,000 IU of vitamin A over two days in adults, a single dose of about 150,000 IU in school-age children, a single dose of 75,000 IU in small (preschool age) children.

Synthetic retinoids (i.e., the acne medication isotretinoin) should not be taken along with vitamin A. These drugs *potentiate* (i.e., increase the potency of) natural vitamin A and its actions in the body. Depending on dosage, they can cause a host of adverse effects, from minor (e.g., skin irritations, redness, rash, and hair loss) to more serious (e.g., exacerbate psoriasis, impair liver function, decrease good HDL cholesterol, and promote anemia). Unlike vitamin A, which causes no problems when the dose is not excessive and is balanced by intake of vitamin D3, isotretinoin, even at low doses, increases the risk of osteoporosis. If you have acne, we recommend you work with a physician certified in functional medicine (www.functionalmedicine.org) to determine and treat its cause(s), naturally and safely.[889 890 891 892]

BONE-HEALTHY ACTION ITEMS

- Eat liver and dairy products, preferably from grass-fed or pasture-raised animals, to get the most vitamin A from your diet.
- Make sure your vitamin A supplement contains retinoic acid, not beta-carotene.
- Base your daily needs for vitamin A on your vitamin D requirements.
- Don't exceed 10,000 IU of vitamin A per day from food and supplements.

The B Vitamins

BONE ESSENTIALS

- Methylation starts and stops thousands of critical-to-life processes, every second, everywhere in your body.
- An optimal supply of 5 B vitamins—folate, B12, B6, riboflavin, and niacin—all in their *activated forms* is essential for the methylation cycle.
- The B vitamins work together to prevent high homocysteine levels, improve magnesium absorption, recycle vitamin K and glutathione, improve our omega-6: omega-3 ratio, support energy cellular production, and promote healthy thyroid function.
- Niacin (B3) boosts the effectiveness of an enzyme that improves blood flow, which is crucial for healthy bones.
- We don't get enough B vitamins from our diet, except for a synthetic form called folic acid. Folic acid in excess promotes colon and breast cancers, depresses immune defenses, and can mask B12 deficiency.

Vitamin B refers to not one, but 8 different vitamins, each designated by a number (i.e., B1, B5, and B7) along with a corresponding name (i.e., thiamine, pantothenic acid, and biotin). If taking a B vitamin supplement, you've likely seen them referred to as *Vitamin B Complex.*

This chapter focuses on 5 of the B vitamins—B9 (folate), B12 (cobalamin), B6 (pyridoxine), B2 (riboflavin), and B3 (niacin)—which play major roles in supporting the health of your bones. They're discussed together, rather than separately, because what they do for your bones can only be understood by looking at *methylation*, a metabolic process constantly occurring in *all* of your cells, in which the actions of these 5 B vitamins are intricately intertwined.

B Vitamins Enable Methylation—a Cellular Process Essential to Life

Methylation is a biochemical reaction that jump starts and stops hundreds of critical-to-life processes everywhere in your body. It's so important that it occurs more than a billion times every second!

Methylation takes place when a *methyl group*—one atom of carbon bound to three hydrogen atoms (CH_3)—gets transferred from one molecule to another. This *one-carbon transfer*, as it's sometimes called in medical literature, sounds like no big deal. However, the results of this methyl group transfer are essential to your continued existence. If the human body were a car, methylation would be the spark plug. Without it, your biochemical engine would stop—not just in your bones, but everywhere.

Proper transcription of DNA depends on methylation. Transcription is the process through which our genetic information contained within our DNA is copied onto messenger RNA. *How important is this process?* It initiates the production of proteins—*all of them* that make up your body's structural elements—plus *all* of your enzymes. These catalyze the reactions that run your metabolism.

When methylation is slowed or blocked, the wrong DNA information (i.e., cancer-causing genes) can get turned on, while health-promoting DNA information (i.e., anti-cancer genes, genes with instructions for health-promoting enzymes) can get turned off. Abnormal methylation increases with aging and is a hallmark of cancer cells. One health-promoting gene specific to bone-building is *bone gamma-carboxyglutamate protein* (BGLAP) which codes for the protein osteocalcin, which brings calcium into your bones.[893][894]

Glutathione production requires methylation. Along with being the body's most important antioxidant, glutathione is used in a key pathway through which the liver clears toxic compounds from our bodies. These include many of those discussed in Part One, including heavy metals (mercury, cadmium, arsenic, and lead), plasticizers, phthalates, pesticides, and many drugs—all of which destroy bone. Plus, glutathione subdues toxins formed from normal bodily processes, like the free radicals produced during energy production in the mitochondria of our cells. When these toxins are not cleared, they can cause the chronic, non-stop inflammation that activates osteoclasts, causing bone loss.

Methylation produces *S-adenosyl methionine* (SAMe), the body's principal methyl group donor. Hundreds of thousands of enzyme reactions involve the transfer of a methyl group. SAMe makes these reactions possible. They're so important and so abundant that SAMe competes with ATP (the energy currency of our body) for the honor of being the number one compound used by our enzymes.[895 896]

The B Vitamins Enable Methylation to Prevent Bone-Damaging Homocysteine Levels

An intermediate step in the methylation cycle produces *homocysteine*, a potential toxin, which is rapidly converted into *methionine*, an essential amino acid. However, if we lack the active forms of the B vitamins needed for methylation, homocysteine doesn't get converted. Instead, this seriously bad-to-the-bone compound accumulates, overfilling the space inside your cells and spilling out into your bloodstream. Homocysteine is highly inflammatory and excessive amounts destroy bone, blood vessels, and brain cells.

When the B vitamins are not provided in their active forms, methylation gets hamstrung. Three *very* unhappy results occur: (1) We no longer produce the methionine needed for SAMe. (2) We produce less glutathione. (3) We produce lots of homocysteine.

Homocysteine, the molecular equivalent of an acid-spray gun, causes bone loss by increasing inflammation, triggering osteoclast production and activity, and further weakening bone by interfering with *collagen cross-linking*. Collagen cross-linking establishes the scaffolding within our bones upon which minerals get deposited. Messing that up seriously lowers bone quality and increases fracture risk.[897 898]

- In people age 65 and over, high homocysteine levels are strongly associated with lowered bone mineral density and increased fracture risk.[899 900 901 902]

- In a population-based study of more than 18,000 men and women in Hordaland, a county in Western Norway, women with high homocysteine (blood levels of 15 micromol/L or greater) were almost 200% more likely to have low BMD compared to those with lower blood levels of homocysteine (less than 9 micromol/L).[903] (Micromol/L is a unit of measure abbreviated as μmol/L.)

- In a study in which men and women were divided into four groups according to their blood levels of homocysteine, risk for hip fracture was almost four times higher for men and twice as high for women in the highest group.[904]

Several *meta-analyses* confirm these findings. One, which included 14,863 subjects, concluded that homocysteine was an independent risk factor for osteoporotic fracture. Another, with 11,511 subjects, estimated a 4% increase in fracture risk for every 1 μmol/L increase in blood levels of homocysteine. Yet another, involving 9 studies with 14,863 participants, found individuals in the highest quartile of blood levels of homocysteine had a 67% greater risk of hip fracture compared to those in the lowest quartile.[905 906 907]

We do need some homocysteine. It's an *essential* player in the methylation cycle, which means it helps us produce SAMe (which keeps our DNA properly methylated) and glutathione (which lowers inflammation and clears toxins). Homocysteine only becomes toxic when we have too much of it, and that happens when we don't have enough of the B vitamins, which all work together in their active forms to keep methylation running smoothly and homocysteine levels low.[908]

So what homocysteine levels are considered too much? In the conventional medicine world (where the *absence of overt disease* is sufficient), a homocysteine blood level of 15 to 30 μmol/L is considered moderately elevated, 30 to 100 μmol/L indicates an intermediate level of risk, and greater than 100 μmol/L indicates severe risk. *Remember the study conducted in Hordaland, Norway mentioned above?* A homocysteine level of just 15 μmol/L increased the risk of low BMD by 200%.

Optimal homocysteine levels are lower than 10 μmol/L—*far* lower according to Joe (Dr. Pizzorno), who has published several papers discussing homocysteine in *Integrative Medicine, A Clinician's Journal*, the PubMed listed journal for which he is the editor in chief. Joe, whose focus is optimal health, not merely the absence of disease, considers optimal homocysteine levels to be 5 to 7 μmol/L.

At elevated levels, homocysteine not only destroys your bones, but also increases your risk of heart attack and stroke because it damages cholesterol, causes blood platelets to stick together, directly injures the linings of your arteries, and impairs your circulation. Plus, this molecular terrorist injures DNA and contributes to cancer and Alzheimer's. So, you have lots of reasons—in addition to the health of your bones—to optimize your methylation![909]

What optimizes methylation? An optimal supply of these 5 B vitamins: folate, B12, B6, riboflavin, and niacin—in their activated (ready to get the job done) forms. Unfortunately, hardly anyone does a good job of activating all the B vitamins. I (Lara) do a lousy job of activating both folate and B6, so I need to take an *active B complex* to get these critical Bs in their active forms.

To understand why this is so important, let's tune in to an episode of *The Methylation Show*, starring all 5 B Vitamins. (See box.) You'll quickly see why you need all of them—in their activated forms. (If you'd rather skip the science, no worries. All you need to know is that the Bs rely on teamwork to get the job done.) Then, we'll take a quick look at the additional ways each B vitamin independently supports the health of your bones.

The Methylation Show, Starring All 5 B Vitamins

We've seen how methylation is critical to producing SAMe, the body's principal methyl group donor that enables hundreds of thousands of enzyme reactions. Without the B vitamins in their active forms, we not only lack the methionine needed to produce SAMe, but we also produce less anti-inflammatory glutathione and lots of highly inflammatory homocysteine.

Methylation puts on quite a show, with a dizzying amount of activity that rivals a Broadway show. And this frenzy is going on in your body constantly. For those who love digging into the details, here's how the active forms of these 5 B vitamins are essential for this to work:

Prologue: The methylation show starts with *Folate* (B9, tetrahydrofolate) and not folic acid. *Tetrahydrofolate* is naturally found in plants, while folic acid is a synthetic man-made precursor with no biological activity. Folic acid has to be changed into tetrahydrofolate using a liver enzyme called *dihydrofolate reductase* before it can be used in the methylation cycle. Some of us can accomplish this successfully though most of us not very well.

Act One: Tetrahydrofolate gets converted into its active form: *5,10-methylenetetrahydrofolate (5,10-MTHF)* with the help of an enzyme called *serine hydroxymethyltransferase (SHMT)*.

- To function, SHMT needs as its cofactor *pyridoxal-5-phosphate* or *P5P (*the active form of *B6)*.

- Converting B6 into its active form of P5P is the job of an enzyme called *pyridoxine phosphate oxidase* (PPO), which itself requires *riboflavin* (in its active form of *flavin mononucleotide* or FMN) as its cofactor.

- **Key Point:** So, the conversion of folate into *5,10-MTHF* requires 2 different B vitamins: B6 and riboflavin, both in their active form.

Act Two: Converting 5,10-MTHF into *5-methylenetetrahydrofolate* (5-MTHF), the principal folate form circulating in the bloodstream, requires an enzyme called *methylenetetrahydrofolate reductase* (MTHFR).

- MTHFR also requires riboflavin as its cofactor.

- Two common gene variations make a poorly functioning MTHFR. Worldwide, at least 24% of us (34% of Caucasians, 10% of Africans) have one (or both) of these variations, meaning you'll have difficulty producing the active form of folate.[910]

- **Key Point:** So, the conversion of 5,10-MTHF into 5-MTHF requires riboflavin and a well-functioning MTHFR enzyme, something many of us lack.

Act Three: 5-MTHF donates its methyl group to *Cobalamin* (B12) changing it into *methylcobalamin* (B12's active form).

Act Four: Methylcobalamin converts *homocysteine* to *methionine*, with the help of the enzyme *methionine synthase* as a catalyst.

Act Five: Methionine is then used to make SAMe, the universal methyl donor for DNA and RNA, proteins, and hundreds of thousands of methylation reactions. SAMe donates its methyl group for one of these many reactions and, in doing so, is converted to *S-Adenosyl Homocysteine* (SAH).

Act Six: SAH is converted to homocysteine by the enzyme *S-adenosyl-L-homocysteine hydrolase* (SAHH).

- SAHH requires Niacin (B3) in the form of *nicotinamide adenine dinucleotide* (NAD+) as its cofactor.

Act Seven: Homocysteine can then go down 2 different pathways, and either be:

1. remethylated back to methionine, via the action of methionine synthase.
   - » This requires the presence of methylcobalamin (B12's active form).
2. used in what's called *the transsulfuration pathway* to produce *cysteine,* which is used to produce glutathione.
   - » Cysteine is produced via the action of a P5P-dependent enzyme called *cystathionine beta-synthase.*
   - » **Key Point:** As in Act One, P5P requires both B6 and riboflavin.

Epilogue: What a three-ring circus! You certainly don't have to remember all this! The take-away here is very simple: for your metabolism to work properly, all of these B vitamins must be present in their active forms.

Other Ways the Active B Vitamins Benefit Your Bones

Just by preventing homocysteine from rampaging your bones and supporting the production (and recycling of) glutathione, the B vitamins have certainly earned their keep.[911] However, the B vitamins play many other important roles, either combined or individually, throughout our bodies.

Improve magnesium's absorption. The active form of B6 (P5P, converted with the help of riboflavin) increases the ability of cells to absorb magnesium. In other words, your ability to absorb magnesium depends on *both* riboflavin and B6 in their active forms.[912][913]

Regenerate vitamin K. A compound called *nicotinamide adenine dinucleotide phosphate* (NADPH), produced by osteoblasts, restores used vitamin K back into its ready-for-action form. That enables K2 to activate the key proteins osteocalcin and matrix Gla protein, which respectively bring calcium into your bones and prevent it from depositing in the heart, blood vessels, and the kidneys. (See Vitamin K, Chapter 5.) The production of NADPH requires niacin and B6 (in its active P5P form, so riboflavin is needed, too). Animals deficient in P5P are unable to heal fractures properly because they cannot effectively recycle their vitamin K2 to help osteocalcin bring calcium into their bones.[914 915]

Improve our ratio of omega-6 to omega-3. P5P is also the required cofactor for an enzyme called *delta-6 desaturase*, a critical enzyme in the pathway through which we produce EPA and DHA from ALA, the type of omega-3 in plants. Several studies show that higher blood levels of P5P are associated with more omega-3 (DHA) and a healthier balance between omega-6 and omega-3, which is *essential* for healthy bones. (See Omega-3 Chapter 5.)

Supports glutathione recycling along with production. We mentioned how the methylation cycle produces glutathione from homocysteine. Specifically, P5P serves as the cofactor for *cystathionine β-synthase*, the enzyme that converts homocysteine to cysteine, which is then used to make glutathione. Another B vitamin, riboflavin (B2) plays two roles here: it's needed for the production of P5P and is also the coenzyme for *glutathione reductase*, the enzyme that restores already used (oxidized) glutathione back into its ready-for-action (reduced) form.

Contribute to energy production: All cells, including our bone cells, require energy to maintain themselves and do their work. Cells produce this energy, called ATP, from within. The active forms of niacin (B3), B12, and riboflavin, all play important roles in ATP production.[916 917 918]

Support healthy thyroid function. Riboflavin is required for the reactions through which iodine is combined with tyrosine to produce thyroid hormones, and also for those through which iodine is recycled to produce more thyroid hormones. A lack of adequate riboflavin increases the risk of hypothyroidism, which promotes bone loss.[919 920 921]

Niacin (B3) Supports Blood Flow and the Delivery of Nutrients and Oxygen to Bone

Niacin, which contributes to energy production and the folate and methylation cycles, plays another extremely important role in bone health. Niacin boosts the effectiveness of an enzyme that improves blood flow. Current research confirms that a healthy blood supply is crucial for healthy bones.

Specifically, niacin increases the activity of an enzyme called *endothelial nitric oxide synthase (eNOS)*. As its name implies, eNOS is involved in the production of nitric oxide (NO) in the endothelium, the lining on the inside surface of our blood vessels. Endothelial NO relaxes vascular smooth muscle, the muscle cells in the lining of our blood vessels, which lowers blood pressure and improves blood flow. This, in turn, improves both the delivery of nutrients to and the removal of wastes from our cells—including those that make up our bones.

Bone turnover and formation require lots of nutrients, delivered via the bloodstream. In fact, bone receives up to 10% of *cardiac output*, the volume of blood being pumped by the heart. When the supply of blood to the bone drops, the delivery of oxygen and other nutrients is lessened, promoting *hypoxia*, a condition where insufficient oxygen reaches tissues. Hypoxia inhibits osteoblast development and bone-forming activity, and increases the production and size of osteoclasts, causing increased bone resorption.[922] [923]

The association between aging, diminished blood flow, and bone loss has only recently become recognized. Now, however, it's well accepted that oxygen delivery to human bone tends to decline with age, and diminished blood flow promotes bone loss.

- A study of older women (average age 74 years) found blood flow to the femur was far lower in the women with osteoporosis compared to those who were osteopenic or had normal BMD. And as blood flow decreased, bone marrow was increasingly replaced by fat, a condition called *sarcopenia* which greatly increases frailty and bone loss.[924] (See Sarcopenia, Chapter 4.)

- Not producing sufficient endothelial NO to relax our blood vessels causes high blood pressure, which also correlates with lower BMD in women. High blood pressure was found to significantly increase the risk for osteoporotic fractures in a very large case-control study (124,655 fracture cases and 373,962 age- and gender-matched controls).[925]

- Insufficient endothelial NO production is a key cause of the reduction in blood flow seen with aging. Research shows that middle-aged and older adults whose diet provides more niacin produce more endothelial NO and have better blood flow.[926] [927]

In addition to niacin (in its NAD+ form), the nitric oxide synthase enzymes use another molecule called *tetrahydrobiopterin* (BH4) to generate NO. BH4 is produced with the help of an enzyme called *dihydrofolate reductase* (DHFR), which also uses niacin (in its NADPH form) as an electron donor. In other words, niacin helps us produce NO via two different pathways.

Produce more NO by avoiding supplements containing folic acid. You may remember from our earlier discussion of the folate cycle, and folic acid, that DHFR is also the enzyme used to convert folic acid (the synthetic, biologically inactive form of folate) into tetrahydrofolate (the biologically active form of folate present in plant foods). DHFR is an enzyme with a limited capacity even in its most effective form. So, folic acid intake of greater than 200 mcg in a single dose is associated with the appearance of unmetabolized folic acid in the bloodstream, made even worse because many of us have inherited slow versions of DHFR.[928] (See box below.)

We want to use our DHFR to produce BN4 and NO, not waste it converting folic acid into folate, which we can easily get by eating vegetables or taking a supplement containing folate, preferably in its active form. So, now you have another reason—supporting healthier blood flow—not to take supplements containing folic acid.

Low Dietary Intakes of B Vitamins and Deficiencies are Common

We've seen the essential roles the B vitamins play related to bone health, as well as enabling the methylation process critical to our metabolic functions. Unfortunately, deficiencies in the B vitamins (except folate as further explained in the next section) are frequently seen in the U.S. population overall and increase dramatically with age.

Abysmally **low dietary intakes of B vitamins were found in high prevalence** in a meta-analysis, published in 2015, of 37 studies conducted in Europe, North America (the U.S. and Canada), Australia, and New Zealand, involving 28,000 adults (age 65 and above). Several B vitamin intakes in the older adults were reported as extremely low (folate 29% to 35%), vitamin B6 (24% to 31%), and riboflavin (31% to 41%).

Reference Daily Intake for B Vitamins		
B Vitamin	Men	Women
Riboflavin	1.3 mg	1.1 mg
Niacin	16 mg	14 mg
Folate	400 mcg	400 mcg
B6 (age 19 to 50)	1.3 mg	1.3 mg
B6 (age 51 and older)	1.7 mg	1.5 mg
B12 (age 14 and older)	2.4 mcg	2.4 mcg

Source: NIH Fact Sheet, Folate (ods.od.nih.gov/factsheets/Folate-HealthProfessional), World's Healthiest Foods (www.whfoods.org)

When we say *low* in the above study, we're talking *below the* Estimated Average Requirement (EAR), an intake level defined as where 50% of people are deficient. The Reference Daily Intake (RDI, see table above), which is supposed to cover the nutrient needs for 98% of the population, is simply the EAR increased by 20%.[929] So, you can see why we aren't big fans of relying upon the RDI recommendations to support optimal health.[930] We'll provide our recommendations for *optimal* levels of the B vitamins later in this chapter.

Other research reveals low dietary levels of specific B vitamins:

• Research utilizing data from the National Health and Nutrition Examination Survey (NHANES) 2005-2006 cycle found 31% of the U.S. population at risk of deficiency for at least one B vitamin or of anemia. *What are the leading causes of anemia?* Insufficiency of folate and/or B12 (in their active forms, whose production requires riboflavin and B6).[931 932 933]

• Low B6 status is quite common in the U.S., due in part to our love affair with refined grains and canned and frozen foods. Approximately 72% of B6 is lost when wheat flour is refined to white flour. Canning of vegetables, meat, fish, and poultry results in losses of 43% to 77% of B6. The B6 content of frozen vegetables is 37% to 45% less than fresh vegetables. B6 binds to proteins during heat processing producing compounds with *anti*-B6 activity.[934]

• Numerous population surveys have revealed B12 deficiency or far-below-optimal status in elders in the U.S. (6% deficient, more than 20% marginal status), Canada (5% deficient), U.K. (5% to 20% deficient), New Zealand (12% deficient, 28% marginal deficiency) and Finland (6% low and 32% borderline).[935]

Riboflavin deficiency should be far less common in the U.S. (just 2%) based on dietary intake.[936] However, dietary intake for this B vitamin may not translate to effective absorption and use by the body. That especially includes elders and anyone with digestive problems resulting in malabsorption, including those using the increasingly popular treatment for obesity, gastric bypass surgery.

- In the United Kingdom, dietary intake data found less than 10% of elders failed to consume recommended amounts. However, the results of biochemical data from labs evaluating riboflavin status in the 2012/2013 and 2013/2014 National Diet and Nutrition Surveys produced a very different picture: suboptimal riboflavin status in 49% and 78% of elders respectively.[937] Large surveys in the United States have found riboflavin deficiency in 10% to 27% of elders.[938]

The discrepancy between the dietary intake data of riboflavin and riboflavin's actual *functional* status in people age 65 and older may indicate that our ability to absorb nutrients decreases as we age, so the amount of riboflavin we need (and also how much B6, B12, niacin, and other nutrients as well) may increase.

Excessive Intake of Folic Acid Harms Our Health

Few of us eat foods rich in natural folate (tetrahydrofolate) such as leafy greens, beans, and Brussels sprouts. Yet, folate insufficiency is rare due to the fortification of processed foods with folic acid. However, this is *not* a good thing!

Unlike natural folate, folic acid is a synthetic precursor for folate which has no biological activity. Before folic acid can be used in the methylation cycle, a liver enzyme called *dihydrofolate reductase* must convert it into tetrahydrofolate. If this conversion doesn't occur, the excessive folic acid in processed foods and many lower quality supplements can cause serious problems.

Making matters worse, about 20% of us have inherited genes that produce less effective variations of this enzyme. putting us at an even higher risk of having high levels of unmetabolized folic acid in our bloodstream.[939] (See Box, SNPs that Affect Your Needs for Certain B Vitamins).

Consuming more folic acid than we can convert to folate has been linked to disease. This synthetic precursor floats around in the bloodstream, where studies show it promotes colon and breast cancers—an estimated 15,000 additional cancers per year in the U.S. alone. Even an amount less than 400 mcg of folic acid per day causes problems.[940 941]

- Since folic acid fortification in processed foods began, North America's downward trend in colorectal cancer incidence has reversed. Many experts now attribute this to excessive folic acid intake.

- The Prostate, Lung, Colorectal, and Ovarian Cancer Screening trial found that women who reported consuming 400 mcg or more of folic acid per day had a 20% greater risk of developing breast cancer. Although folic acid aids in normal DNA replication, researchers hypothesize that, in malignant cells, excess folic acid may cause cell proliferation.[942]

Unmetabolized folic acid has been shown to depress our immune defenses. A study by Canadian researchers in Ottawa, in collaboration with colleagues from the Fred Hutchinson Cancer Research Center in Seattle, WA, evaluated dietary folate and supplemental folic acid intakes in 105 healthy, postmenopausal women. Unmetabolized folic acid, detected in the blood of 78% of fasting participants, was inversely related to natural killer cell cytotoxicity (the ability of immune cells to kill their targets). In other words, this measure of immune function averaged 23% lower in the women with detectable folic acid in their blood. Furthermore, this inverse relation was stronger among women older than 60 and worsened as blood concentrations of unmetabolized folic acid increased.[943 944]

High folic acid intake can mask anemia due to vitamin B12 deficiency. This delays a diagnosis of B12 deficiency, which can cause irreversible neurological damage if not treated early. In a recent NHANES study involving close to 2,000 seniors, a combination of low vitamin B12 status and high blood levels of folic acid (>59 nmol/L) was associated with more than triple the risk of having anemia.[945]

Add folic acid as another reason to stay away from processed foods that harm our health. And make sure you avoid supplements that contain folic acid (discussed more below).

Certain Drugs and Genetic Variations Increase Your Needs for the B Vitamins

Our low intake and absorption of the B vitamins—critical for strong bones—puts us at the risk of deficiency, a problem that worsens as we age. On top of that, many of us have greater needs due to: (1) commonly used drugs that deplete B vitamins and (2) common genetic variations that impact the function of our enzymes, increasing our B vitamin needs.

1. **Various medications reduce the usable amount of certain B vitamins**, such as:

   Vitamin B12, which is depleted by *acid-blockers* and *metformin*:

   » **Acid-blocking medications,** including proton pump inhibitors (PPIs) and H2-receptor antagonists, suppress production of stomach acid, without which we cannot liberate nutrients from our food, including the B vitamins. Plus, these medications cause the lining of the stomach to atrophy. The end result is nutrient malabsorption, particularly that of B12, which is found only in animal-derived foods (meats, eggs, and dairy products).[946]

   » B12 requires stomach acid for its release plus the help of a carrier called *intrinsic factor*, which ferries B12 the entire length of the small intestine before it binds to receptors that enable its absorption into the bloodstream. The cells in the lining of the stomach that produce and release stomach acid, called parietal cells, are also responsible for secreting intrinsic factor. PPIs and H2-blockers prevent the secretion of both stomach acid and intrinsic factor, effectively preventing the absorption of B12. Not surprisingly, in case-control studies, these acid-blocking medications have been associated with up to 4.5 times higher risk of vitamin B12 deficiency.[947]

   - Recently, in the U.S., a large community survey (25,956 cases and 184,199 controls) found that the long-term use (>2 years) of H2-receptor antagonists and PPIs was associated with a 25% to 65% greater risk of a subsequent diagnosis of vitamin B12 deficiency.[948]

   - Their prevention of B12 absorption is one reason why acid-suppressing drugs lower bone density and increase the risk of fracture not just in elders but even in young adults. A population-based study of 124,799 cases and 605,643 controls found PPIs increase young adults' (aged 18 to 29 years) risk of fracture by 39%.[949][950][951]

» **Metformin**, which is used to manage pre-diabetes, type 2 diabetes, and polycystic ovary syndrome, causes vitamin B12 deficiency by interfering with the special receptors at the end of the small intestine to which the B12-intrinsic factor complex binds, thus preventing B12's absorption.[952]

Vitamin B6 is depleted by *anticonvulsants* and *oral contraceptives:*

» **Anticonvulsants**, particularly the class called *enzyme-inducing anti-epileptic drugs* (such as phenytoin and carbamazepine), cause B6 deficiency so severe that B6 levels were undetectable or nearly so in 30% of the patients evaluated. Enzyme-inducing anti-epileptic drugs are thought to deplete B6 by increasing its elimination in urine, either by increasing the activity of enzymes that prepare B6 for urinary excretion or by forming a complex with B6 that is then eliminated in the urine.[953]

» **Oral contraceptives** (i.e., *the Pill*) have adverse effects on vitamins and minerals which have been investigated in many studies beginning back in the 1960s. The consistent results caused The World Health Organization (WHO) to issue a report that oral contraceptives cause depletions of numerous key nutrients, including key B vitamins (folate, riboflavin, B6, and B12). Oral contraceptives inhibit folate's absorption, increase its excretion in urine, and increase the activity of the enzymes that prepare folate for elimination. These drugs also block B12's binding to *transcobalamin*, its carrier in the bloodstream, thus preventing B12's delivery throughout the body.[954]

2. **Your genetic inheritance may increase your needs for certain B vitamins**. SNPs (variations in our genes) that result in our production of less effective enzymes impact our B vitamin needs. The four best-studied SNPs are:

» MTHFR C677T and A1298C, which affect the ability to use folate

» rs70991108, which affects the ability to use folate and produce nitric oxide

» TCN2 C776G, which affects the ability to use B12

For details on how these variations, some of which are quite common, affect your needs and strategies to correct for those you may have, see the below box.

Genetic Variations that Affect Your Needs for Certain B Vitamins

Several common SNPs (genetic variations) affect our production or use of B vitamins, including a couple which involve the *methyltetrahydrofolate reductase* (MTHFR) enzyme, which plays an important role in the folate and methylation cycles. We produce a MTHFR enzyme that is far less effective if our genes are affected by one of two SNPs: **MTHFR C677T and A1298C** (though to a lesser degree). Individuals carrying either of these SNPs have lower BMD and are at greatly increased risk of fractures, as confirmed by meta-analyses of very large studies. MTHFR C677T alone more than doubles fracture risk.[955 956 957 958]

- **These two SNPs are very common.** About 50% of people carry at least one *mutant allele* (mutated gene) for MTHFR C677T (also called rs1801133), and 35% carry at least one mutant allele for MTHFR A1298C (rs1801131). That means 85% of people have SNPs that result in an MTHFR enzyme with below-normal activity.

A slow MTHFR interferes with methylation, increasing levels of bone-destructive homocysteine and decreasing production of bone-protective glutathione. I (Lara) have inherited the mutant versions of *both* of these SNPs, each of which increases my risk for osteoporosis, cardiovascular disease, and dementia.

How did I correct for these SNPs and overcome my reduced ability to produce the active form of folate (5-MTHF)?

1. **By eating plenty of folate-rich foods.** Fully saturating my slow MTHFR enzyme with lots of folate helps improve its activity. The reason for this is a foundational law in biochemistry called the Michaelis constant (KM), which shows that when an enzyme is badly formed (as is my MTHFR), it will be less active in part because of its lessened ability to bind to the substrate it acts upon (in this case, folate). Supplying plenty of folate enables more to become bound, which lets the enzyme work better.

2. By taking an *active B complex* to get all the B vitamins in their ready-for-action forms.

Another common SNP affects the gene that produces *dihydrofolate reductase*, the enzyme that converts folic acid to folate and also helps us improve blood flow by producing nitric oxide.

- **rs70991108: Twenty percent are homozygous for this SNP**, meaning they've inherited both alleles that decrease the activity of their dihydrofolate reductase enzyme. A less effective dihydrofolate reductase enzyme is less able to convert biologically *inactive* folic acid to biologically *active* folate and won't produce blood-flow-increasing nitric oxide.

Studies show that older individuals with this SNP are at increased risk of having high levels of unmetabolized folic acid in the bloodstream, a potentially very dangerous outcome. If you are among the 1 in 5 people whose genetic inheritance includes rs70991108, eat a diet rich in leafy greens and legumes, and take supplements containing folate, not folic acid, which should be avoided.

About 20% of the population carry a SNP affecting *transcobalamin*, a protein required for the transport, cellular uptake, and utilization of cobalamin (B12):

- **TCN2, rs1801198** (also called 776G>C) results in a reduced ability to bind B12. Since the *fix* for this problem is getting plenty of B12, so at least some of it binds to transcobalamin, the B12 needs for 20% of the population are likely significantly higher than the RDI. One study of elderly individuals with low B12 status found that a dose of 500 mcg/d was not sufficient to normalize the B12 status in 8% to 23% of participants, a portion who may have been carriers of TCN2 776G>C.

If B12 is not available in its active form (methylcobalamin), homocysteine accumulates. In the same way, a compound called *methylmalonic acid* accumulates when *adenosylcobalamin* (another important form of B12) isn't available for its use in energy production in our mitochondria.

When B12 (as adenosylcobalamin) isn't available, levels of a compound called methylmalonic acid accumulate in our cells. It spills into the bloodstream and is eliminated in urine, making it a useful marker of B12 insufficiency. People with SNPs in

TCN2 776 have been found to have higher levels of urinary methylmalonic acid. The *fix* for this is supplemental B12 in the form of adenosylcobalamin.[959][960]

Is Your Diet Providing You with the B Vitamins Your Bones Need?

Keep a food diary for five to seven days, then use the tables below to see how much of the various B vitamins your *normal* diet is providing. In the next section, we share our recommendations for *optimal* levels and what to look for in a B vitamin supplement (which you will likely need).

Best Food Sources of B9 (Folate)		
Food	Serving Size	B9 (mcg)
Soy beans, edamame, organic, cooked	½ cup	311
Cranberry beans, organic, cooked	½ cup	183
Asparagus, organic, cooked from fresh	6 spears	149
Pinto beans, organic, cooked,	½ cup	147
Garbanzo beans, organic, cooked	½ cup	141
Lettuce, romaine, organic, raw	1½ cups	136
Spinach, organic, cooked	½ cup	131
Black beans, organic, cooked	½ cup	128
Navy beans, organic, cooked	½ cup	127
Red kidney beans, organic, cooked	½ cup	115
Brussels sprouts, organic, cooked	1 cup	94
Artichoke, organic	1 (128 grams)	90
Great Northern beans, organic, cooked	½ cup	90
Cranberry beans, organic, cooked	½ cup	183
Soybeans, edamame, organic, cooked	½ cup	311
Peanuts, organic, dry roasted, 1 ounce	1 ounce	41
Egg, free-range, 1 large, hard-boiled	22	22
Halibut, cooked	3 ounces	12
Crab, Dungeness	3 ounces	36
Orange, organic, fresh	1 small	29
Papaya, raw, cubed	½ cup	27
Banana, organic	1 medium	24

Best Food Sources of B9 (Folate)

Food	Serving Size	B9 (mcg)
Cantaloupe, organic	1 wedge	14
Milk, organic, grass fed, whole	1 cup	12

Best Food Sources of B12 (Cobalamin)

Food	Serving Size	B12 (mcg)
Sardines	3.2 ounces	8.11
Salmon, wild-caught, Alaskan, broiled	4 ounces	5.67
Tuna, yellow-fin	4 ounces	4.66
Cod	4 ounces	2.62
Shrimp	4 ounces	1.88
Scallops	4 ounces	2.44
Lamb, organic, grass fed	4 ounces	2.51
Beef, organic, grass fed	4 ounces	1.44
Yogurt, organic, grass fed, whole milk	1 cup	0.91
Cow's milk, organic, grass fed	½ cup	0.55

Best Food Sources of B6 (Pyridoxine)

Food	Serving Size	B6 (mcg)
Tuna, yellowfin	4 ounces	1.18
Turkey, pasture-raised, light meat, roasted	4 ounces	0.92
Beef, organic, grass fed	4 ounces	0.74
Chicken, pasture-raised, breast, baked	4 ounces	0.68
Salmon, wild-caught Alaskan, broiled	4 ounces	0.64
Sweet potato, organic	1 cup	0.57
Potatoes, organic	1 cup	0.54
Sunflower seeds, organic	¼ cup	0.47
Spinach, organic, cooked	1 cup	0.44
Banana, organic	1 medium	0.43

Best Food Sources of B2 (Riboflavin)		
Food	Serving Size	B2 (mg)
Soybeans, organic, cooked	1 cup	0.49
Tempeh, organic, cooked	4 ounces	0.40
Spinach, organic, cooked	1 cup	0.42
Beet greens, organic, cooked	1 cup	0.42
Asparagus, organic, cooked	1 cup	0.25
Mushrooms, Crimini, organic, raw	1 cup	0.35
Eggs, organic, free-range, hard-boiled	1 large	0.26
Yogurt, organic, grass-fed, whole milk	1 cup	0.35
Almonds, organic, sliced, raw	¼ cup	0.23
Turkey, pasture-raised, light meat, roasted	4 ounces	0.23

Best Food Sources of B3 (Niacin)		
Food	Serving Size	B3 (mg)
Tuna, yellow-fin, baked	4 ounces	25.03
Chicken, pasture-raised, breast, roasted	4 ounces	15.55
Turkey, pasture-raised, light meat, roasted	4 ounces	13.32
Salmon, wild-caught, Alaskan, broiled	4 ounces	9.02
Lamb, grass-fed, lean, roasted	4 ounces	8.05
Beef, grass-fed, strip steak, cooked	4 ounces	7.06
Sardines, Atlantic, canned	3.2 ounces	4.76
Peanuts, organic, raw	¼ cup	4.40
Shrimp, large, steamed	4 ounces	3.04
Brown rice, organic, long-grain, cooked	1 cup	2.98

Source for all of the above tables: NIH Fact Sheet, Folate (ods.od.nih.gov/factsheets/Fo-late-HealthProfessional), World's Healthiest Foods (www.whfoods.org)

Optimal Levels of B Vitamins and What to Look for in a Supplement

As with many nutrients, the Recommended Dietary Allowances (RDAs) for the five B vitamins are largely insufficient. Our B vitamin needs increase as we age and are often depleted by certain drugs. Add to this the fact that several common SNPs significantly affect our B vitamin needs, and you won't be surprised to learn that deficiencies in all of the B vitamins are frequently seen in the U.S. population overall and increase dramatically with age.

See below the dosages we recommend for optimal health. The table also provides the RDA for comparison, along with dosage levels used in studies. Stay below the safe upper limit for daily consumption set for folic acid, niacin, and B6.

Optimal Dose Range for B Vitamins					
B Vitamin	RDI for Men	RDI for Women	Safe Upper Limit	Researched Doses	Recommended Dose
Folic acid*	400 mcg		1,000 mcg	0.5 to 5.0 mg	Less than 400 mcg
Folate	400 mcg		None	0.5 to 5.0 mg	400 mcg as MTHF
B6	1.3 mg <50		100 mg	10 to 200 mg	25 mg as P5P
	1.7 mg	1.5 mg			
B12	2.4 mcg		None	100 to 1,000 mcg	500 mcg as methylco-balamin
Riboflavin	1.3 mg	1.1 mg	None	15 to 50 mg**	10 mg as riboflavin-5-phosphate
Niacin	16 mg	14 mg	35 mg	250 to 500 mg/d	100 mg as inositol hexanicotinate***

*Individuals who have inherited the rs70991108 SNP for the dihydrofolate reductase enzyme should not consume supplemental folic acid.

**The maximum dose of riboflavin that can be absorbed at one time is 25 mg, so if more is used, it should be in divided doses.

***Do not use time-release niacin, a formulation that was developed to minimize flushing, but which has been reported to cause reversible liver damage in large doses (1-3 grams/day). Use inositol hexanicotinate, a form of niacin that does not cause flushing; nor has it been found to cause liver damage in doses of 2 to 4 grams per day, which are the doses of this form of niacin used in the research.

Source: Nutritional Medicine, Vitamin B6...[961]; Vitamins and the Brain...[962]

Choose a B vitamin supplement that provides the activated forms of folate, B6, and B12. Most of us have inherited SNPs that greatly lessen our ability to convert these vitamins into their active forms. Therefore, we suggest supplementing with 5-MTHF (folate), P5P (B6), and methylcobalamin (B12), so you have the forms needed to enable methylation and bone-supporting functions.

Do not take supplements containing folic acid: Many Americans have unacceptably high levels of unmetabolized folic acid. Of those taking folic acid-containing supplements, 80% have detectable levels of unmetabolized folic acid in their blood. Particularly in older adults, high blood levels of unmetabolized folic acid are associated with signs of B12 deficiency, including cognitive impairment and anemia. Older women, a group research shows are consuming folic acid above the UL, are also more susceptible to vitamin B12 deficiency because of malabsorption issues and may be covering up anemia caused by lack of B12 with excessive folic acid intake.

Take a *full-spectrum* active B complex to avoid *The Folate Trap*. Remember our discussion of *The Methylation Show*? During the first stage of the methylation cycle, a methyl is added to folate to produce 5-methyl-THF, which can then transfer the methyl group to B12, converting it into methylcobalamin to continue the cycle.

- *But what happens if B12 is not available?* The concentration of 5-MTHF continues to rise, though with nowhere to hand off the available methyl groups. This metabolic dead-end situation is called the *folate trap* (or methyl trap) and shuts down the methylation cycle. Even if you have B12, the folate and methylation cycle can become derailed if you lack folate (or the B6, riboflavin, and niacin needed to convert THF to 5-MTHF). If you're taking a supplement containing the active form of folate (5-MTHF), you must always supplement with B12. Note that B12 supplementation can increase folate requirements and aggravate folate insufficiency. And folate supplementation increases B6 and riboflavin requirements.

In short, *all of these B vitamins* are required for proper function and healthy bones.[963]

B Vitamins Safety

The B vitamins are water-soluble, so any excess is rapidly excreted in urine. All are well accepted to be safe at much higher doses than the RDA (with one exception, folic acid as discussed below). However, a daily safe upper limit has been set for the following 3 B vitamins:

- **Niacin:** The upper limit for niacin is 35 mg/d in the U.S. and Canada, due only to niacin's ability to cause temporary skin flushing at doses greater than 100 mg. However, long-term daily consumption of 1,000 mg or more has caused nausea, vomiting, diarrhea, and (very rarely) liver damage.

- **Vitamin B6:** The upper limit for B6 is 100 mg/d (about 75 × the RDA). This level was set because of a few case reports of *reversible* sensory neuropathy (numbness or tingling, typically in the feet or hands) following doses *greater than 1,000 mg/d* taken for *extended periods*. However, multiple clinical trials have demonstrated a *complete lack* of such effects, even when participants consumed up to *750 mg/d* for a number of *years*.

- **Folic acid and folate:** The upper limit for both is generally set at 1,000 mcg/day because increasing folate *by itself* can mask the symptoms of vitamin B12 deficiency. That includes nerve damage, which can become irreversible if this deficiency is not treated.

As we saw earlier, folic acid presents the greatest concern. Doses greater than 400 mcg/d can result in high levels of unmetabolized folic acid floating around in the bloodstream, which accumulating evidence indicates may lower immune function and promote cancer. Natural folate, however, has not been found to cause harm. The most important takeaways from all this is: Avoid supplements containing folic acid! And ensure your B12 status is adequate.[964][965]

BONE-HEALTHY ACTION ITEMS

- Use a food diary to determine your dietary intake of B vitamins.
- Take a full-spectrum, active B supplement to get all of the B vitamins in their active forms.
- Choose supplements with folate and avoid those containing folic acid.
- Medications and genetics can affect your B vitamin status. Consider testing. (See Lab Tests, Chapter 10.)

Vitamin C

BONE ESSENTIALS

- Vitamin C plays critical roles in producing osteoblasts and synthesizing collagen.
- Studies show vitamin C helps us maintain BMD as we age and reduce the risk of hip and other fractures.
- Our risk for vitamin C deficiency increases as we age, and for those who are overweight, smoke, or are exposed to second-hand smoke or other environmental toxins.

During the great sea voyages of the 15th to 18th centuries, the lack of vitamin C (a condition later named scurvy) killed an estimated two million seamen. Scurvy ravages the body and mind within months, causing blistering skin, previously healed bones to rebreak, and more gruesome symptoms we'll spare you from here. Our point is simply that you need vitamin C.[966]

While most animals and plants can synthesize this essential vitamin, some mammals, including humans require a dietary source. While the RDA amount of vitamin C is enough to prevent a disease-causing deficiency, research shows you need 10 to 20 times that amount (or more) to produce a host of benefits for healthy bones.

What Vitamin C Does for Your Bones

Vitamin C, a powerful antioxidant, neutralizes the two major types of free radicals: reactive oxygen species (ROS) and reactive nitrogen species (RNS). Plus, vitamin C recycles other antioxidants, including vitamin E and glutathione, so they can be used again. (See Vitamin E, Chapter 7.)

Glutathione is so essential that our cells produce it. Without adequate glutathione, they die. Not only is glutathione an antioxidant, but it works in the liver where it converts many extremely dangerous toxins into water-soluble compounds we can eliminate in urine.[967] Estrogen boosts glutathione production, so postmenopausal women produce less. Vitamin C helps restore glutathione to premenopausal levels.[968 969 970 971]

Vitamin C is required for collagen formation. Vitamin C is the co-factor for the *dioxygenase enzymes*, which are required for our synthesis of collagen. Since more than 90% of the protein in the bone matrix is collagen, vitamin C is an essential nutrient for healthy bones.

Vitamin C boosts osteoblast production and activity. Vitamin C stimulates the production of mesenchymal stem cells (MSCs), the precursor cells for osteoblasts, and promotes their development into mature osteoblasts. Then, it increases osteoblasts' production of:

- **bone alkaline phosphatase**, an enzyme involved in new bone formation
- **osteocalcin**, the protein that, once activated by vitamin K2, binds calcium and brings it into our bones
- **osteopontin**, a protein that helps osteoclasts develop their ruffled borders, so they can anchor to the mineral matrix in bone and begin bone resorption. Remember, before new healthy bone can be laid down, old, brittle, or damaged bone must be removed.
- **osteonectin**, a protein osteoblasts secrete during bone formation that binds calcium, initiating mineralization and the formation of hydroxyapatite crystals
- **runt-related transcription factor 2** (RunX2 a.k.a. core-binding factor subunit alpha-1 [CBF-alpha-1]), a protein without which osteoblast differentiation cannot occur
- **bone sialoprotein** (BSP), which constitutes approximately 8% of all non-collagen proteins found in bone. BSP directs the formation of the first apatite crystals produced as new bone is developed. These apatite crystals are the inorganic component of bone tissue and give bones their ability to withstand compression without breaking.[972][973]

If you smoke or are exposed to secondhand smoke, vitamin C is especially important for your bones. Cigarette smoke harms bone, in part, through nicotine's effects on both MSCs and mature osteoblasts. Except at very low levels, nicotine inhibits MSC development into osteoblasts and blocks mature osteoblasts' production of key proteins used to build new bone, including osteocalcin and collagen type I. Vitamin C greatly increases the amount of nicotine needed to inhibit osteoblast activity.[974]

Vitamin C Helps Maintain BMD as We Age

Studies have shown associations between vitamin C consumption at levels above the RDA and higher bone density for both postmenopausal women and aging men:

- A group of 334 elderly men (average age 75) were followed for four years. Those with the highest total (dietary and supplemental) vitamin C intake lost the least bone mineral density (BMD).[975]

- In another study, men with the highest dietary vitamin C intake (above 300 mg/day) had significantly less bone loss than men in the lowest group of vitamin C intake, who were consuming 106 mg/day, a clear indication that the current RDA of 90 mg for men is far from optimal.[976]

- A study of 1,196 postmenopausal women (age 50 years and over) found strong associations between dietary vitamin C intake and bone mineral density at all sites evaluated: the lumbar spine, femoral neck, and total hip. The women with osteoporosis consumed far less dietary vitamin C (less than 46 mg/d) than did those without osteoporosis (who consumed *at least* 94 mg/d). For those women age 50 to 59 years or 70 years or older who were also found deficient in vitamin D, consuming less than 100 mg/d of vitamin C correlated with a 79% increase in risk for osteoporosis![977]

Vitamin C is associated with a lower risk of hip and other osteoporotic fractures. The longest trial reported to date is the Framingham Osteoporosis Study, in which 366 men and 592 women (average age of 75) were followed for 15 to 17 years. Study participants were divided into 3 groups according to their total vitamin C intake (dietary and supplemental). Those in the group consuming the most vitamin C (an average of 313 mg/d) had a 69% lower risk of hip fracture compared with the group consuming the least vitamin C intake (an average of 94 mg/d).[978]

How Much Vitamin C Do We Need?

The RDA for vitamin C, 75 mg/day for adult women and 90 mg/day for adult men, is inadequate. You may have noticed in the research above that higher amounts than this were needed for beneficial effects. These amounts were set back in 1996 using healthy volunteers. In addition, vitamin C gets used up much more rapidly not just in acute illness, but with chronic inflammation, which affects the majority of us over age 50 and plays a major role in osteoporosis.[979 980 981 982]

Our prehistoric ancestors are thought to have consumed 2.3 grams or more of vitamin C daily, and many of today's leading clinicians believe doses ranging from 1,000 to 2,000 mg/d are optimal for most people. This level of vitamin C intake is quite safe: the UL (tolerable upper limit) for vitamin C is 3,000 mg/d, and the research evidence suggests that intakes up to 4,000 mg/d are well tolerated in the general population.[983 984]

What increases your need for vitamin C and risk of deficiency?

- **Being overweight.** Excess adipose (fat) tissue is not an inert storage depot for extra calories; it spews out signaling molecules called *adipokines*, which increase free radical production, thus increasing your needs for vitamin C.[985]

- **Exposure to environmental toxins.** In addition to cigarette smokers, those exposed to secondhand smoke or other environmental toxins (e.g., smog, lead, mercury, cadmium, arsenic, pesticide residues, benzene, BPA, phthalates, plasticizers, and many more) are at increased risk for vitamin C deficiency. Discussing each of these would take another book—fortunately, Joe has recently published one: *The Toxin Solution.*

- **Aging.** As we age, our liver cells produce fewer of the proteins that help us transport vitamin C around the body (called the *sodium-dependent vitamin C transporters* or SVCTs).[986 987]

- **Taking oral contraceptives.** Oral contraceptives decrease blood levels of vitamin C and also deplete other nutrients: folate; vitamins B2, B6, B12, and E; and the minerals magnesium, selenium, and zinc. The good news is that supplementing with vitamins C and E can lessen some of oral contraceptives' adverse effects on your antioxidant status, which would otherwise increase your risk for cardiovascular disease and osteoporosis.[988 989]

Can We Get Enough Vitamin C from Diet?

The recommended 5 servings per day of fruits and vegetables provide only around 200 mg of vitamin C. And few Americans consume even that. Furthermore, the amount of vitamin C in produce depends upon its quality and freshness. Fresh fruits and vegetables can take a week to 10 days to get to your grocery store, losing much of their vitamin C en route. The vitamin C content of prepared foods is even lower because food processing greatly decreases vitamin C content.[990]

Add as much dietary vitamin C to your menu as possible. Then, use the chart below to determine how close you are to achieving an optimal daily intake of 1,000 to 2,000 mg.

Best Food Sources of Vitamin C		
Fruit	**Serving Size**	**Vitamin C (mg)**
Acerola cherry	1 cup	1,644
Papaya	1 medium	168
Strawberries	1 cup	85
Orange, naval	1 medium	82
Pineapple	1 cup	79
Kiwi	1 2-inch fruit	64
Mango	1 cup	60
Cantaloupe	1 cup	59
Grapefruit, pink	½ medium	38
Raspberries	1 cup	32
Lemons & limes	¼ cup	24
Blueberries	1 cup	14
Avocado	1 cup	15
Banana	1 medium	10
Kale	1 cup, chopped	80
Brussels sprouts	1 cup	75
Sweet potato	1, medium	40
Beet greens	1 cup	36
Collards	1 cup	35
Swiss chard	1 cup	32
Potato	1 cup	17
Onion	1 cup	11
Beets	1 cup	6

Source: World's Healthiest Foods (bit.ly/WHF-VitaminC)

What to Look for in a Vitamin C Supplement

If you're like most of us, your dietary intake of vitamin C is likely to be below 1,000 to 2,000 mg/d. If so, consider taking supplemental vitamin C to achieve this level or more based on your specific needs. Here are our recommendations for getting the most out of your supplement:

Vitamin C is best taken in several smaller doses throughout the day. As you consume more at once, the fractional absorption of vitamin C decreases. When 200 mg is consumed, 100% is absorbed. When 1,250 mg is taken all at once, less than 50% is absorbed.[991] Products with a smaller amount of vitamin C per tablet or capsule, or those in powder form, will allow you to better customize your dosage.

Ascorbic acid is the form of vitamin C we recommend. Vitamin C is offered in different formulations, designed to improve bioavailability, reduce stomach upset, or otherwise improve effectiveness. We'll explain more about those varieties below, though most have not shown a significant difference over ascorbic acid or have other downsides.

Ascorbic acid supplements are 100% vitamin C, so the amount shown on the label is the amount of vitamin C they deliver per dose. They tend to be the least expensive supplemental form. Though an *acid*, it's a very weak one that doesn't cause stomach upset for most people. Those highly sensitive to acid may experience gas or loose stools when taking larger amounts. However, the reaction can easily be prevented by taking 3 to 6 smaller doses throughout the day, with meals or snacks. As mentioned, this improves absorption over a larger dose anyway.

Ascorbic acid is also the preferable choice over buffered versions when taking large doses (3,000 mg/d) of vitamin C, such as to fight infections, such as colds or flu. Taking several 1,000 mg doses of a mineral ascorbate (discussed next) could result in excessive consumption of sodium, calcium, or magnesium.

Vitamin C is also available in the following forms:

- **Mineral ascorbates (buffered vitamin C)** contain ascorbate ions bound to a mineral—typically calcium, sodium, or magnesium. Since they are not acidic, they are less likely to cause gastrointestinal distress. Stomach acid (hydrochloric acid) breaks down and further converts the mineral ascorbates into ascorbic acid and the previously bound mineral. That's one of the reasons stomach acid is required for healthy bones. For this same reason, if you are taking an acid-blocking medication, your ability to digest and absorb vitamin C from a mineral ascorbate will be impaired.

Mineral ascorbate supplements differ in the amount of minerals and vitamin C they contain. You'll need to check the label to see the amount of vitamin C and other minerals you're getting.[992]

Sodium ascorbate should not be used by anyone with high blood pressure or chronic kidney disease. High salt intake increases blood pressure in susceptible individuals (those who have chronic kidney disease, are older than age 50, or are African-American), accelerates loss of kidney function and protein loss in the urine in CKD patients, increases water retention (edema) in individuals with kidney or heart failure, and in population studies, has been shown to increase blood pressure as well as the risk of stroke or heart attack.[993]

- **Ascorbic acid with vitamin C metabolites (Ester-C®).** One company offers calcium ascorbate accompanied by small amounts of vitamin C metabolites, which are claimed to increase vitamin C's bioavailability. These metabolites include dehydroascorbic acid (oxidized ascorbic acid), calcium threonate, and trace levels of xylonate and lyxonate.

  One small study involving 36 participants found Ester-C slightly improved vitamin C concentrations in leukocytes (an average of 7.73 µg/mL compared to 6.37 µg/mL seen with ascorbic acid), but there were no differences in Tmax (the time it takes for maximal concentration to be reached) or Cmax (the highest concentration reached in the blood after a dose is given). Plasma vitamin C concentrations seen with Ester-C and ascorbic acid were similar, increasing rapidly during the first 4 hours post-dose, peaking at 4 hours then dropping. Other studies have also reported no difference in plasma vitamin C concentrations after a single dose of 1,000 mg vitamin C given in the form of Ester-C or ascorbic acid. The rate of urinary excretion was not checked in this study, but in others, has not differed between Ester-C and ascorbic acid tablets.[994]

- **Vitamin C with bioflavonoids.** In animal studies, vitamin C's absorption and transport to organs are significantly increased by bioflavonoids such as hesperidin, rutin, and catechin, which are naturally present in flavonoid-rich fruits and vegetables. However, human studies have shown little difference between the bioavailability of synthetic vitamin C and that from different fruits, fruit juices, and vegetables.

Overall, the research suggests that when supplementing with vitamin C, we can save money and simply use inexpensive ascorbic acid in tablet or powder form.[995]

Vitamin C Safety

Reviews of the medical research conducted by different authors have consistently found that vitamin C is safe at intakes of 2,000 mg/d. Numerous studies of vitamin C supplementation have provided no substantive evidence to support concerns about safety other than occasional gastrointestinal upset or mild diarrhea. Similar to unabsorbed magnesium, (see Magnesium, chapter 5), unabsorbed vitamin C can cause mild osmotic diarrhea by drawing water into the bowels. The UL for vitamin C, set primarily to avoid osmotic diarrhea, is 3,000 mg/d.[996]

On various websites, you're likely to see a list of hypothetical adverse effects, including claims that vitamin C might increase oxalate and kidney stone formation, increase uric acid concentrations and risk of gout, cause excess iron absorption, reduce vitamin B12 concentrations, induce *rebound* scurvy, or exert pro-oxidant effects. These have been examined in detail and found to have *no substantive basis*. According to the most current review of the research, published by the Linus Pauling Institute at Oregon State, "There is no reliable scientific evidence that large amounts of vitamin C (up to 10 grams/day in adults) are toxic or detrimental to health."[997]

Vitamin C does have some interactions with drugs:

- **Aluminum-containing antacids**: If taken at the same time as aluminum hydroxide medications, vitamin C may increase absorption of aluminum, a neurotoxin known to contribute to the development of Alzheimer's disease and osteoporosis.[998]

- **Propranolol**: Do not take vitamin C for at least 2 hours before or after taking propranolol. Taking 2 grams of vitamin C thirty minutes before taking propranolol reduced its bioavailability. (Propranolol is a beta-blocker used to manage high blood pressure, irregular heart rate, hyperthyroidism, performance anxiety, and essential tremors. It's also used to prevent migraine headaches and further heart problems in individuals with angina or who have had a previous heart attack.)

- **Proton-pump inhibitors**: One capsule prevents stomach acid production for up to 24 hours, also preventing absorption and decreasing blood levels of vitamin C (and other nutrients).

- **Tetracyclines**: Do not take vitamin C at the same time as tetracycline. Administration of 500 mg of vitamin C along with 250 mg of tetracycline increased the blood level of the drug by 3- to 15-fold after 2 hours.

- **Warfarin**: Large doses of vitamin C may increase the dosage of warfarin required. Only 2 case reports have suggested this possibility, though err on the side of caution. For best absorption of vitamin C, you should be taking smaller doses (250 to 500 mg) several times a day anyway. These lower amounts have never been suggested to interfere with warfarin dosage.[999]

BONE-HEALTHY ACTION ITEMS

- For full benefits, get the clinician-recommended 1,000 to 2,000 mg/d of vitamin C from diet and supplements.
- Take vitamin C in several doses of 250 to 500 mg throughout the day for better absorption.
- We recommend taking ascorbic acid, the least expensive form of supplemental vitamin C.

Vitamin E

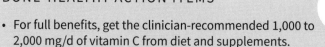

BONE ESSENTIALS

- Natural vitamin E is a family of 8 interactive compounds—4 tocopherols and 4 tocotrienols— which protect the *lipids* (fats) in our bodies against damage by free radicals.
- Most vitamin E supplements contain only alpha-tocopherol, which is not only less effective but, at high doses, can increase inflammation and promote bone loss.

- Natural vitamin E (mixed tocopherols and tocotrienols) has been shown to benefit bone mineral density.
- Elders (age 65 and older) whose diets provide about 550 IU/d of *natural* vitamin E have significantly better immune responses and resistance to infectious diseases.

Vitamin E is an antioxidant that protects the *lipids* (fats) in our bodies against damage by free radicals. Lipids play a critical role as structural components of cell membranes. Our neurons are loaded with lipids— the human brain is nearly 60% fat.[1000] The omega-3 and omega-6 essential fatty acids are lipids. So is cholesterol, which is *essential* for your body to produce vitamin D and make hormones like estrogen, testosterone, and adrenal hormones.

By protecting lipids against free radical damage, vitamin E helps protect our bones from the excessive activation of osteoclasts that cause bone loss.[1001 1002 1003]

Vitamin E is a Family of 8 Interactive Compounds— Not Just Alpha-tocopherol

Most supplements provide vitamin E in the form of *alpha-tocopherol*. However, the vitamin E found naturally in foods consists of *tocopherols* and *tocotrienols,* 4 varieties of each differentiated by a Greek letter prefix: alpha (α-), beta (β-), gamma (γ-) or delta (δ-). Each of these 8 versions of vitamin E has both unique and complementary biological actions. Consider the two different basic types of free radicals our bodies must neutralize:

- α-*tocopherol* can stop *reactive oxygen species (ROS).*
- γ-*tocopherol* is required to defuse *reactive nitrogen species (RNS).*

Furthermore, vitamin E only works part-time as an antioxidant; many of its benefits, particularly its beneficial effects on our bones, are due to the actions that each of the eight vitamin E isomers has on the enzymes and signaling molecules directing what goes on inside our cells.

High-dose α-tocopherol is not only less effective but can increase inflammation. High dose α-tocopherol suppresses blood levels of γ-tocopherol, causing them to drop by 30% to 70%. This promotes inflammation because γ-tocopherol disarms RNS, a class of free radicals that α-tocopherol cannot. Gamma-tocopherol, though not α-tocopherol, lowers levels of *C-reactive protein*, a key marker associated with cardiovascular disease and bone loss. (See Lab Tests, Chapter 10.)[1004 1005 1006 1007]

Studies demonstrate that α-tocopherol alone:

- **stimulates osteoclast activity and bone resorption, and induces osteoporosis**. These adverse effects are significant and occur rapidly. In an 8-week study, animals that were fed high dose α-tocopherol alone had a 20% decrease in bone mass caused by an increase in osteoclast size and bone resorption.[1008]

- **decreases blood levels of bone-specific alkaline phosphatase (BSAP)**. In postmenopausal women, vitamin E supplementation—in the form of α-tocopherol alone—decreases blood levels of BSAP, an enzyme involved in the formation of new bone. A study involving 497 postmenopausal women (average age 65) found that the 45% who used vitamin E (α-tocopherol only) supplements had significantly lower blood levels of γ-tocopherol and lower bone-specific alkaline phosphate levels. The authors noted that α-tocopherol supplementation suppressed γ-tocopherol, and that decrease itself might negatively affect bone formation.[1009]

- **interferes with vitamin K's bone-building effects.** α-tocopherol increases the rate at which vitamin K is excreted from the body and lessens vitamin K1's conversion to vitamin K2. Alpha-tocopherol and vitamin K1 compete for the use of the same enzymes, including the enzyme (UBIAD1) that changes vitamin K1 into the MK-4 form of K2. Vitamin K2 is the form that activates two proteins regulating our use of calcium: osteocalcin, which brings calcium into bone, and matrix Gla protein, which prevents calcium from depositing in soft tissues. (See Vitamin K, Chapter 5.) When too much α-tocopherol is present, our ability to produce K2 is undercut.[1010 1011 1012]

Natural Vitamin E is Associated with Higher BMD and Lower Fracture Risk

Studies looking at dietary increases of vitamin E show several positive effects on bone mass and strength. Note that these studies often use α-tocopherol as a measure. However, because the vitamin E is from diet (not supplements), we know the foods provide the full complement of tocopherols and tocotrienols.

- A study involving 2,178 women (aged 40 to 75) found those whose diets contained the most vitamin E had the highest BMD—an average greater BMD of 2.5% in the lumbar spine, 3.06% in the total hip, 3.41% in the intertrochanter (upper femur), and 3.54% in the neck of the femur. Similar positive associations were observed between BMD at each of the studied bone sites and blood levels of α-tocopherol (the only vitamin E compound checked although dietary vitamin E was being studied). Average BMD levels were 1.24% to 4.83% greater in the women whose blood levels of α-tocopherol were highest. Since vitamin E naturally provided in foods delivers 5 times as much γ-tocopherol as α-tocopherol, a high level of α-tocopherol from food indicates an even higher level of γ-tocopherol.[1013]

- A large epidemiologic study looked at the possible association between dietary intake of α-tocopherol (and therefore of all the natural vitamin E compounds) and fracture risk in 61,433 perimenopausal women. When vitamin E intake was lower than 5 mg/d, the risk for hip fracture increased 86%, and the risk for any fracture increased 20%.[1014][1015]

- A study involving 232 postmenopausal women found those with osteoporosis had much lower blood levels of vitamin E than those with healthy bones.[1016]

How Much Vitamin E Do You Need?

The Recommended Dietary Allowance (RDA) for vitamin E is currently set at 15 mg/d (22 IU/d) of α-tocopherol for adults (aged 19 and older).[1017] Current evidence *strongly* suggests that the RDA is far too low to protect against the increasing free radical damage typically seen with aging or to support healthy immune function, which is typically compromised as we age.[1018][1019][1020]

Recommended dosages range from 150 IU to 400 IU of α-tocopherol per day or even higher in the peer-reviewed medical literature, though no consensus has been reached about the exact daily intake of vitamin

E for optimal health protection. The medical researchers publishing the most current papers on vitamin E believe that the scientific evidence is strong enough to recommend daily intakes of at least 150 IU of α-tocopherol per day.[1021]

Since foods rich in vitamin E contain 5 times as much γ-tocopherol as α-tocopherol, this translates to an intake of mixed tocopherols and tocotrienols of as much as 750 IU per day. While this amount may sound high, research in healthy elders shows that 4 months of supplementation with 800 IU of vitamin E (α-tocopherol) per day had no adverse effects.[1022] Furthermore, a solid body of peer-reviewed medical literature has demonstrated that vitamin E is safe in amounts up to 1600 IU/day, significantly above the Food and Nutrition Board's upper limit of 1,000 IU for α-tocopherol.[1023] [1024]

If you are not regularly consuming vitamin E-rich foods, you are likely to be deficient in this important bone-health nutrient. In several studies, more than 40% of elderly participants (aged 65 to 98 years) were found to have intakes of vitamin E less than 10 mg per day (just two thirds of the seriously inadequate RDA). In other studies, data have shown that elderly people, as well as laboratory and farm animals, benefited from diets that contain *more than five times the RDA* of vitamin E for their species. For humans, that translates to 110 IU/d of α-tocopherol or 550 IU/d mixed tocopherols (5 times as much). The people and animals had significantly better immune responses and increased resistance to infectious diseases compared to non-supplemented controls.

This makes sense as our immune cells (T cells and B cells) are enriched with vitamin E to protect themselves against the free radicals (ROS and RNS) these cells produce to destroy pathogens. Both T and B cells are produced inside our bones. T-cells originate from bone marrow and mature in the thymus; B-cells originate and mature in bone marrow.[1025]

Your need for vitamin E is greater if you are taking a bisphosphonate. If you are taking a nitrogen-bisphosphonate, your need for γ-tocopherol will be increased as these drugs greatly depress levels of both γ-tocopherol and CoQ10. Nitrogen-containing bisphosphonates include pamidronate/APD, neridronate, olpadronate, alendronate, ibandronate, risedronate, and zoledronate.[1026]

Best Food Sources of Vitamin E and What to Look For in a Supplement

The chart below shows the best food sources of vitamin E. While the amounts listed are for α-tocopherols, these foods contain natural vitamin E, which provides mixed tocopherols and tocotrienols. Therefore, getting at least 150 IU/d of α-tocopherol from the oils, seeds, vegetables, and fruit on the list should provide the recommended amount of mixed tocopherols and tocotrienols.

Best Food Sources of Vitamin E		
Food	Serving Size	Vitamin E (IU* per serving)
Wheat germ oil	1 tablespoon	30.3
Sunflower seeds, dry roasted	1 ounce	11
Almonds, dry roasted	1 ounce	10
Sunflower oil	1 tablespoon	8.3
Safflower oil	1 tablespoon	6.8
Hazelnuts, dry roasted	1 ounces (~¼ cup)	6.4
Peanuts	1 ounce	4.5
Peanut butter	2 tablespoons	4.3
Peanuts, dry roasted,	1 ounces (~¼ cup)	3.2
Corn oil	1 tablespoon	5.6
Spinach	1 cup	5.6
Swiss chard	1 cup	4.9
Asparagus	1 cup	4.0
Shrimp	4 ounces	3.7
Broccoli	1 cup	3.5
Beet greens	1 cup	3.8
Olives	1 cup	3.3
Olive oil	1 Tablespoon	2.8
Chili peppers	2 teaspoons	3.0
Collard greens	1 cup	2.4
Bell peppers	1 cup	2.2

*To convert from IU to milligrams: for vitamin E, 1 IU is the biological equivalent of about 0.67 mg (natural) d-alpha-tocopherol, or 0.9 mg of (synthetic) dl-alpha-tocopherol

Source: NIH Fact Sheet, Vitamin E (ods.od.nih.gov/factsheets/VitaminE-HealthProfessional/#en4); World's Healthiest Foods, Vitamin E (https://bit.ly/WHF-VitaminE)

You'd still need quite a bit of wheat germ or other oils to get this amount from diet alone, so supplementation may be necessary. When selecting a vitamin E supplement, keep in mind the following:

- **Avoid supplements that provide only α-tocopherol.** Some include this in high enough amounts to actually promote bone loss!

- **Look for mixed tocopherols and tocotrienols.** Your vitamin E supplements should provide a similar ratio of tocopherols as is present in vitamin E-rich foods, which is 5:2:1 (5 γ-tocopherol: 2 δ-tocopherol: 1 α-tocopherol). However, this may not match exactly as the amounts of tocopherols and tocotrienols in foods vary, thus so will a supplement derived from such foods.

- **Choose a natural form of alpha-tocopherols over synthetic.** Your supplement bottle is likely to include either *natural* d-alpha-tocopherols or *synthetic* dl-alpha-tocopherol. Natural α-tocopherols are biologically active, thus capable of affecting membrane-resident enzymes and cellular signaling. The synthetic version may function as an antioxidant but is composed of 87.5% otherwise non-biologically active compounds. Therefore, we recommend you select the natural d-alpha-tocopherols form.[1027]

Vitamin E Safety

Natural (mixed tocopherols and tocotrienols) vitamin E is very safe. As noted above, a solid body of peer-reviewed medical literature has demonstrated that natural vitamin E is safe in amounts up to 1,600 IU/day.[1028]

BONE-HEALTHY ACTION ITEMS

- If you are not regularly consuming oils, seeds, vegetables, and fruit naturally rich in vitamin E, you are likely to be deficient.
- Avoid supplements that provide the synthetic form, dl-α-tocopherol.
- Avoid supplements that provide only α-tocopherol.
- Consume 400 to 800 IU daily of mixed tocopherols and tocotrienols to support the health of your bones and immune system.

Conclusion Part Two

Calcium and vitamin D are most often credited with supporting strong bones. Thankfully, more people are getting the word about the critical role vitamin K2 plays in directing calcium to our bone, rather than our soft tissue and organs. However, you now understand the vital role that more than a dozen nutrients play, including essential omega-3 oils, minerals such as strontium, and others we need in minute amounts, like zinc and copper. You've seen how healthy bones need a combination of vitamins from A to K.

These same nutrients that benefit your bone also boost your body. Getting enough of the vitamins, minerals, and healthy fats we need has become more difficult due to our society's approach to food production and the predominance of processed, packaged foods. Tragically, this has left many of us short of even the inadequate RDI levels, let alone the optimal amounts our bones—and bodies—need.

As you get older, how many times have you been told to accept whatever physical decline you're experiencing as a natural part of aging? Balderdash! Do try to be polite about it, but do NOT accept this! These are the nutrients your bones *must* have for health. Furthermore, these nutrients are essential for keeping you healthy overall. Use the chart below as a starting point and review this section to determine your specific needs. Take advantage of readily available lab tests to check for nutrient insufficiencies, inflammation, hormone levels, and other measures to identify what's causing your bone loss.

Then plan, like us, to enjoy strong bones—and vibrant overall health— all the way until age 120 (the supposed maximum human lifespan).

Nutrients Required to Build and Maintain Healthy Bones

Note: Dosages are the total from diet and supplements combined.

Minerals	Calcium	1,200 to 1,500 mg/d
	Magnesium	600 to 750 mg/d (calcium to magnesium ratio of 2:1)
	Boron	3 to 6 mg/d
	Zinc	15 to 30 mg/d
	Copper	1 to 2 mg/d (zinc to copper ratio of 15:1)
	Manganese	5 mg/d
	Silicon	40 mg/d
	Selenium	200 mcg/d
	Iodine	150 mcg to 1 mg/d (required for thyroid hormone production; monitor TSH, fT4, fT3, rT3)
	Strontium citrate	680 mg/d if osteoporosis, osteopenia (340 mg/d to maintain)
Vitamins	Vitamin D3	2,000 to 5,000 iu/d (an amount sufficient to produce 25(OH)D blood level of 60 to 80 ng/mL)
	Vitamin K1	1,000 to 5,000 mcg/d
	Vitamin K2 (MK-7)	100 to 180 mcg/d (360 mcg/d used in CKD, cardiovascular, postmenopausal osteoporosis studies with no adverse reactions)
	Vitamin A	Comparable amount to that of vitamin D
	B Vitamins	Active B Complex, 1 capsule daily (should include activated forms of B6, B12, folate, riboflavin, and niacin)
	Vitamin C	1,000 to 2,000 mg/d
	Vitamin E (mixed tocopherols and tocotrienols)	400 IU/d
Essential Fatty Acids	EPA/DHA	2.6 grams (or more, sufficient to result in omega-6 to omega-3 ratio of 4:1 or less)
Protein	organic legumes, pastured animals, free-range chicken, wild-caught fish	1.2 g/kg of body weight, balanced by at least 1,200 mg calcium

PART THREE

Tools to Support Healthy Bones

By now, you realize that maintaining strong, healthy bones requires a host of nutrients—vitamins, minerals, fats, and protein—often working closely together. You also know about the threats our bones face regularly from our SAD diet, heavy metals, and other common toxins. Hopefully, you've already begun implementing some of the simple strategies we shared to avoid or mitigate these dangers.

Now, we'll help you build on that foundation by sharing tools that enable you to implement a bone-health plan that works specifically for you! First, we lay out the basic principles of a bone-building diet, so you can create recipes (or adapt your favorites) to provide the nutrients missing from the average diet. And we give you some smoothie recipes that make getting a powerhouse of bone-building nutrients easy and delicious.

We touched earlier on the benefits of exercise for your bones and beyond. We'll share our favorite weight-bearing exercises—barre3, Pilates, and yoga—including modifications you can make to suit your fitness level. Lara will even demo some of the moves for you.

Finally, we provide the resources you need to help pinpoint any specific challenges. The last chapter is your guide to the readily available diagnostic scans and lab tests that can give you crucial insight on your vitamin status; hormone levels; digestive, parathyroid, kidney, liver, and thyroid function; and other factors specific to your needs for strong, healthy bones.

CHAPTER 8

How to Create a Bone-Building Diet

Throughout this book, we've shared what foods (or *food-like substances*) destroy your bones and which you can eat to continuously rebuild and maintain the health of your bones. Here's where we pull everything together.

We're not going to tell you exactly what to eat. That's not effective. *In all the diet and recipe books you own, how many of the diet plans—in which every day is structured and every recipe is laid out for every meal—have you followed?* Probably none. I (Lara) just scan the recipes and adapt the ones that appeal to me, so they fit the principles of a bone-building diet. This is how I use cookbooks and the staggering array of recipes on the web. So, that's what we want to share with you: the basic principles of a bone-building diet. Plus, we'll share a few outrageously delicious smoothie recipes that will make meeting your fruit and vegetable goals so easy!

Key Principles of a Bone-Building Diet

Promotes a slightly alkaline pH (i.e., slightly above 7). Our cellular machinery—all the enzymes whose activity makes up our metabolism, including the metabolism in the cells of our bones—work best at a slightly alkaline pH. They do not work well at an acidic pH. And an acidic pH promotes bone loss. We are not talking about the acidity of the foods, but rather their effect on body pH.

What promotes a slightly alkaline metabolic pH? A plant-based diet, like a Mediterranean-type diet, which is heavy on fresh vegetables, whole fruits, legumes, nuts, and seeds. And lighter on grains (even whole grains). While grains themselves are not acid inducing, they are typically so high in salt that they impair the ability of our kidneys to excrete excess acid. Get sufficient protein, ideally derived from organically grown legumes, pastured animals, free-range chickens, and wild-caught fish. Your daily goal is 1.2 to 1.5 g/kg of body weight (typically, 25 to 35 grams, 3 times per day). And protein must be balanced by sufficient calcium, at least 1,200 mg daily total from food and supplements combined. That will offset any loss of calcium resulting from consuming meat, dairy, or fish-derived protein.

Does not promote inflammation. Dietary triggers of inflammation include the ultra-processed *Frankenfoods* that make up most of the aptly named SAD (standard American diet). The SAD contains heaps of refined sugars, highly processed fats, and refined grains. Wheat promotes inflammation in everyone, not just those with celiac disease, so you should minimize your consumption of even organic whole wheat.

All processed foods promote inflammation in a mind-boggling number of ways (see Part One). They're likely to contain GMOs (genetically modified organisms), too much salt, numerous chemicals, phosphate additives, pesticide residues, and heavy metals (e.g., cadmium, which high phosphate fertilizers used in conventional agriculture deposit in the soil). This bone-destructive mix is then canned or packaged in plastic, which adds plasticizers like BPA (or BPS, BPF, BPZ, or BPAF), which migrate from the lining of cans or plastic wrap or plastic containers into the food. These are endocrine disruptors that promote thyroid disorders and obesity. In sum, processed foods contain the perfect ingredients for bone loss. Avoid them.

Provides the proper ratio of omega-6: omega-3 fatty acids to fight inflammation. The ratio of omega-6: omega-3 in your diet should be no higher than 4:1. The SAD ratio provided by processed foods is 20:1. The SAD is way too high in omega-6 fatty acids, specifically the pro-inflammatory arachidonic acid (AA). AA is present in far greater amounts in products derived from conventionally raised animals and farmed fish than those from pastured animals, free-range chickens, or wild-caught fish. Also, choose smaller, shorter-lived species of fish (e.g., Alaskan salmon or sardines) to minimize their heavy metal content (e.g., mercury). Plus, this can help avoid the plastics that are now being found in the flesh of fish—and the humans who eat them. Do not eat farmed fish, which will contain so much omega-6 that the omega-3 they do provide will not be effectively utilized. Plus, they will contain pesticide residues and possibly antibiotics.

Eat meat and dairy products derived from pastured or free-range animals whose diet is supplemented with organically grown hay and whole grains. These products contain more omega-3s, plus the meats contain an anti-inflammatory fat called conjugated linoleic acid, both of which will provide balance for the AA they contain. Conventionally raised animals will not only contain far more inflammatory omega-6 and far less omega-3 (or none) but may also contain inflammation-producing antibiotic, pesticide, and hormone residues.

Eat full-fat dairy products—except for cow's milk. Vitamin K is fat soluble. When the fat is reduced, vitamin K is removed. Consume no more than 8 oz. of cow's milk daily. Cow's milk contains lactose, which our bodies break down into glucose and D-galactose, a sugar so inflammatory it's used in animal studies to rapidly and prematurely age the animals.

Use cold-pressed, organic extra-virgin olive oil, and other organic, cold-pressed oils. Do not buy processed, heated, or hydrogenated oils. They promote inflammation and the vitamin K they contain will have been changed into a form called dihydrophylloquinone. Your body cannot use this form to produce vitamin K2.

Provides optimal protein to maintain muscle mass and prevent sarcopenia. As mentioned above, you want to consume 1.2 to 1.5 grams of protein/kg of body weight, the amount now recommended to prevent sarcopenia in elders. Depending on your weight, this translates to approximately 20 to 35 grams of protein at each of 3 meals over the course of the day.

> **Example:** Lara weighs 108 pounds or 49 kg. So she needs at least 59 grams (49 x 1.2 grams) of protein daily. Since she is very active, exercising at least an hour every day, she tries to consume around 73.5 grams (49 kg x 1.5 grams) of protein daily. Joe weighs 165 pounds (75 kg), so he requires 90 to 112.5 grams of protein daily.

Provides a rainbow of nutrient-dense, fiber-rich plant foods. A variety of organically grown plant foods is essential. You should be consuming a minimum of 10 servings of vegetables and 4 servings of fresh fruit every day. Yes, you can! Just one 8-ounce glass of any of Emma's Amazing Smoothies (see recipes below) will provide 5 vegetable and 2 fruit servings.

The nutrient content of conventionally grown foods has dropped greatly in the last 50 years. Organically grown foods provide far more minerals and protective, anti-inflammatory phytochemicals than chemically grown foods. What's more, they don't contain GMOs, or bone-busting cadmium or pesticide residues. The nutrient composition of each plant is different. More variety delivers a wider spectrum of anti-inflammatory phytochemicals as well as vitamins, minerals, and fiber, to support good elimination and a healthy microbiome in your gut.

Let your dietary habits work *for,* not against, you! What we eat is largely a matter of habit. When cooking, most people rely upon 12 to 15 tried and true recipes that are quick and easy to prepare and produce reliable, satisfying meals. Use the principles above to adapt your current favorites and to develop new recipes that work for—not against—your bones and overall health.

We know getting optimal amounts of fruits and vegetables can be challenging, so we're providing a way to make it simple, quick, and *so* delicious: 6 smoothies created for you by Dr. Emma Gasinski, PT, DPT, RYT. Start with these and create your own. If getting enough protein is a challenge, add a scoop of your favorite protein powder. Each of these recipes will make 6 cups (8 ounces each). We drink at least a cup every day. Any left over will keep in the refrigerator for one more day. We *promise* your vitality will soar within a week.

Emma's Amazing Smoothies

The following recipes are all vitamin, mineral, phytochemical, and fiber-rich bone-building goodness! Use all organic ingredients if possible. Prep time is just 5 to 10 minutes, blending time 3 minutes, and clean-up time 2 minutes. Total time: just 15 minutes.

The instructions are the same for each recipe. Add all ingredients to a high-speed blender. Add 4 to 5 cups (or however much will fit) of ice-cold water. Blend low speed to start. Gradually increase to full speed and blend for 2 minutes or until smooth. Drink at least 8 ounces right away. Transfer the remainder to a glass container (we use Mason jars) and refrigerate until the following day.

Orange Drink	
Ingredients	
Greens, frozen (spinach, kale, arugula, swiss chard, and beet greens)	3 to 4 cups
Zucchini, sliced, frozen	1 medium size
Carrots, chopped	2 cups
Lemon, zested and juiced	1 whole
Turmeric	pinky size piece
Ginger	thumb-size piece
Black pepper	¼ teaspoon
Flaxseed	generous 2 tablespoons
Coconut flakes	¼ cup
Medjool dates (be sure to pit if needed)	3 to 4
Navel orange, everything but the peel	1
Mango, frozen	1 cup
Non-dairy unsweetened milk of choice	1 cup

Violet Drink
Ingredients

Cauliflower, broken into pieces and frozen	1 head
Zucchini, sliced, frozen	1 cup
Cucumber, skin peeled if not English cucumber, sliced, frozen	1
Coconut flake	¼ cup
Lemon, zested and juiced	½ a lemon
Medjool dates (be sure to pit if needed)	3 to 4
Flaxseed	2 tablespoons
Blueberries, frozen	2 cups
Cherries, frozen	½ to 1 cup
Non-dairy unsweetened milk of choice	1 cup

Red Drink
Ingredients

Greens, frozen (spinach, kale, arugula, swiss chard, and beet greens)	3 to 4 cups
Flaxseed	generous 2 tablespoons
Zucchini, sliced, frozen	1 medium size
Carrots, chopped	2 medium size
Lime, zested and juiced	1
Ginger	thumb-size piece
*Red beets, cut in half or quarters	2 small or 1 medium
Dates, Medjool or Halawi (be sure to remove pits if needed)	3
Navel orange, everything but the peel	1
Strawberries, frozen	1 ½ cups
Raspberries, frozen	1 cup
Non-dairy unsweetened milk of choice	1 cup

*Spend some romantic time with your beloved and enjoy the improved blood-delivery side effect of beets!

Cherry Drink
Ingredients

Greens, frozen (spinach, kale, arugula, swiss chard, and beet greens)	3 to 4 cups
Beet, cut in half or quarters	1 medium size
Zucchini, frozen	1 cup
Basil	8 to 10 leaves
Toasted almonds	¼ cup
Flaxseed	generous 2 tablespoons
Lime, zested and juiced	1
Medjool dates (be sure to pit if needed)	3 to 4
Cherries, frozen	2 cups
Non-dairy unsweetened milk of choice	1 cup

Green Drink
Ingredients

Greens, frozen (spinach, kale, arugula, swiss chard, and beet greens)	3 to 4 cups
Zucchini, frozen	1 cup
Flaxseed	generous 2 tablespoons
Cucumber, skin peeled if not English cucumber, sliced, frozen	1
Celery, cut into bite-size pieces	3 to 4 stalks
Green apples, cored	2
Ginger	thumb-size piece
Lemon, zested and juiced	1 whole
Ice water	6 cups

Pineapple Drink

Ingredients

Greens, frozen (spinach, kale, arugula, swiss chard, and beet greens)	3 to 4 cups
Zucchini, frozen	1 cup
Flaxseed	generous 2 tablespoons
Cucumber, skin peeled if not English cucumber, sliced, frozen	1
Cilantro, stems and leaves	1 small bunch
Ginger	thumb-size piece
Lime, zested and juiced	1
Coconut, unsweetened, shredded	¼ cup
Pineapple, frozen	2 cups
Ice water	6 cups

CHAPTER 9

Exercises that Build Bone Safely

We all know how much exercise benefits your overall health. Regular exercise helps you keep your heart and circulatory system healthy and maintain a healthy body weight. Plus, nothing clears out stress hormones like a really good workout!

Exercise is also essential for your bones. The right types of exercise activate osteocytes, the type of cells within your bones that respond to mechanical loading (weight-bearing exercise) by initiating bone renewal. In this section, we share our favorite, most effective bone-building exercises:

1. barre3
2. Pilates
3. yoga (especially Iyengar Yoga)

All are appropriate for women and men of all ages and fitness levels and can be easily modified to suit your individual needs.*

Important Note: Before starting any fitness program, consult your physician or other healthcare professional to determine if it's right for your needs. All exercises and physical activities, even those modified to be safer, carry inherent risks of physical injury, particularly for those with a personal or family history of high blood pressure or heart disease, or for those who have ever experienced chest pain, smoke, have high cholesterol, are obese, or have a bone or joint problem. If you experience faintness, dizziness, pain, or shortness of breath at any time while exercising you should stop immediately.

barre3

Incorporates Yoga, Pilates, and Ballet Exercises

barre3 allows you to build strength using functional movements that require balance, control, and muscle strength, so you can move with ease and grace in real-life situations. The exercise patterns equalize the strength between the right and left sides of your body and strengthen the muscles in the back of your body to match those in the front. Most of us spend our days sitting, using a computer, and looking down at our phones. This promotes imbalance and puts you at risk for injuries. barre3 is functional training that corrects this, restores balance, and prevents injuries. Here's one example:

barre3 squats: Working on your squat form—to make sure your glutes are firing, your abs are supporting your lower back, and your spine is long—will help you throughout your day. *How?* Just think of all the times you need to bend to put something down or pick something up. Or every time you get up from a couch or get out of your car. This is why barre3 offers *functional training*.

In contrast, exercises using movements you'd normally never do are *not* functional training. Machines that isolate a single muscle don't promote functional fitness. Take the leg press, which eliminates engaging your core muscles since you don't need to keep yourself stable. In real life, you don't rest your back against a board when you bend down to pick up something. Contrast that to a squat—a move you make every time you lower yourself into or get up from a chair—that engages your legs, back and abdominal muscles.

Our bodies are meant to move, but our modern lifestyle is increasingly sedentary. *The result?* Major muscle groups suffer from lack of daily use, and imbalances develop in the body that cause pain and lead to injury. Your moves during barre3 counter common imbalances that increase your risk of fracture, including:

Rounded, tight shoulders/chest: Sitting, working at the computer, and watching TV promote the tendency for the upper back to round. Over time, the muscles in the front of the chest and shoulders tighten and shorten producing the rounding in the spine that eventually becomes that classic sign of osteoporosis—the dowager hump. Imbalances in the muscles of the shoulders and chest create tension and pain in the upper back and neck, promote vertebral wedging, and increase the risk of spinal wedging, compression, and injury.

barre3 classes include stretches and strength-based exercises that open up the front of the chest and strengthen the upper-back muscles to keep you open and erect. Here's one you can try right now:

- **Chest Stretch:** Reach your hands back like a cape. If it feels good, interlace your fingers and draw the back of the shoulders down and toward each other. Take three to five deep breaths and release. Seems simple, but this is a highly effective stretch that opens shortened, tight chest muscles by activating the upper-back muscles, which then lengthen and release the front of your chest.

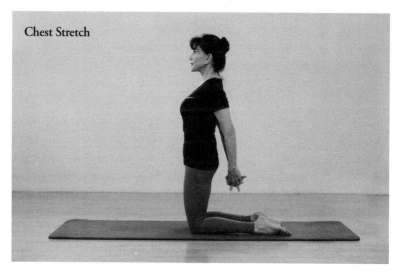

Chest Stretch

- **Lazy glutes:** Sitting too much also creates imbalances in your hips and core. Your muscles are meant to contract then lengthen. When you sit and sit and sit, your gluteal muscles get stuck in a lengthened state. Over time, they forget how to contract. Also, you're literally sitting on nerves. After a while, they stop responding, making it harder for your glutes to receive the message to wake up and engage when they need to. When you stand and get moving again, your glutes don't activate correctly, so your lower-back muscles have to kick in to do the work your glutes are supposed to be doing when you're standing and walking. Your lower-back muscles are key players in supporting your core, but they're not big enough to take over the job of your glutes—the largest most powerful muscles in your body—so you end up with lower-back tension and pain. barre3 provides many functional moves that get your glutes back online. Here's an example:

- **Bridge Lifts:** Lifting your butt off the ground is exactly what your glutes are designed to do. If you feel this more in your hamstrings or lower back, your glutes need help waking up. To gently activate them, slow down, work in a smaller range, and focus your attention on lifting from the back of your hips. You can also give your glutes a good poke, a little *time-to-wake-up* message. Go ahead and try! (Hey, if you don't want to grab your butt, neither will the guy or gal in your life.) Plus, barre3 is online. No one will see you.

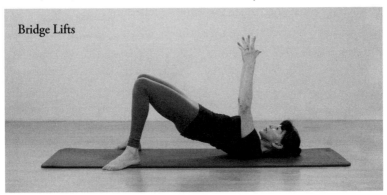

Bridge Lifts

Your core (the muscles that support and elongate your torso). When your core is strong and balanced, it supports the stability and mobility of your spine and hips. Every barre3 posture and movement engages your core. A great example here is:

- **Plank**: Whether you're holding your plank against the wall, on your elbows, or full length out on the floor, gravity is pulling your whole torso toward the ground. All of your core muscles—your abs and all the muscles that support your rib cage, spine, back, and hips—must lift against gravity and stabilize your body. When you hold this and fully exhale, you activate the deepest layer of your ab wall, which then sends a signal to all your other core muscles to engage and *brace*. Try it. When you stand back up, you'll still feel lifted and taller.

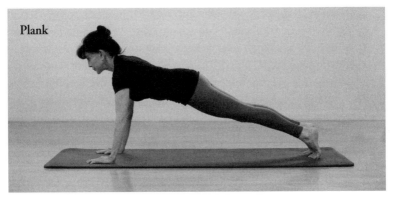

Plank

Lack of movement in your hip joint. To be well nourished and agile, your hip joints need to be flexed, extended, and lengthened to the back, to the side, turned out, turned in, and rotated in complete circles. barre3 moves the hip joint in all directions in every class, developing the strength and mobility your hips need to support you in your everyday life. Our example here is:

- **Diamond**: And these diamonds are definitely a girl's best friend. Diamonds work rotation in your hips. As you move your top leg up and down, you increase your hip mobility while strengthening your outer glutes and deep hip muscles. And you're turning on all your supportive core muscles, too.

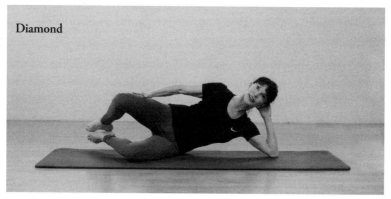

Diamond

barre3 exercises follow a 3-step sequence. Each step in the barre3 sequence tells your bones to grow stronger:

- **First, an isometric hold.** You simply get into proper alignment and contract your muscles to stay in that position without moving. Your muscles start to fire. Often, they will fatigue *more* quickly than when moving. You're engaging both large and small stabilizer muscles, which may even start to quiver because you'll be working to the point of failure, which is where your muscles send your bones the signals to grow stronger. barre3 helps get you right to your edge—wherever that happens to be—safely, without straining tendons or ligaments and risking injury. Plank pose is a great example of an isometric hold.

- **Second, once your muscles are firing correctly in a hold, barre3 layers on one-inch, pulsing movements.** This is called *Partial Range of Motion*, and it's a serious strength builder. You fatigue the muscle faster and dramatically increase strength because these tiny but powerful movements help you get an incredible deep-muscle burn. Once again, that brings you to your edge, notifying your bones it's time to build, with no negative pain in your joints.

- **Third, you get dynamic and energetic movement, which gets your heart pumping, and boosts your endorphins.** After the first two steps, you'll crave these wonderful, large range of motion moves that send fresh oxygen to your muscles and use your joints' full range of mobility. These functional moves reinforce your ability to move in smart, safe ways all day long.

Put them all together and the magic really happens! You're building balanced strength, lengthening and supporting your spine, waking up the muscles that support your hips, increasing hip joint mobility, and creating beautiful posture.

barre3 is safe and effective. Classes begin with deep, grounding breaths that help you shift into a more self-aware state, better able to tune in to how your body is feeling. As you begin each barre3 posture (or move), the instructor explains what muscle groups are being targeted, what sensations you will be feeling, and areas in your body where you should not be feeling tension, like your neck or lower back. You'll have time to see how the move feels in your body, so if it's not working for you, the instructor can give modifications that target the same muscles.

If a posture feels great and challenging, wonderful—go to your bone-building edge! If it causes tension in areas that should feel at ease, it's time to modify. barre3 instructors show options for how to shift the posture, so it suits your body's needs and how to substitute another posture that will get you just as deep into your muscles. For example, if doing a Plank on the floor causes tension in your low-back or pain in your wrists, you'll lose engagement in your core, and the posture will be ineffective.

If you modify the posture—coming down to your elbows or taking your Plank against the wall or a chair or countertop—you'll allow your entire core to engage. No pain, just gain. The modifications offered for every barre3 exercise let you get the benefits without hurting your body. And, if you do barre3 every day, you'll likely want to modify often. Our bodies feel different day to day, and it's good to explore new layers within each posture to learn more, send slightly different signals to your bones, and break plateaus. After a barre3 workout, you'll feel taller, more energized, stronger, and more aware—better than when you started.

Pilates
Builds Bone Safely, Effectively, and Beautifully

Pilates teaches you how to strengthen your stabilizing muscles. You have two main types of muscles: large muscles that move you (mobilizing muscles) and smaller muscles that support your skeleton (stabilizing muscles). In daily life as well as during exercise moves, the mobilizing muscles—which are bigger, more exterior, and stronger—tend to take over. We neglect the smaller, interior muscles that stabilize our spine and hip joints. However, these are the very muscles that, when activated, most directly attach to bone and stimulate strengthening. For strong, fracture-resistant bones, you must learn how to zero-in on these smaller interior muscles, ensuring they remain strong and active.

Pilates works from the core outward. Your *core muscles* are the stabilizers that support the trunk of your body and surround the space where your organs reside. These are the muscles that enable you to maintain an erect, graceful, and pain-free posture in all the functional movements that get you through your normal day (or a walk, hike, or any workout). Core strengthening focuses on these key muscles that support your spine and pelvis (your multifidi, transversus abdominis, internal and external obliques, and psoas). In the hip joint, your core muscles include your deep lateral hip rotators (such as the piriformis). In your rib cage and shoulder girdle, the core muscles include your serratus anterior and rotator cuff muscles. Don't worry—you don't have to know the names of these muscles to get the benefits of Pilates, but visualizing your deep, core muscles working can help you activate them and get the most out of your practice.

Pilates helps you strengthen your stabilizing core muscles, so you can hold your body properly and get the most out of resistance exercises. You don't want to *just* lift weight. You already do this carrying in the groceries or lifting the mattress to put on fresh sheets when you're making the bed. (And you can injure yourself doing these things if your postural alignment is off.) Basic resistance exercises make it easy for your large mobilizing muscles to take over. Here's an example:

- **Squats**. If you do these quickly without focus, your quadriceps—the muscles on the front of your thighs—take over, and you never engage your deep hip stabilizers, the muscles you need to strengthen to stabilize your hip and protect against hip fracture. To do that, you want to target the muscles that attach to the upper portion of your femur, which your DEXA report calls your *femur neck*, because that's where fragility hip fractures typically occur.

If your core is unstable, your body may try to compensate by arching your lower back too much. (Your butt will stick out and your stomach will pooch out—not attractive!) Or you will hike up one side of your hips putting pressure on your lumbar spine. Or you'll stress your knee joints. All three of these actions increase your risk of pain and injury. The muscles you want to light up are your lateral hip rotator muscles. To turn them on and create the desired pull at the top of your thigh, you must first stabilize your pelvis and spine. *What does this?* Your core muscles. So, strong bones start with a strong core, and that's the primary focus of Pilates.

Pilates teaches you to activate your core muscles and develop well-balanced, beautiful body alignment, both of which are essential to build and maintain beautiful bones. When you walk, squat, climb stairs, or get up from a chair, you're lifting your own weight. If your posture is off, you won't be zeroing in on the muscles that most benefit your bones. Instead, you'll be creating imbalanced-movement habits that increase your risk of an aching neck, shoulders, hip, or back—or even a fragility fracture. For this reason, it's best to start Pilates with the help of an experienced instructor. Your first session will involve a postural analysis that identifies your imbalances and serves as the foundation for a safe, corrective exercise plan. This plan will restore not just balance and stronger bones, but your ease and beauty in movement.

Modifications can make Pilates safe and effective. Standard Pilates classes include a lot of forward bending (flexion) exercises you will want to avoid—at least until your spine is no longer osteoporotic. However, it's easy to modify exercises so you target the same muscles in a way that lets you safely build bone. For example, the standard form of the signature Pilates exercise the *Hundred* flexes the upper body up off the floor while fully extending the legs in the air. This is too much flexion for someone at risk of compression fracture. Instead, you can do this:

- **Hundred (modified):** With your head and shoulders resting on the mat, lift your legs into a right-angle, bent-knee position by using your core, while maintaining a stable, balanced pelvis. By pumping your arms, you will dynamically challenge your abdominal muscles— without inappropriately challenging your spine. As your core muscles strengthen, Pilates will continue to challenge you. You can hold weighted balls in your hands or extend your legs straight out at an angle of about 80 to 90 degrees. When this becomes easy—and it will—you can place a *Magic Circle* (a resistance ring also called a Pilates Ring) around the outside of your mid-to-lower calves. Pressing your legs out against the Magic Circle will add even more challenge and load.

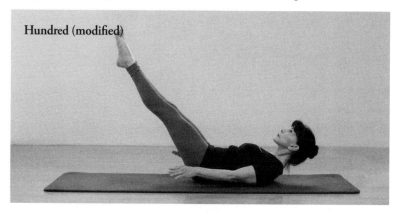

Hundred (modified)

Some Pilates exercises involve a seated position and normally flex the spine forward in a *C curve*. Some examples you can modify include:

- Half Roll Back, **Roll Up**, **Saw**, and Neck Pull: You'll want to modify these exercises to maintain a more neutral, erect spine and hinge at the hip joint instead of curving (flexing) your spine forward. These modifications are not *easier*, just safer. This adjustment will challenge the spinal extensors in your back and abdominal muscles as well as the muscles of your hip, safely promoting strong bones in both areas. Plus, mastering these exercises will give you a beautifully erect posture and lend grace and control to your every forward-leaning movement.

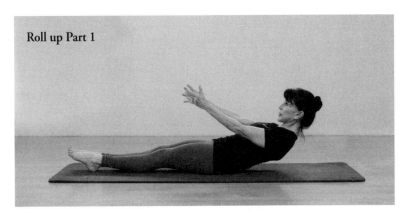

Roll up Part 1

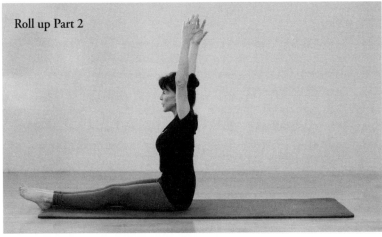

Roll up Part 2

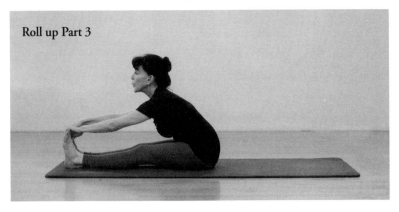

Roll up Part 3

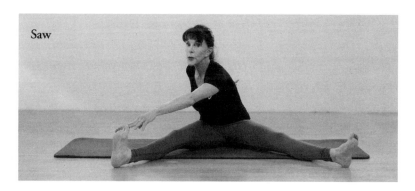

Saw

Pilates exercises, such as the Breaststroke, **Swimming**, and **Single Leg Kick**, also include a progression to their performance that will strengthen your back extensors, further supporting your spine. As you grow stronger, it's a good idea to check in periodically with your instructor, both for new exercises and to ensure your form is correct. This way, you get the very best results from your workouts.

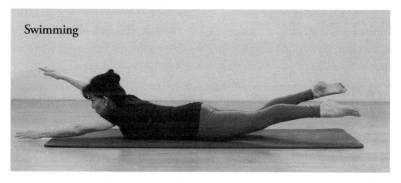

Swimming

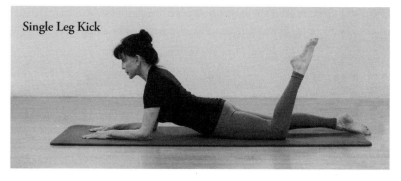

Single Leg Kick

A few Pilates exercises should be avoided by people with osteoporosis. Exercises that require flexion, such as the Rolling Like a Ball, Cat Stretch, Seal, and Jack Knife should be avoided—not forever, just until your bones' health has been restored! A special cautionary note: If you are taking a bisphosphonate or denosumab, even if your DEXA shows increased bone density, don't add flexion exercises back in! Your bones may have the right density but may not have good resiliency. To check for resilience, you will need to have your TBS run. Until your TBS shows good bone quality, flexion exercises are not advised! (See Lab Tests, Chapter 10.)

Yoga
Activates Sensor in Bone that Initiates Bone-Building

Yoga builds fracture-free bones by producing muscle contractions that activate osteocytes in areas most susceptible to fracture. Osteocytes, the most abundant type of bone cell, are mechanosensors. They respond to the mechanical loading produced when a muscle pulls on a bone by secreting biochemical signals that initiate the bone renewal process in both osteoblasts and osteoclasts.[1029]

Why is yoga especially effective for bone-building compared to other forms of exercise? Yoga, particularly the more slow-moving, precise style of Iyengar Yoga, tasks us with holding the body in novel positions. These are positions we generally don't visit in our day-to-day activities or during other forms of exercise for an extended period of time. The effort required to hold these unusual positions applies mechanical force to the entire body in ways that other forms of exercise do not. The *extended-period-of-time* piece is also key here. Research shows that levels of bone-building markers begin to increase when mechanical force is applied for at least 12 seconds, but that holding a pose for longer than 72 seconds does not produce any further benefit.

Beyond this, yoga has further indirect bone-health effects. It can help improve posture, balance, coordination, strength, and mobility—all key benefits for preventing a fall. Yoga also promotes a sense of peace and well-being, helping to alleviate the inflammatory effects of chronic stress.[1030] [1031]

A pioneer in the application of yoga for a multitude of medical conditions is Dr. Loren Fishman, Medical Director of Manhattan Physical Medicine & Rehabilitation and student of B.K.S. Iyengar. In 2005, excited by the potential bone-health effects of yoga, Dr. Fishman began putting theory to test by conducting a small pilot study in his office involving 11 subjects and 7 controls with either osteopenia or osteoporosis. These subjects practiced a sequence of 12 yoga poses daily for 2 years. At the end of the study, the subjects who practiced yoga had better bone mineral density in the spine and hips compared to the controls.[1032]

This led to a large-scale study published in 2016, this time with 227 active participants. These participants were on average 68 years old and 83% of them had either osteopenia or osteoporosis. After 2 years of practicing the 12 poses consistently, participants showed promising results. They reported bone density gains in the spine, hips, and femur.[1033] Fishman is now conducting a third, more robust study to again show that properly chosen yoga poses can support strong bones. See the box for Dr. Fishman's 12 poses and photos of selected poses below.

Dr. Fishman's 12-Pose Sequence

1. Vrksasana (Tree Pose)
2. Trikonasana (Triangle Pose)
3. Virabhadrasana II (Warrior II Pose)
4. Parsvakonasana (Side-Angle Pose)
5. Parivrtta Trikonasana (Twisted Triangle Pose)
6. Salabhasana (Locust Pose)
7. Setu Bandhasana (Bridge Pose)
8. Supta Padangusthasana I (Reclining Hand-to-Big-Toe Pose I)
9. Supta Padangusthasana II (Reclining Hand-to-Big-Toe Pose II)
10. Marichyasana II (Straight-Legged Twist)
11. Matsyendrasana (Bent-Knee Twist)
12. Savasana (Corpse Pose)

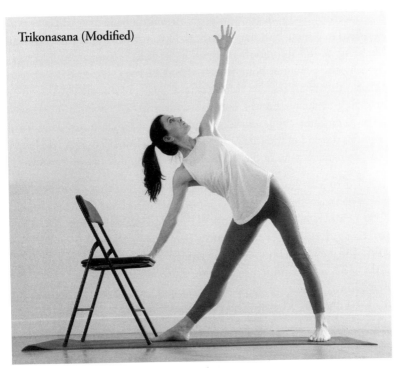

Trikonasana (Modified)

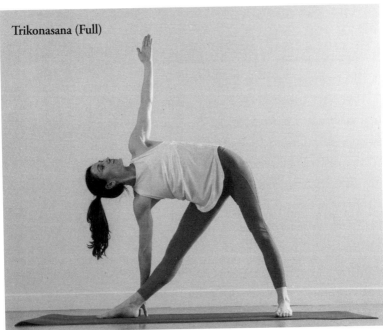

Trikonasana (Full)

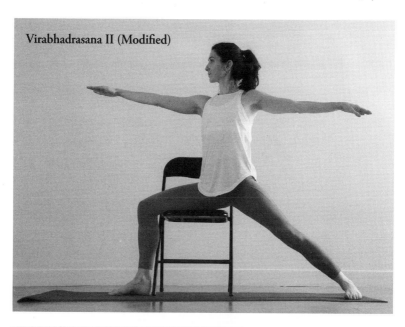

Virabhadrasana II (Modified)

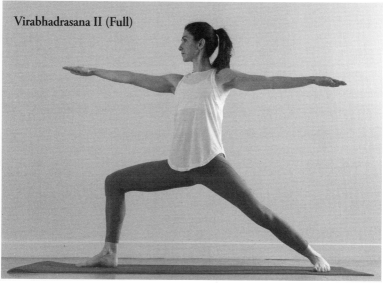

Virabhadrasana II (Full)

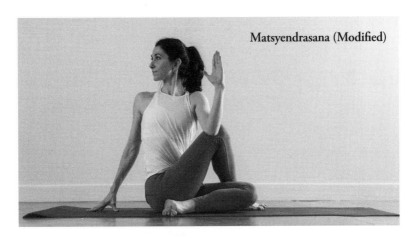

Matsyendrasana (Modified)

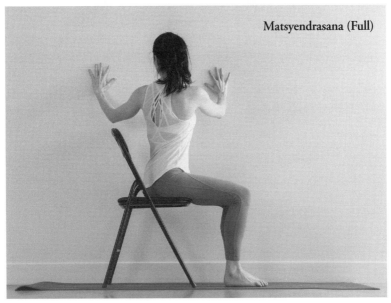

Matsyendrasana (Full)

When practicing yoga to improve bone health, here are some key things to keep in mind:

- **Avoid spinal flexion.** As mentioned earlier, spinal flexion, which pulls the spine into a *C curve*, causes weight to concentrate at the front vertebral body, making it vulnerable to fracture. While there are many suitable yoga poses for increasing bone strength, some traditional poses require deep-forward folding which is not safe for those with osteoporosis or osteopenia. The 12-pose yoga sequence

Dr. Fishman designed for his study provides a great sampling of poses that are both safe and effective.

- **Twist with care.** While osteoporosis patients are often warned against twisting, Dr. Fishman explains that nothing strengthens the spine quite like a good twist—and it CAN be practiced safely. Twist with a straight spine (avoid rounding the shoulders inward) and use core strength to deepen a twist, rather than relying on force from the arms and legs.

- **Hold the pose.** Stay in a yoga posture log enough to stimulate protein synthesis. Protein synthesis starts after 12 seconds and continues to 72 seconds. Fishman suggests a 30-second hold for each pose.

- **Exert yourself.** While there are many calming and relaxing aspects of yoga, when using this practice for bone strengthening you want to maximize mechanical force. So, for each 30-second hold, fully engage your muscles as hard as you can. This will make all of the difference.

- **Modify when needed.** While you do need to exert yourself to stimulate protein synthesis, this does not mean you must practice the *full* version of each yoga pose. It can take time and practice to build up the strength and flexibility required to perform the full version of each pose. Luckily, props and modifications can be used to ease your body into it—meaning you can reap the bone-health benefits of yoga right away, without risking injury. See sample modifications below and check out the full modified versions of Dr. Fishman's 12-Pose Sequence (bit.ly/FishmanYoga).

Be aware that studio classes will commonly incorporate forward folding, so it's best to learn from an instructor qualified to teach yoga for osteoporosis to start. That way, you can learn the basics of a safe practice and modify it to suit your needs.

CASES FROM THE COMMUNITY

The Community is a sponsored group of more than 17,000 men and women supporting each other to build stronger bones naturally.
(www.algaecal.com/community)

Debra's Story

Debra didn't see this coming. Living in snowy New England, she skied regularly and had no reason to think her bones were thinning—until a fall on the slopes left the active 51-year-old with a broken hip.

She was dumbfounded. A broken hip…in her 50s! *How could that happen from a fall that seemed relatively minor?* Then, she remembered the broken wrist she suffered a while back. At the time, she thought it was a freak accident. Since she had no indicators for osteoporosis, her doctor never ordered a DEXA scan. But connecting the dots, she realized her bones might not be as strong as she had once believed.

Debra did her research and decided she wanted a natural approach for building her bone. Trained as a psychologist, she joined *The Community*, asked the right questions, and dug deep into many of the studies I (Lara) shared. "I got quite an education from everyone," she quipped, "almost like getting my second Ph.D."

At my suggestion, Debra sought out a functional medicine doctor, who prescribed hormone replacement therapy to address early menopause. While she already ate a healthy, organic diet, she realized it wasn't providing all the nutrients she needed. She began taking plant-based calcium (AlgaeCal), plus strontium citrate and, after checking her vitamin D levels, added an extra 1,000 mg of vitamin D3.

After 4 to 6 months, Debra noticed her back felt stronger, and she no longer had pain. She returned to an active schedule: tennis and weight training, each twice per week, plus daily hikes with her dog. Debra says she is committed to maintaining her bones, so she can continue to play, romp, enjoy life, and be able to lift her future grandkids. Plus, living in a cold climate, she wants resilient bones, so she doesn't have to fear dire consequences from a slip on an icy patch of ground.

Lara's Take: Too often, a broken bone after a minor fall reveals osteoporosis. Debra did the right things to seek out information, identify the supplemental nutrients she needed, and address her early menopause, during which bone loss increases.

See details on supplements for calcium on page 135 and strontium citrate on page 273. Learn more about bioidentical hormone replacement therapy (BHRT) on page 265 and determining vitamin D levels on page 176. Statements regarding the products above have not been evaluated by the Food and Drug Administration. These products are not intended to diagnose, treat, cure, or prevent any disease.

CHAPTER 10

Identifying What's Off, Lab Tests for Bone Health

By now, you know what healthy bones need and the factors that can derail the remodeling process. There are a lot of them! Of course, the most important ones are those causing YOUR bone loss and how to fix them! This is like solving a mystery and the guidance in the earlier sections of this book provides clues to point you in the right direction.

That's where lab tests come in! Fortunately, we have access to a multitude of inexpensive tests that can help pinpoint nutritional deficiencies or causes of bone loss (many more than when Lara was solving the mystery of her faulty vitamin D receptors). Discuss running the tests you feel are important for you with your doctor.

Important Note: Normal reference ranges vary by laboratory, so ALWAYS check the reference range provided on your lab report! We provide some examples below, though recommend you always work with your doctor or other healthcare professional qualified to interpret your individual results. When lab tests utilize a blood sample, most require that blood be drawn while fasting 8 to 12 hours. Carefully read the instructions you receive before testing or call the lab to check.

About Website Addresses: For some of the tests below, we've provided website resources. We've shortened longer links to be more user friendly. To reach these sites, enter the links (which begin with bit.ly) into your browser and you will be redirected to the site indicated.

Determine Your Risk of Fracture

Dual-energy X-ray Absorptiometry (DEXA or DXA) Scan

Measures bone mineral density (bone quantity) in the most common fracture sites: spine, hip, and sometimes wrist.

- The T-score indicates how your Bone Mineral Density (BMD) compares to that of a healthy 30-year-old woman.

T-Score Range	Bone Density
-1 or higher	normal bone density
Between -1.0 to -2.5	considered osteopenia
-2.5 or less	indicates osteoporosis

- The Z-score compares your BMD to others in your age group. If you're 50 or older, a Z-score of 2.0 or greater is considered normal. We suggest you ignore your Z score, since you don't want to be *normal* in this case. After age 50, it's *normal* for 34% of women to have osteopenia or osteoporosis. And 53% have osteopenia or osteoporosis after age 65.

DEXA, by itself, is inadequate because it reports only bone quantity. DEXA does not measure the health of your bones' internal microarchitecture (i.e., their quality) which is a key determinant of bone strength and resistance to fracture.

Trabecular Bone Score (TBS)

Measures trabecular bone microarchitecture or bone quality and thus bones' ability to resist fracture. Trabecular bone is the most metabolically active type of bone.

- Low-impact fractures from osteopenia and osteoporosis most commonly occur in the upper femur, which is at least 50% trabecular bone, and the vertebrae, which are 90% trabecular bone. That's why improvement shows up first in the spine.

- TBS is run by scanning your DEXA images with a special software program that reveals the number of trabeculae present and how well connected they are. *Are they present as discrete rods or rods joined to form stable, supportive plates?* Knowing this tells you about the ability of your bones to resist fracture.

The next time you're scheduled for a DEXA, make sure the facility also offers TBS. See the sample report (page 385-387) provided by Media-Maps Group, the company that created and provides TBS software to medical facilities and use this online directory to find a center that offers TBS (www.medimapsgroup.com/find-a-clinic-with-tbs).

Fracture Risk Assessment Tool (FRAX®)

FRAX is a World Health Organization-sponsored, country-specific, fracture risk assessment tool that combines BMD at the femoral neck (or total hip) with other risk factors for fracture, like gender and ethnicity, to predict a person's 10-year probability of having a fragility fracture in the hip, spine, forearm, or shoulder. The FRAX tool is a computer-driven algorithm available online (www.shef.ac.uk/FRAX).

To calculate your FRAX score, you'll answer 12 questions about yourself and provide the results from your most recent DEXA, specifically the BMD of the neck of your femur, which will be given in grams per centimeter squared (g/cm2) on your DEXA report.

You are considered at risk if you have **either** of the following:

- low bone mass (T-score between -1.0 and -2.5 at the femoral neck or spine) AND a 10-year probability of a hip fracture greater than or equal to (≥) 3%; or
- a 10-year probability of a major osteoporosis-related fracture ≥ 20%.

Trabecular Bone Score (TBS) Sample Report

Patient:	▓▓▓▓▓		
Patient ID:	279537	Date of birth - Age:	▓▓▓▓▓ - 55 years
Height - Weight - BMI:	151.5 cm - 62.5 kg - 27.2 kg/m²	Gender - Ethnicity:	Female - White
Referring physician:	▓▓▓▓▓	Acquisition date:	03/02/2015

BONE HEALTH REPORT

(1) TBS Mapping

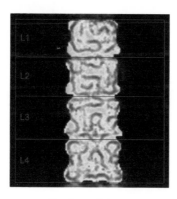

Non-diagnostic image

(2) TBS Spine Results

TBS L1-L4 = 1.212 - Degraded microarchitecture

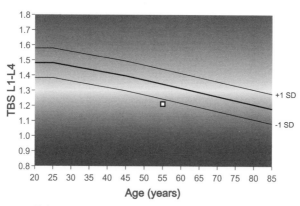

Reference population: USA (NHANES / Medimaps) - White

continued next page

(3) Fracture Risk Assessment

Osteoporosis is a systemic skeletal disease characterized by low bone mass and microarchitectural deterioration of bone tissue, with a consequent increase in bone fragility and susceptibility to fracture.[1]

The TBS is derived from the texture of the DXA image and has been shown to be related to bone microarchitecture and fracture risk. It provides information independent of BMD.

		BMD T-score*		
		Normal	Osteopenia	Osteoporosis
TBS**	Normal			
	Partially degraded			
	Degraded		▫	

* BMD T-score is the min value of spine, total hip and femoral neck
** Spine TBS L1-L4 Normal microarchitecture > 1.31; Degraded ≤ 1.23

Low risk	Medium risk	High risk	Very High risk

Color coded Bone Health categories based on Fracture Risk[2]

(4) Therapeutic Decision Tools

The FRAX® 10-year probability of fracture:

Type of Fracture	Risk	Risk adjusted*
Major Osteoporotic	24 %	26 %
Hip	1.9 %	2.3 %

* Adjusted for TBS [3]. Validated only for Caucasian and Asian women and men. Refer to local guidelines before using these values.
Reported Risk factors: parent fractured hip, glucocorticoids

The BMD T-score:

Bone Site	BMD T-score	BMD T-score adjusted*
Spine	-2.3	-3.7
Femoral Neck	-2.1	-2.8
Total Hip	-1.6	-2.3

* Adjusted for ethnicity, gender and TBS [4]. Validated for Caucasian women only
The greyed cell is the minimum value of the 3 sites.

TBS osteo

(5) Detailed Spine Results

Region	TBS	TBS Z-score	BMD (g/cm²)	BMD T-score
L1	1.238	-	0.765	-1.5
L2	1.210	-	0.857	-1.6
L3	1.253	-	0.788	-2.7
L4	1.145	-	0.778	-3.1
L1-L4	1.212	-1.3	0.796	-2.3
L1-L3	1.234	-1.4	0.804	-1.9
L1-L4(L3)	1.198	-1.2	0.799	-2.1
L1-L4(L2)	1.212	-1.2	0.778	-2.5
L2-L4	1.203	-1.4	0.805	-2.5
L1-L2	1.224	-1.4	0.813	-1.5
L1-L3(L2)	1.246	-1.3	0.778	-2.1
L1-L4(L2L3)	1.191	-1.1	0.772	-2.4
L2-L3	1.232	-1.6	0.820	-2.2
L2-L4(L3)	1.177	-1.3	0.814	-2.4
L3-L4	1.199	-1.3	0.783	-2.9

(6) Conclusion

The Lumbar spine TBS is 1.212 which suggests a degraded microarchitecture compared to reference population.

The patient's associated major osteoporotic fracture risk, based on the combined results of BMD and TBS, is in the High risk zone.

Furthermore, the minimum BMD T-Score, either adjusted by the gender, the ethnicity and the TBS or not adjusted, positions the patient in the Osteoporosis category equivalent.

The patient's FRAX results should be interpreted in regard to the intervention thresholds provided by national medical guidelines.

Final decision regarding diagnostic or therapeutic recommendations should include BMD, TBS, additional clinical risk factors as well as the clinical context of the patient.

(7) Notes & References

Date of analysis: 03/02/2015 – TBS iNsight version 3.1.1
DXA: Discovery A #84322 – File: PA15302A.p11

1. Consensus Development Conference, Am J Med 94, 646-650 (1994)
2. Adapted from J. Bone Miner. Res. 26, 2762–2769 (2011)
3. Calcif Tissue Int. 96, 500-509 (2015)
4. Adapted from Osteoporos Int. 29, 751-758 (2018)

Source: Sample report provided by Medimaps group (www.medimapsgroup.com). Report typically provided in full color to best illustrate TBS mapping and other results.

See if Your Bones are Rebuilding

Bone Turnover Markers (Serum CTx, PINP)

CTx is a marker of bone resorption. PINP is a marker of bone formation. Ideally, both markers should be within the reference ranges seen in healthy premenopausal women.

Quite a few studies have now attempted to establish standard reference ranges for serum CTx and PINP by collecting data on healthy, young premenopausal women between the ages of 35 and 45 when bone remodeling is low and balanced. The most recent review of the research, published in 2017 by the IFCC-IOF Working Group for Standardization of Bone Marker Assays (WG-BMA), reports reference ranges for serum CTx as 114 to 628 ng/L and PINP as 16.3 to 78.2.

- Postmenopausal women losing too much bone typically have a CTx of 500 to as much as 1,000 pg/mL! The ranges given for CTx and PINP vary from lab to lab and are also quite wide, so it's most useful to run this lab initially to get a baseline and then run it again after 3 to 6 months of following your treatment plan to compare results.

- What you want to see is a balance between CTx and PINP. This is indicated by CTx below 500 and PINP in the mid to upper third of its reference range.

- For accurate test results, blood samples for CTx should be collected in the morning hours at approximately the same time and while fasting. Sample collection conditions for PINP are less critical as PINP has minimal circadian variability and is not affected by food intake, but it's easiest to have blood drawn for CTx and PINP at the same time.[1034] [1035]

24-Hour Urine Calcium

Calcium is excreted in both urine and feces. Ordinarily, 98% of calcium that passes through the kidneys is reabsorbed. If a 24-hour urine reports more than 200 mg of calcium for a woman or more than 250 mg for a man, the kidneys are losing more calcium than they should be, and that increases your risk for osteoporosis and kidney stones.

Increased urinary calcium excretion (hypercalciuria) may be due to:

- Consuming more than a total of 1,500 mg of calcium daily from food, supplements, and medications. Many over-the-counter antacids contain calcium carbonate. Each pill or chew will contain at least 200 mg and some contain more than 1,000 mg.

- Taking a diuretic, many of which increase calcium loss in urine.

- Consuming too much supplemental vitamin D. Your 25(OH)D result should not be greater than 80 ng/mL.

- Kidney Dysfunction: See Kidney Dysfunction under *What's Causing Your Bone Loss.*

- *BUN/Creatinine Ratio:* BUN measures the amount of urea nitrogen, a waste product of your liver's breakdown of cellular proteins that is sent into the bloodstream, removed by glomerular filtration in your kidneys, and excreted in urine. Creatinine is a breakdown product of creatine phosphate in muscle, usually produced at a fairly constant rate, removed from your blood by glomerular filtration, and excreted in urine.

  » Normal BUN levels are around 7 to 20 mg/dL (2.5 to 7.1 mmol/L).

  » Normal ratio of BUN to creatinine falls between 10:1 and 20:1.

- Hyperparathyroidism: In addition to a 24-hour urine calcium, run tests for *ionized calcium* (not just serum calcium) along with *intact PTH (iPTH).*

  » Ionized calcium is the unbound, metabolically active calcium in your bloodstream and is a more sensitive marker of primary hyperparathyroidism (PHPT). Serum calcium can be in normal range (10.1 mg/dL or less) when ionized calcium is elevated. The normal range for ionized calcium in adults is 4.64 to 5.28 mg/dL.

  » Intact PTH is the biologically active form of parathyroid hormone. Although lab reference ranges for normal can run from 15 to 65 pg/mL, if your serum calcium levels are at the upper end of the range (9 to 10) or higher, iPTH should be suppressed (i.e., should be less than 20 pg/mL).

Levels of iPTH peak during sleep hours and are lowest during mid-morning to late afternoon hours, so the earlier you can get into the lab for your blood draw, the better.

What's Causing Your Bone Loss?

Nutrient Insufficiencies

- **Vitamin D**: 25(OH)D (*aka* calcidiol) is the form in which vitamin D circulates in your bloodstream. *Blood levels of 25(OH)D should be checked twice yearly, in late winter and late summer, and dosage adjusted, if indicated, to remain in optimal range of 60 to 80 ng/mL.*

- **Vitamin K2 (unOC)**: Uncarboxylated (or undercarboxylated) osteocalcin is inactive osteocalcin, which has not been activated by vitamin K2 and therefore cannot bring calcium into your bones. If you are taking a vitamin K2 supplement providing 100 mcg of MK-7, but your unOC levels are still high, this means you require more vitamin K2 to activate your vitamin K-dependent proteins.[1036]

- **Vitamin A (serum retinol)**: Blood levels of retinol should fall within the range of: Mayo Clinic (32.5 to 78.0 mcg/dL); LabCorp (22.0 to 69.5 mcg/dL); and Quest Diagnostics (38 to 98 mcg/dL). Values above 120.0 mcg/dL indicate possible toxicity. Fast 8 to 12 hours prior to blood sample collection. Do not consume alcohol for 24 hours prior to collection.

- **Magnesium (RBC)**: Red blood cell levels should fall within the range of: LabCorp (4.2 to 6.8 mg/dL) and Quest Diagnostics (4.0 to 6.4 mg/dL).

- **Selenium (RBC)**: Red blood cell levels should fall within the range of: Quest Diagnostic (120 to 300 mcg/L; bit.ly/Quest-Sel); Doctor's Data (greater than 100 micromoles/L; (bit.ly/DD-Sel)

- **B vitamins**:
  - » *Homocysteine*, if elevated, may indicate folate, B6, or B12 deficiency. EMB consult range, (0 to 12 micromol/L; bit.ly/EMB-homocy). Dr. Pizzorno's recommendation for optimal range is 6 to 10 micromol/L. Mayo Clinic range varies depending upon age (bit.ly/Mayo-homocy). Fast 8 to 12 hours prior to blood sample collection.[1037 1038]
  - » *RBC Folate* indicates long-term folate status (during the last 3 months), so it's a better choice than serum folate which reflects recent dietary intake. RBC folate is widely available (i.e., LabCorp: bit.ly/LC-folate). Biotin interferes with the RBC folate assay.

» *Serum B12.* B12 deficiency is defined by the CDC as either a low serum vitamin B12 (<200 pg/mL) or elevated methylmalonic acid (>0.271 μmol/L). Serum B12 continues to be widely used but measures the total amount of B12 in your blood, while only 20% of the B12 in your bloodstream is metabolically active. For this reason, serum B12 can underreport the true prevalence of B12 deficiency. Research has shown that up to 40% of older people can have normal serum vitamin B12 but low metabolic status. Serum B12 should be combined with methylmalonic acid testing.

» *Methylmalonic Acid* (MMA) is a better functional marker of B12 status because it accumulates in urine when B12 is insufficient. If elevated, MMA indicates adenosyl B12 deficiency. However, MMA acid may also be elevated when kidney function is impaired, and loss of kidney function is common in elders. Reference range: Mayo Clinic (< or = 040 nmol/L); LabCorp (0 to 378 nmol/L); Quest Diagnostics (87 to 318 nmol/L).

The combination of the following two lab tests will check functional markers for all of the vitamins listed above. Test kits provide complete instructions for test preparation and proper use of the kit to provide samples:

• Genova Diagnostics: *Fat-Soluble Vitamins Profile*, serum (requires a blood draw): Checks A (retinol), D (total 25(OH)D)—also 25(OH) D2 and 25(OH)D3—E (alpha tocopherol only) and K2 (undercarboxylated osteocalcin). (bit.ly/GDX-vita)

• Genova Diagnostics: *NutrEval FMV* (first morning urine; bit.ly/ GDX-fmv)

Kidney Dysfunction

Glomerular filtration rate (GFR) typically declines with age, even in people without kidney disease. The estimated GFR (eGFR) calculation measures your level of kidney function taking age into account. At any age, however, a GFR below 60 for three months indicates possible kidney disease.[1039]

Age	Normal eGFR Range
young adults	90 to 120
50 to 59	93
60 to 69	85
70 and older	75

Digestive Dysfunction

- **Dysbiosis:** Genova Diagnostics offers 2 stool tests that can be helpful:
  - » *Comprehensive Digestive Stool Analysis 2.0 (CDSA 2.0)* includes functional markers of digestion/absorption, inflammation/allergic response, and the gut microbiome (bit.ly/GDX-cdsa).
  - » *GI Effects Comprehensive Profile – Stool* is an even more comprehensive test (bit.ly/GDX-Gi-Eff).

Markers for *H. pylori, C. difficile,* and zonulin can be added to either test. Do not take antimicrobials, proton pump inhibitors, or bismuth preparations for 2 weeks prior to testing. Test kits provide detailed instructions.

- **Hypochlorhydria**
  - » Home test: Dissolve a quarter teaspoon of bicarbonate (i.e., baking soda) in 1/4 to 1/2 cup of water, and drink on an empty stomach. If you have adequate levels of stomach acid, the baking soda and stomach acid will create a chemical reaction that produces carbon dioxide gas which causes belching. You should experience belching within 3 to 5 minutes after drinking the solution. A belch after this time (or not at all) may highlight a low level of stomach acid. To increase accuracy, take the test on 5 consecutive mornings and pull all outcomes together.[1040]
  - » *Heidelberg Test*: This test is conducted in your doctor's office. You swallow a supplement-sized capsule, which contains a micro-sensor that measures the pH of the stomach acid. Its findings are relayed by radio signal to a receiver positioned on top of your clothing over your stomach. The capsule is tethered on a string, which allows the capsule to remain in the correct position until the end of the test. While being tested, you swallow a solution

of bicarbonate (i.e., baking soda and water) or a standard test meal, which stimulates the gastric juices to reestablish acidity. As the healthy stomach cells continue to secrete hydrochloric acid (HCl), the pH gradually moves back into the acidic range. The rate at which the pH changes from alkaline back to acid, as you consume bicarbonate solution several times, accurately shows your stomach's ability to produce HCl. After the test, you're given water to drink, which opens the throat allowing the capsule to be gently lifted out by its attached tether.

Liver Dysfunction

Liver Function Test/Description	Ranges*
TSB (total serum bilirubin) tests for a pigment created as the body's normal process of breaking down old red blood cells. Elevated levels may indicate liver damage or disease.	A normal amount (approximate) is 1.2 mg/dL for adults. (Lower levels are usually not a concern.)
ALT (alanine transaminase) tests for an enzyme in the liver whose levels rise when its cells are being damaged. Also called alanine aminotransferase (ALAT).	Greater than 40 U/mL indicates liver damage or toxin exposure.
AST (aspartate aminotransferase) is an enzyme that can increase due to a damaged liver (or other organ).	Range for women: 8 to 43 U/L
GGT (gamma-glutamyl transferase) is an enzyme found mostly in the liver that helps metabolize toxins.	Range for women: 5 to 36 U/L. Levels above 25 U/L may indicate excessive alcohol consumption or exposure to environmental toxins.

*Normal results may vary by lab and can be affected by certain foods, medications or strenuous exercise.

Blood Sugar Control Dysfunction

- *Hemoglobin A1c* and *Pentosidine* are AGEs (advanced glycation end products). Elevated levels correlate with increased fracture risk in adults with type 2 diabetes. Even in postmenopausal women who do not have type 2 diabetes, higher levels of pentosidine are associated with higher risk of vertebral fractures.[1041] [1042] [1043]

- *HOMA Index* (insulin resistance): A calculated measure of insulin resistance which is associated with increased AGE formation in the bone matrix, which increases fragility.[1044]

Metabolic Acidosis

- *24-Hour Urine Citrate:* Urinary citrate is a major inhibitor of kidney stone formation due in part to binding of calcium in urine. Low urine citrate levels are a risk for kidney-stone formation. Several metabolic disorders are associated with low urine citrate. Any condition that lowers renal tubular pH or intracellular pH may decrease citrate excretion (e.g., metabolic acidosis, increased acid ingestion, hypokalemia, or hypomagnesemia).

  Low urinary citrate promotes kidney stone formation and growth, and responds to therapy by correcting acidosis, hypokalemia, or hypomagnesemia; by altering diet; or increasing consumption of citrate and potassium. Reference range: 420 to 1,191 mg/24 hours. Any value less than the mean (about 805 mg/24 hours) represents a potential risk for kidney-stone formation and growth. (Mayo Clinic: bit.ly/Mayo-Citr).

Thyroid Dysfunction (Hypothyroidism, Hyperthyroidism, Subclinical Hypothyroidism)

- *Thyroid Stimulating Hormone* (TSH; milliunits per liter): Healthy thyroid function is a midrange: women between 0.46 to 4.68 mIU/L and men between 0.5 to 4.59 mIU/L
  - » <0.10 mIU/L is considered low, hyperthyroid suspect.
  - » 0.10 to 0.29 mIU/L is considered borderline low.
  - » >4.2 mIU/L is considered high, hypothyroid suspect.
- *Free T4:* Mayo Clinic range (0.9 to 1.7 ng/dL)
  - » Elevated values suggest hyperthyroidism or too high a dose of levothyroxine or Armour® thyroid
  - » Low values suggest hypothyroidism, particularly if TSH is in normal range.
- *Free T3:* Mayo Clinic range (80 to 200 ng/dL), Cleveland Clinic range (5.0 to 11 µg/dL)

» Values above the reference range suggest hyperthyroidism or too high a dose of levothyroxine, T4 (or T3 if prescribed).

» Values below the reference range of the lab used suggest hypothyroidism, if TSH and T4 are in normal range, low T3 suggests euthyroid sick syndrome.

Thyroid Stimulating Hormone (TSH) Outside Normal Range	Potential Indications
TSH Low	• Hyperthyroidism (Free T4 and/or free T3 will be elevated.) • Too high a dose of levothyroxine or Armour® Thyroid. (Free T4 and possibly T3 will be elevated.) • Medication use (i.e., metformin and glucocorticoids) that suppresses TSH secretion (Free T4 and free T3 will be low.) • Pituitary function suppressed and not secreting TSH (secondary hypothyroidism). (Free T4 and T3 will also be low.) • Pituitary dysfunction may be due to medications that cause hyperprolactinemia: benzodiazepines, SSRIs, opioid pain medications.
TSH Slightly Elevated	• May be a protective response to maintain stable thyroid hormone levels with aging. • May indicate subclinical hypothyroidism.
TSH Significantly Elevated	• If T4 and T3 are also elevated, this suggests hyperthyroidism. • Could indicate Graves' disease (autoimmune) disease. • Could be caused by pituitary dysfunction causing excessive secretion of TSH, possibly due to a benign growth.

• *Thyroperoxidase* (TPO) *Antibodies*: Mayo Clinic normal range (<9.0 IU/mL)

» TPO is an enzyme involved in the production of thyroid hormone in the thyroid gland. Autoimmune reactions produce antibodies to TPO and thus prevent thyroid hormone synthesis.

» Values above 9.0 IU/mL suggest Hashimoto's autoimmune thyroiditis, the most common form of primary hypothyroidism, but elevations in TPO antibodies may also be seen in Graves' disease (hyperthyroidism).

» In patients with subclinical hypothyroidism, the presence of

TPO antibodies is associated with an increased risk of progressing to hypothyroidism.

- Autoimmune Activity Indicators
  » *Anti-thyroid antibodies* (TSI, TSH receptor antibody): If elevated, suggest autoimmune (hypothyroidism/Hashimoto's).
  » *Anti-thyroglobulin, anti-thyroid peroxidase antibodies*: If elevated, suggest autoimmune (hyperthyroidism/Graves' disease).
- Subclinical Hypercortisolism (due to incidental adenoma)
  » *Dexamethasone Challenge:* Dexamethasone (1 mg) administration followed by checking cortisol levels a few hours later. A cortisol level ≥ 1.8 to 2.0 mcg/dL (55 nmol/L) identifies patients likely to have an adrenal incidentaloma. Note that the range depends upon the dosage used and when the samples are collected. We are recommending a lower range than commonly accepted as normal.
  » Following this, *late night cortisol* may be measured. If cortisol remains high, then a blood test for adrenocorticotropic hormone (ACTH) may be run. If ACTH is high, this suggests Cushing's disease, which is most often caused by a non-cancerous tumor on the pituitary gland rather than the adrenal gland. If the result is only a slight increase in ACTH, this strongly suggests subclinical hypercortisolism.
  » A reduction in bone formation is suggestive of subclinical hypercortisolism. This can be checked by lab tests that check *blood levels of osteocalcin* and *bone alkaline phosphatase*. Low levels in these markers of bone formation suggest an adrenal incidentaloma.
  » Most individuals with subclinical hypercortisolism can be cured. If due to glucocorticoid medications, these can often be slowly decreased. If caused by an adrenal incidentaloma tumor, it may be treated by a combination of surgery, chemotherapy, and/or radiation.

Rheumatoid Arthritis (RA)

- *Antinuclear Antibodies (ANA).* Your immune system normally makes antibodies to help you fight infection. Antinuclear antibodies, however, often attack your body's own tissues, targeting each cell's nucleus. The presence of ANA is an abnormal test result, but many people have +ANA with no disease

- *Rheumatoid Factors (RF)* are proteins produced by your immune system that can attack healthy tissue. Normal range is 0 to 20 iu/ml. Higher levels can be due to autoimmune diseases, such as rheumatoid arthritis, also chronic infection or vaccinations. Once the RF level is elevated, it can remain so even if the condition goes into remission.

- *Anti-cyclic Citrullinated Peptide (anti-CCP)*. A level greater than 20 units is suggestive of RA and more specific than rheumatoid factor.

Food Intolerance

- IgG Food Antibodies: Genova Diagnostics (bit.ly/GDX-FoodSen)
- Celiac and Gluten Sensitivity: This lab includes Total IgA, tTG IgA, DGP IgA, EMA IgA, Anti-Gliadin IgG, and IgA. Genova Diagnostics (bit.ly/GDX-GlutSen)
- Elimination/Rechallenge Diet: This is the gold standard for checking possible food intolerance: a diet that temporarily removes main allergens and problematic foods (wheat/gluten, dairy, sugar, alcohol, refined, and packaged foods) and is a whole-foods diet. After several weeks, potential problem foods are reintroduced one by one to *rechallenge* the body. Those that provoke symptoms are again removed from the diet, possibly rechallenged later. You can download Dr. Liz Lipski's excellent Comprehensive Elimination Diet plan for free. (bit.ly/LizElimDiet)

Environmental Toxins

- *Gamma-Glutamyltransferase (GGT, also reported as GGTP)* is an enzyme primarily produced in the liver that has in the past been used to help diagnose hepatitis. When the liver is inflamed, it leaks enzymes into the blood. However, within the normal range, levels rise in response to alcohol, environmental toxins, and oxidative damage. Normal range for adults is 5 to 40 U/L (bit.ly/UCSF-ggt). Mayo Clinic reference range for women: 5 to 36 U/L, for men: 8 to 61 U/L (bit.ly/Mayo-ggt). We recommend GGT be below 25 since a level of 30 is associated with an 8-fold increased risk for diabetes.[1045]

- *Doctor's Data Urine Toxic Metals Challenge Test* evaluates body load of heavy metals, including cadmium, lead, and mercury. This test requires two urine specimens, a baseline urine followed by administration of a chelator and collection of a second urine about 6 hours later (bit.ly/DD-metals). Challenge testing should only be done in collaboration with a knowledgeable healthcare professional.

- *Great Plains GPL-Tox Profile* (Toxic Non-Metal Chemicals) screens for body load of many—but not all—toxic chemicals and endocrine disruptors such as organophosphate pesticides, phthalates (plasticizers), benzene, xylene, vinyl chloride, pyrethroid insecticides, acrylamide, perchlorate, diphenyl phosphate, ethylene oxide, acrylonitrile, and more (bit.ly/GPL-tox).

Indicators of Chronic Inflammation:

- *Erythrocyte Sedimentation Rate* (*ESR,* also called *sed rate*) can reveal inflammatory activity in your body. When your blood is placed in a tall, thin tube, red blood cells (erythrocytes) gradually settle to the bottom. Inflammation can cause the cells to clump. Because these clumps are denser than individual cells, they settle to the bottom more quickly. The more quickly red blood cells fall in a test tube in one hour, the greater the inflammatory response of your immune system.

- *High sensitivity C-reactive protein (hsCRP):* CRP, a protein whose levels rise in the blood in response to inflammation, is a known predictor of risk for cardiovascular disease and, more recently, for fracture. There are two different tests for C-reactive protein: *CRP* and *hs-CRP.* CRP, the standard test, measures a much wider, higher range but does not capture the lower ranges, which are what you want to check to see if low-level, chronic inflammation is contributing to your bone loss. hs-CRP accurately detects these lower concentrations.

  » *Healthy* people whose hs-CRP results are in the high end of the normal range (above 3.0 mg/L) have 1.5 to 4 times the risk of having a heart attack compared to those whose hs-CRP values are 1.0 mg/L or less, and a meta-analysis of 10 studies found fracture risk increased at least 60% in those in the upper tertial (i.e., those with the highest hsCRP).[1046]

  » If you have an inflammatory condition, like arthritis or periodontal disease, you should have CRP, not hs-CRP run. Your CRP levels will be too high to measure using hs-CRP.

» Because hs-CRP is a marker of inflammation, it is important that you are not just getting over a cold, flu, other infection, or injury when you run this test. Also, don't take nonsteroidal anti-inflammatory medications (e.g., aspirin, ibuprofen, or naproxen) which can temporarily reduce CRP levels and give a falsely lowered estimate of risk. Statins can also interfere with accurate assessment of hsCRP.

» Women on conventional hormone replacement (but not bio-identical hormone replacement) have been shown to have elevated hs-CRP levels, yet another reason to use BHRT and not HRT.

- *Homocysteine:* A highly inflammatory compound produced during methylation, a necessary process occurring all the time in our cells, homocysteine is either immediately converted into other, harmless compounds with the help of the activated B vitamins, or accumulates, spills out into the bloodstream, and causes damage to all it touches, including our bones.

» A normal blood level of homocysteine in the blood is less than 15 micromol/L. Optimal level is 6 to 10 micromol/L.[1047]

» Risk for fracture in individuals with elevated homocysteine is increased by at least 60%.[1048]

» If your homocysteine levels are elevated, your genetic inheritance may include one or more slow enzymes for the conversion of the B vitamins into their activated forms, in which case, you may wish to supplement with an *active B complex.*

- *NMR LipoProfile* includes LDL particle number (LDL-P), small LDL particle number (small LDL-P), HDL particle number (HDL-P), LDL particle size, as well as standard cholesterol test analytes (LDL-C, HDL-C, triglycerides, and total cholesterol), and also LP-IR, an indicator of risk for insulin resistance. Life Extension (bit.ly/LE-nmr); Labcorp (bit.ly/LC-nmr).

Hormone Insufficiency

- Bio-identical Hormone Replacement Therapy (estrogens, progesterone, testosterone, DHEA): Run one of the below labs both before and soon after initiating BHRT treatment, so a prescription that meets your specific needs can be made and then annually to confirm dosages remain accurate and safe.

  » *24-Hour Comprehensive Urine Hormone Panels:* Meridian Valley Labs (MVL)

  » *DUTCH* (Dried Urine Test for Comprehensive Hormones)

  Either of these two lab tests can be used to fully and accurately assess your levels of sex hormones (estrogens, progesterone, testosterone, and DHEA) and estrogen's metabolites, so you can confirm that your estrogens are being metabolized to produce safe, anti-inflammatory derivatives, not those that could increase risk of breast cancer. Both tests also check the adrenal hormones, cortisol, and cortisone.

  The main differences between the MVL test and DUTCH are (1) which analytes are checked and (2) how the urine samples are collected and sent in:

  » The MVL test reports the *Estrogen Quotient*, which gives you a very good indication of whether you are at risk for breast cancer, includes thyroid hormones as well, and you can request that growth hormone be added.

  » The DUTCH test does not include thyroid hormones, growth hormone, or the Estrogen Quotient. It does include melatonin and some nutritional organic acids the MVL test does not.

  » For the MVL test, you collect your urine in the jug provided for a full 24 hours, then fill several vials (also provided) with samples that you send to the lab.

  » For the DUTCH test, you collect a urine sample at either 4 or 5 specified times beginning at dinnertime on the first day and ending with a final sample taken 2 hours after waking on the following day. You dip a filter paper collection device into each urine sample, let them dry for a full 24 hours, and then mail the fully dried collection devices to the lab.

Closing Thoughts

Throughout this book, we've described study after study, hundreds in all. Each one represents the dedication, diligence, and patience of many researchers all over the world. A great thank-you is due to all of these pioneers whose investigations provide insight and solid data for what *actually* works to help people build and strengthen their bones. Without their rigorous work, the bone-saving material in the book would not be possible.

Joe thanks the brave men and women who, for over a century, have kept alive the important concepts of healthful living: eating organic rather than chemically-grown foods, using safe and effective nutritional supplements rather than just dependence on drugs, and believing and supporting doctors of natural, integrative, and functional medicine. He's also grateful to his patients for the trust they have placed in him during what is often among the most challenging and uncertain times in their lives.

Lara thanks *The Community*, whose stories you've heard here. While publishing articles and presenting at conferences is a great honor, she most loves being able to help thousands of women and men who are facing challenges similar to what she experienced some three decades ago. Connecting on social media, through live videos, and via messaging in real time to educate so many people and give them hope and direction is truly a blessing.

Finally, we both thank you for exploring this book and having the dedication to read it to the end. We appreciate your trust in us, and, more importantly, trusting your own intuition, which told you to follow the natural approach to improve your bone health—despite pushback from friends, family, and societal norms.

Now comes the most important part—following through. Put the material you read here into action in your life. Never forget that you were born preapproved to have healthy bones. Three life-affirming actions—good nutritional support, protecting yourself against harmful compounds in your diet and environment, and regular exercise—work together to support your body's inborn drive towards the healthy, balanced remodeling process that is your birthright.

You'll discover that the same actions that support your healthy bones ultimately support a healthy you!

Index

References

1   Emkey RD, Emkey GR. Calcium metabolism and correcting calcium deficiencies. Endocrinol Metab Clin North Am. 2012 Sep;41(3):527-56. Epub 2012 May 30. PMID: 22877428

2   Pizzorno J, Frassetto LA, Katzinger J. Diet-induced acidosis: is it real and clinically relevant? Br J Nutr. 2010 Apr;103(8):1185-94. Epub 2009 Dec 15. PMID: 20003625

3   Pizzorno J, Frassetto LA, Katzinger J. Diet-induced acidosis: is it real and clinically relevant? Br J Nutr. 2010 Apr;103(8):1185-94. Epub 2009 Dec 15. PMID: 20003625

4   Shariati-Bafghi SE, Nosrat-Mirshekarlou E, Karamati M, et al. Higher Dietary Acidity is Associated with Lower Bone Mineral Density in Postmenopausal Iranian Women, Independent of Dietary Calcium Intake. Int J Vitam Nutr Res. 2014;84(3-4):206-17. PMID: 26098484

5   Pizzorno J, Frassetto LA, Katzinger J. Diet-induced acidosis: is it real and clinically relevant? Br J Nutr. 2010 Apr;103(8):1185-94. Epub 2009 Dec 15. PMID: 20003625

6   Groenendijk I, Boeft L, Loon L, et al. High Versus low Dietary Protein Intake and Bone Health in Older Adults: a Systematic Review and Meta-Analysis. Comput Struct Biotechnol J. 2019 Jul 22;17:1101-1112. eCollection 2019. PMID: 31462966

7   Park Y, Choi J, Hwang H. Protein supplementation improves muscle mass and physical performance in undernourished prefrail and frail elderly subjects: a randomized, double-blind, placebo-controlled trial. Randomized Controlled Trial Am J Clin Nutr. 2018 Nov 1;108(5):1026-1033. https://academic.oup.com/ajcn/article/108/5/1026/5201551

8   TC, Frankenfeld CL. Dietary Protein Intake above the Current RDA and Bone Health: A Systematic Review and Meta-Analysis. J Am Coll Nutr. 2017 Aug;36(6):481-496. Epub 2017 Jul 7. PMID: 28686536.

9   Emkey RD, Emkey GR. Calcium metabolism and correcting calcium deficiencies. Endocrinol Metab Clin North Am. 2012 Sep;41(3):527-56. Epub 2012 May 30. PMID: 22877428

10 Dawson-Hughes B, Harris SS. Calcium intake influences the association of protein intake with rates of bone loss in elderly men and women. Am J Clin Nutr. 2002 Apr;75(4):773-9. PMID: 11916767

11 Heaney RP. Protein and calcium: antagonists or synergists? Calcium intake influences the association of protein intake with rates of bone loss in elderly men and women. Am J Clin Nutr. 2002 Apr;75(4):609-10. PMID: 11916747

12 Sahni S, Cupples LA, McLean RR, et al. Protective effect of high protein and calcium intake on the risk of hip fracture in the Framingham offspring cohort. J Bone Miner Res. 2010 Dec;25(12):2770-6. doi: 10.1002/jbmr.194. Epub 2010 Jul 26. PMID: 20662074

13 Yuna Zhong, Catherine A Okoro, Lina S Balluz. Association of total calcium and dietary protein intakes with fracture risk in postmenopausal women: the 1999-2002 NHANES. PMID: 19230618

14 L. Wu,1,2 B. J. C. Luthringer,1 F. Feyerabend, et al. Increased levels of sodium chloride directly increase osteoclastic differentiation and resorption in mice and men. 2017 Aug 29. PMID: 28849275

15 https://www.cdc.gov/heartdisease/sodium.htm

16 https://www.cdc.gov/heartdisease/sodium.htm

17 The nature and significance of the relationship between urinary sodium and urinary calcium in women. J Nutr. 1993 Sep;123(9):1615-22. PMID: 8360790

18 Breslau NA, McGuire JL, Zerwekh JE, et al. (1982) The role of dietary sodium on renal excretion and intestinal absorption of calcium on vitamin D metabolism. J Clin Endocrinol Metab. 1982 Aug;55(2):369-73. PMID:6896338

19 Tsanzi E, Fitch CW, Tou JC. Effect of consuming different caloric sweeteners on bone health and possible mechanisms. Nutr Rev. 2008 Jun;66(6):301-9. PMID: 18522618

20 Tsanzi E, Fitch CW, Tou JC. Effect of consuming different caloric sweeteners on bone health and possible mechanisms. Nutr Rev. 2008 Jun;66(6):301-9. PMID: 18522618

21 Lemann Jr J, Lennon EJ, Piering WR, et al. Evidence that glucose ingestion inhibits net renal tubular reabsorption of calcium and magnesium in man. J Lab Clin Med. 1970 Apr;75(4):578-85. PMID: 5444345

22 Thom JA, Morris JE, Bishop A, et al. The influence of refined carbohydrate on urinary calcium excretion. Br J Urol. 1978 Dec;50(7):459-64. PMID: 572722

23 Urine Calcium: Laboratory Measurement and Clinical Utility http://www.medscape.com/viewarticle/732914

24 Baldini V, Mastropasqua M, Francucci C, et al. Cardiovascular disease and osteoporosis. J Endocrinol Invest. 2005;28(10 Suppl):69-72. PMID: 16550727

25 Rathinavelu S, Guidry-Elizondo C, Banum J, et al. Molecular Modulation of Osteoblasts and Osteoclasts in Type 2 Diabetes.J Diabetes Res. 2018 Nov 4;2018:6354787. eCollection 2018. PMID: 30525054

26 Liu C, Broe K, Zhou Y, et al. Visceral Adipose Tissue Is Associated With Bone Microarchitecture in the Framingham Osteoporosis Study. J Bone Miner Res. 2017 Jan;32(1):143-150. Epub 2016 Sep 6. PMID: 27487454

27 Mantovani A, Sani E, Fassio A, Colecchia A, Viapiana O, Gatti D, Idolazzi L, Rossini M, Salvagno G, Lippi G, Zoppini G, Byrne CD, Bonora E, Targher G. Association between non-alcoholic fatty liver disease and bone turnover biomarkers in post-menopausal women with type 2 diabetes. Diabetes Metab. 2019 Sep;45(4):347-355. Epub 2018 Oct 10. PMID: 30315891.

28 Diabetes Metab. 2019 Sep;45(4):347-355. Epub 2018 Oct 10. PMID: 30315891

29 Reginster J, Beaudart C, Buckinx F, et al. Osteoporosis and sarcopenia: two diseases or one? Curr Opin Clin Nutr Metab Care. 2016 Jan;19(1):31-6. PMID: 26418824

30 Wang Y, Beydoun MA, Min J, Xue H, Kaminsky LA, Cheskin LJ. Has the prevalence of overweight, obesity and central obesity levelled off in the United States? Trends, patterns, disparities, and future projections for the obesity epidemic. Int J Epidemiol. 2020 Jun 1;49(3):810-823. PMID: 32016289; PMCID: PMC7394965

31 Dilzer A, Park Y. Implication of conjugated linoleic acid (CLA) in human health. Crit Rev Food Sci Nutr. 2012;52(6):488-513. PMID: 22452730

32 Lawson RE, Moss AR, Givens DI.The role of dairy products in supplying conjugated linoleic acid to man's diet: a review. Nutr Res Rev. 2001 Jun;14(1):153-72. PMID: 19087420

33 Benbrook CM, Butler G, Latif MA, et al. Organic production enhances milk nutritional quality by shifting Fatty Acid composition: a United States-wide, 18-month study. PLoS One. 2013 Dec 9;8(12):e82429. eCollection 2013. PMID: 24349282

34 Dhiman TR, Nam SH, Ure AL. Factors affecting conjugated linoleic acid content in milk and meat. Crit Rev Food Sci Nutr. 2005;45(6):463-82. PMID: 16183568

35 Booth SL, Lichtenstein AH, O'Brien-Morse M, et al. Effects of a hydrogenated form of vitamin K on bone formation and resorption. Am J Clin Nutr. 2001 Dec;74(6):783-90. PMID: 11722960

36 Dietz WH1, Scanlon KS. Eliminating the use of partially hydrogenated oil in food production and preparation. JAMA. 2012 Jul 11;308(2):143-4. PMID: 22782414

37 Kontogianni MD1, Melistas L, Yannakoulia M, et al. Association between dietary patterns and indices of bone mass in a sample of Mediterranean women. Nutrition. 2009 Feb;25(2):165-71. Epub 2008 Oct 11 PMID: 18849146

38 Hagiwara K, Goto T, Araki M, et al. Olive polyphenol hydroxytyrosol prevents bone loss. Eur J Pharmacol. 2011 Jul 15;662(1-3):78-84. Epub 2011 Apr 27. PMID: 21539839

39 Franco MN, Galeano-Díaz T, Sánchez J, De Miguel C, Martín-Vertedor D. Total phenolic compounds and tocopherols profiles of seven olive oil varieties grown in the south-west of Spain. J Oleo Sci. 2014;63(2):115-25. PMID: 24500102

40 Kruger MC1, Coetzee M, Haag M, et al. Long-chain polyunsaturated fatty acids: selected mechanisms of action on bone. Prog Lipid Res. 2010 Oct;49(4):438-49. Epub 2010 Jun 17. PMID: 20600307

41 Yuan J, Akiyama M, Nakahama K, et al. The effects of polyunsaturated fatty acids and their metabolites on osteoclastogenesis in vitro. Prostaglandins Other Lipid Mediat. 2010 Jun;92(1-4):85-90. Epub 2010 Apr 13. PMID: 20394833

42 Kajarabille N, Díaz-Castro J, Hijano S, et al. A new insight to bone turnover: role of ω-3 polyunsaturated fatty acids. ScientificWorldJournal. 2013 Nov 4;2013:589641. PMID: 24302863

43 Casado-Díaz A, Santiago-Mora R, Dorado G, et al. The omega-6 arachidonic fatty acid, but not the omega-3 fatty acids, inhibits osteoblastogenesis and induces adipogenesis of human mesenchymal stem cells: potential implication in osteoporosis. Osteoporos Int. 2013 May;24(5):1647-61. Epub 2012 Oct 27. PMID: 23104199

44 Kelly OJ, Gilman JC, Kim Y, et al. Long-chain polyunsaturated fatty acids may mutually benefit both obesity and osteoporosis. Nutr Res. 2013 Jul;33(7):521-33. Epub 2013 Jun 10. PMID: 23827126

45 Casado-Díaz A, Santiago-Mora R, Dorado G, et al. The omega-6 arachidonic fatty acid, but not the omega-3 fatty acids, inhibits osteoblastogenesis and induces adipogenesis of human mesenchymal stem cells: potential implication in osteoporosis. Osteoporos Int. 2013 May;24(5):1647-61. Epub 2012 Oct 27. PMID: 23104199

46 Lee SM, An WS. Cardioprotective effects of ω -3 PUFAs in chronic kidney disease. Biomed Res Int. 2013;2013:712949. Epub 2013 Apr 4. PMID: 23653897

47 Kajarabille N, Díaz-Castro J, Hijano S, et al. A new insight to bone turnover: role of ω-3 polyunsaturated fatty acids. ScientificWorldJournal. 2013 Nov 4;2013:589641. PMID: 24302863

48 Guebre-Egziabher F, Debard C, Drai J, et al. Differential dose effect of fish oil on inflammation and adipose tissue gene expression in chronic kidney disease patients. Nutrition. 2013 May;29(5):730-6. Epub 2013 Jan 30. PMID: 23375525

49 Fasano A., Linus Pauling Award Acceptance Speech, IFM Symposium, May 2012, Houston, TX

50 El Asmar R, Panigrahi P, Bamford P, Berti I, Not T, Coppa GV, Catassi C, Fasano A. Host-dependent activation of the zonulin system is involved in the impairment of the gut barrier function following bacterial colonization. Gastroenterology. 2002 Nov;123(5):1607-15. PMID: 12404235

51 Roszkowska A, Pawlicka M, Mroczek A, Bałabuszek K, Nieradko-Iwanicka B. Non-Celiac Gluten Sensitivity: A

Review. Medicina (Kaunas). 2019 May 28;55(6):222. PMID: 31142014; PMCID: PMC6630947.

52 Yuan Z, Liu D, Citations: Zhang L, et al. Mitotic illegitimate recombination is a mechanism for novel changes in high-molecular-weight glutenin subunits in wheat-rye hybrids. PLoS One. 2011;6(8):e23511. Epub 2011 Aug 22. PMID: 21887262

53 Molnár-Láng M, Kruppa K, Cseh A, et al. Identification and phenotypic description of new wheat: six-rowed winter barley disomic additions. Genome. 2012 Apr;55(4):302-11. Epub 2012 Mar 23. PMID: 22439846

54 Leduc V, Moneret-Vautrin DA, Guerin L, et al. Anaphylaxis to wheat isolates: immunochemical study of a case proved by means of double-blind, placebo-controlled food challenge. J Allergy Clin Immunol. 2003 Apr;111(4):897-9. PMID: 12704375

55 Battais F, Richard C, Jacquenet S, et al. Wheat grain allergies: an update on wheat allergens. Eur Ann Allergy Clin Immunol. 2008 Nov;40(3):67-76. PMID: 19334370

56 Denery-Papini S, Bodinier M, Larré C, et al. Allergy to deamidated gluten in patients tolerant to wheat: specific epitopes linked to deamidation. Allergy. 2012 Aug;67(8):1023-32. Epub 2012 Jun 28. PMID: 22737987

57 Catassi C, Sapone A, Fasano A, et al. Non-Celiac Gluten sensitivity: the new frontier of gluten related disorders. Nutrients. 2013 Sep 26;5(10):3839-53. PMID: 24077239

58 Sapone A, Lammers KM, Fasano A, et al. Divergence of gut permeability and mucosal immune gene expression in two gluten-associated conditions: celiac disease and gluten sensitivity. BMC Med. 2011 Mar 9;9:23. PMID: 21392369

59 Sapone A, Bai JC, Fasano A, et al. Spectrum of gluten-related disorders: consensus on new nomenclature and classification. BMC Med. 2012 Feb 7;10:13. Review. PMID: 22313950

60 Gaddini G, Turner R, Grant K, et al. Alcohol: A Simple Nutrient with Complex Actions on Bone in the Adult Skeleton. Alcohol Clin Exp Res. 2016 Apr;40(4):657-71. Epub 2016 Mar 12. PMID: 26971854 https://www.ncbi.nlm.nih.gov/pmc/articles/PMC4918769/

61 https://blog.udemy.com/alcohol-content-of-beer/

62 https://winefolly.com/tips/the-lightest-to-the-strongest-wine/

63 Maurel DB, Boisseau N, Benhamou CL, et al. Alcohol and bone: review of dose effects and mechanisms. Osteoporos Int. 2012 Jan;23(1):1-16. Epub 2011 Sep 17. PMID: 21927919

64 Mobasheri A, Shakibaei M.Osteogenic effects of resveratrol in vitro: potential for the prevention and treatment of osteoporosis. Ann N Y Acad Sci. 2013 Jul;1290:59-66. PMID: 23855466

65 Maurel DB, Boisseau N, Benhamou CL, et al. Alcohol and bone: review of dose effects and mechanisms. Osteoporos Int. 2012 Jan;23(1):1-16. Epub 2011 Sep 17. PMID: 21927919

66 Du L, Li S, Qi L, et al. Metabonomic analysis of the joint toxic action of long-term low-level exposure to a mixture of four organophosphate pesticides in rat plasma. Mol Biosyst. 2014 Mar 13. [Epub ahead of print] PMID: 24626741

67 C Demur, B Métais, C Canlet, et al. Dietary exposure to a low dose of pesticides alone or as a mixture: the biological metabolic fingerprint and impact on hematopoiesis. PMID: 23528616

68 Siddarth M, Datta SK, Mustafa M, et al. Increased level of organochlorine pesticides in chronic kidney disease patients of unknown etiology: role of GSTM1/GSTT1 polymorphism. Chemosphere. 2014 Feb;96:174-9. Epub 2013 Nov 9. PMID: 24216264

69 Josephy PD. Genetic variations in human glutathione transferase enzymes: significance for pharmacology and toxicology. Hum Genomics Proteomics. 2010 Jun 13;2010:876940. PMID: 20981235

70 Montagnani A, Gonnelli S. Antidiabetic therapy effects on bone metabolism and fracture risk. Diabetes Obes Metab. 2013 Sep;15(9):784-91. Epub 2013 Feb 24. PMID: 23368527

71 Montagnani A, Gonnelli S, Alessandri M, et al. Osteoporosis and risk of fracture in patients with diabetes: an update. Aging Clin Exp Res. 2011 Apr;23(2):84-90. PMID: 21743287

72 Schwartz AV, Sellmeyer DE. Diabetes, fracture, and bone fragility. Curr Osteoporos Rep. 2007 Sep;5(3):105-11. PMID: 17925191

73 Yamamoto M. Secondary osteoporosis or secondary contributors to bone loss in fracture. Bone metabolic disorders in patients with diabetes mellitus. [Article in Japanese] Clin Calcium. 2013 Sep;23(9):1327-35. PMID: 23999370

74 Varenna M, Manara M, Galli L, et al. The association between osteoporosis and hypertension: the role of a low dairy intake. Calcif Tissue Int. 2013 Jul;93(1):86-92. Epub 2013 May 8. PMID: 23652773

75 Fehérvári M, Sarkadi H, Krepuska M, et al. Bone mineral density is associated with site-specific atherosclerosis in patients with severe peripheral artery disease. Calcif Tissue Int. 2013 Jul;93(1):55-61. Epub 2013 Apr 6. PMID: 23564349

76 Fehérvári M, Krepuska M, Csobay-Novák C, et al. [Prevalence of osteoporosis in patients with severe peripheral artery disease].[Article in Hungarian] Orv Hetil. 2013 Mar 10;154(10):369-75. PMID: 23461977

77 Palacios S, Neyro JL, Puertas JC, et al. Clinical profile of Spanish postmenopausal women with a diagnosis of osteoporosis and risk factors for endometrial pathology, breast cancer, and cardiovascular disease. Menopause. 2013 Aug;20(8):852-9. PMID: 23481116

78 Tankó LB, Christiansen C, Cox DA, et al. Relationship between osteoporosis and cardiovascular disease in postmenopausal women. J Bone Miner Res. 2005 Nov;20(11):1912-20. Epub 2005 Jul 18. PMID: 16234963

79 Uribarri J, Calvo MS. Dietary phosphorus intake and health. Am J Clin Nutr. 2013 Dec 31. [Epub ahead of print] PMID: 24381089

80 Uribarri J, Calvo MS. Dietary phosphorus excess: a risk factor in chronic bone, kidney, and cardiovascular disease? Adv Nutr. 2013 Sep 1;4(5):542-4. PMID: 24038251

81 Calvo MS, Moshfegh AJ, Tucker KL. Assessing the health impact of phosphorus in the food supply: issues and considerations. Adv Nutr. 2014 Jan1 5(1): 104-13. PMID:24425729

82 Calvo MS, Moshfegh AJ, Tucker KL. Assessing the health impact of phosphorus in the food supply: issues and considerations. Adv Nutr. 2014 Jan 1;5(1):104-13. PMID: 24425729

83 Calvo MS, Tucker KL. Is phosphorus intake that exceeds dietary requirements a risk factor in bone health? Ann N Y Acad Sci. 2013 Oct;1301(1):29-35. PMID: 24472074

84 Chang AR, Lazo M, Appel LJ, Gutie´rrez OM, Grams ME. High dietary phosphorus intake is associated with all-cause mortality: results from NHANES III. Am J Clin Nutr. 2014 Feb;99(2):320-7. Epub 2013 Nov 13. PMID: 24225358

85 Uribarri J, Calvo MS. Dietary phosphorus excess: a risk factor in chronic bone, kidney, and cardiovascular disease? Adv Nutr. 2013 Sep 1;4(5):542-4. PMID: 24038251

86 Fernando GR, Martha RM, Evangelina R. Consumption of soft drinks with phosphoric acid as a risk factor for the development of hypocalcemia in postmenopausal women. J Clin Epidemiol. 1999 Oct;52(10):1007-10. PMID: 10513764

87 Johansen DL, Eiken PA. [Cola as a possible cause of secondary hyperparathyroidism]. Ugeskr Laeger. 2002 Sep 9;164(37):4290-1. PMID: 12362872 [Article in Danish]

88 Kristensen M, Jensen M, Kudsk J, et al. Short-term effects on bone turnover of replacing milk with cola beverages: a 10-day interventional study in young men. Osteoporos Int. 2005 Dec;16(12):1803-8. Epub 2005 May 11. PMID: 15886860

89 Calvo MS, Moshfegh AJ, Tucker KL. Assessing the health impact of phosphorus in the food supply: issues and considerations. Adv Nutr. 2014 Jan 1;5(1):104-13. PMID: 24425729

90 Meeker JD, Ferguson KK. Relationship between urinary phthalate and bisphenol A concentrations and serum thyroid measures in U.S. adults and adolescents from the National Health and Nutrition Examination Survey (NHANES) 2007-2008. Environ Health Perspect. 2011 Oct;119(10):1396-402. Epub 2011 Jul 11. PMID: 21749963

91 Huang H, Pan W, Chang J, et al. Does exposure to phthalates influence thyroid function and growth hormone homeostasis? The Taiwan Environmental Survey for Toxicants (TEST) 2013. Environ Res 2017 Feb;153:63-72. Epub 2016 Nov 29. PMID: 27907809

92 Park C, Choi W, Hwang M, et al. Associations between urinary phthalate metabolites and bisphenol A levels, and serum thyroid hormones among the Korean adult population—Korean National Environmental Health Survey (KoNEHS) 2012-2014. Sci Total Environ. 2017 Apr 15;584-585:950-957. Epub 2017 Jan 31. PMID: 28153396

93 Min K, Min J. Urinary phthalate metabolites and the risk of low bone mineral density and osteoporosis in older women. J Clin Endocrinol Metab. 2014 Oct;99(10):E1997-2003. Epub 2014 Jul 22. PMID: 25050905

94 Hwang J, Min K, Choi K, et al. Bisphenol A reduces differentiation and stimulates apoptosis of osteoclasts and osteoblasts Life Sci. 2013 Sep 17;93(9-11):367-72. Epub 2013 Jul 27. PMID: 23900028

95 Chin K, Pang K, Mark-Lee W. A Review on the Effects of Bisphenol A and Its Derivatives on Skeletal Health. Int J Med Sci. 2018 Jun 22;15(10):1043-1050. eCollection 2018. PMID: 30013446

96 Thent Z, Froemming G, Muid S. Bisphenol A exposure disturbs the bone metabolism: An evolving interest towards an old culprit. Life Sci. 2018 Apr 1;198:1-7. Epub 2018 Feb 10. PMID: 29432759

97 Johns L, Ferguson K, Cantonwine D, et al. Urinary BPA and Phthalate Metabolite Concentrations and Plasma Vitamin D Levels in Pregnant Women: A Repeated Measures Analysis. Environ Health Perspect. 2017 Aug 31;125(8):087026. PMID: 28934718 https://www.ncbi.nlm.nih.gov/pubmed/?term=28934718

98 https://silentspring.org/news/fresh-food-diet-reduces-levels-hormone-disruptors-bpa-and-dehp

99 Rudel R, Gray J, Engel C, et al. Food packaging and bisphenol A and bis(2-ethylhexyl) phthalate exposure: Findings from a dietary intervention. Environmental Health Perspectives, 119:914-920. doi:10.1289/ehp.1003170 PMID: 21450549

100 Rudel R, Ackerman J, Dodson R. 2011. Dietary Intervention and DEHP Reduction: Rudel et al. Respond. Environmental Health Perspectives, 119(9):a380-a381. doi:10.1289/ehp.1103852R

101 Everett ET. Fluoride's effects on the formation of teeth and bones, and the influence of genetics. J Dent Res. 2011 May;90(5):552-60. Epub 2010 Oct 6. PMID: 20929720

102 Whitford GM. Intake and metabolism of fluoride. Adv Dent Res. 1994 Jun;8(1):5-14. PMID: 7993560

103 Bergandi L, Aina V, Malavasi G, et al. The toxic effect of fluoride on MG-63 osteoblast cells is also dependent on the production of nitric oxide. Chem Biol Interact. 2011 Apr 25;190(2-3):179-86. Epub 2011 Feb 15. PMID: 21329685

104 Bergandi L, Aina V, Garetto S, et al. Fluoride-containing bioactive glasses inhibit pentose phosphate oxidative pathway and glucose 6-phosphate dehydrogenase activity in human osteoblasts. Chem Biol Interact. 2010 Feb 12;183(3):405-15. Epub 2009 Nov 27. PMID: 19945446

105 Song YE, Tan H, Liu KJ, et al. Effect of fluoride exposure on bone metabolism indicators ALP, BALP, and BGP. Environ Health Prev Med. 2011 May;16(3):158-63. Epub 2010 Oct 2. PMID: 21431799

106 Everett ET. Fluoride's effects on the formation of teeth and bones, and the influence of genetics. J Dent Res. 2011 May;90(5):552-60. Epub 2010 Oct 6. PMID: 20929720

107 DePaula CA, Pan Y, Guzelsu N. Uniform partial dissolution of bone mineral by using fluoride and phosphate ions combination. Connect Tissue Res. 2008;49(5):328-42. PMID: 18991086

108 Wright JV. Fight tooth decay and dramatically slash or even eliminate dental cavities for a lifetime! Nutrition & Healing. Vol. 19, Issue 3, May 2012.

109 delishably.com/beverages/Fluoride-Content-in-Black-Tea-White-Tea-and-Green-Tea-Tea-Health-Benefits-and-Dangers

110 Jha SK, Mishra VK, Sharma DK, et al. Fluoride in the environment and its metabolism in humans. Rev Environ Contam Toxicol. 2011;211:121-42. PMID: 21287392

111 Rosin A. The long-term consequences of exposure to lead. Isr Med Assoc J. 2009 Nov;11(11):689-94. PMID: 20108558

112 Obeng-Gyasi E. Sources of lead exposure in various countries. Rev Environ Health. 2019 Mar 26;34(1):25-34. PMID: 30854835

113 Rosin A. The long-term consequences of exposure to lead. Isr Med Assoc J. 2009 Nov;11(11):689-94. PMID: 20108558

114 Khalil N, Cauley JA, Wilson JW, et al. Relationship of blood lead levels to incident non-spine fractures and falls in older women: the study of osteoporotic fractures. J Bone Miner Res. 2008 Sep;23(9):1417-25. PMID: 18410230

115 Rosin A. The long-term consequences of exposure to lead. Isr Med Assoc J. 2009 Nov;11(11):689-94. PMID: 20108558

116 Chang WJ, Joe KT, Park HY, Jeong JD, Lee DH.The relationship of liver function tests to mixed exposure to lead and organic solvents. Ann Occup Environ Med. 2013 May 21;25(1):5. PMID: 24472152

117 Beier EE, Maher JR, Sheu TJ, et al. Heavy metal lead exposure, osteoporotic-like phenotype in an animal model, and depression of Wnt signaling.Environ Health Perspect. 2013 Jan;121(1):97-104. Epub 2012 Oct 19. PMID: 23086611

118 Rosin A. The long-term consequences of exposure to lead. Isr Med Assoc J. 2009 Nov;11(11):689-94. PMID: 20108558

119 Chang WJ, Joe KT, Park HY, Jeong JD, Lee DH.The relationship of liver function tests to mixed exposure to lead and organic solvents. Ann Occup Environ Med. 2013 May 21;25(1):5. PMID: 24472152

120 Mumford SL, Dasharathy SS, Pollack AZ, et al. Serum uric acid in relation to endogenous reproductive hormones during the menstrual cycle: findings from the BioCycle study. Hum Reprod. 2013 Jul;28(7):1853-62. Epub 2013 Apr 5. PMID: 23562957

121 Jin T, Nordberg G, Ye T, et al. Osteoporosis and renal dysfunction in a general population exposed to cadmium in China. Environ Res. 2004 Nov;96(3):353-9. PMID: 15364604

122 https://www.osha.gov/pls/oshaweb/owadisp.show_document?p_table=STANDARDS&p_id=10036

123 Satarug S, Garrett SH, Sens MA, Sens DA. Cadmium, environmental exposure, and health outcomes. Cien Saude Colet. 2011 May;16(5):2587-602. PMID: 21655733 Republished from Environ Health Perspect. 2010 Feb;118(2):182-90

124 Gallagher CM, Kovach JS, Meliker JR. Urinary cadmium and osteoporosis in U.S. Women >or= 50 years of age: NHANES 1988-1994 and 1999-2004. Environ Health Perspect. 2008 Oct;116(10):1338-43. Epub 2008 Jun 13. PMID: 18941575

125 James KA, Meliker JR. Environmental cadmium exposure and osteoporosis: a review. Int J Public Health. 2013 Oct;58(5):737-45. Epub 2013 Jul 23. PMID: 23877535

126 Alfvén T, Elinder CG, Carlsson MD, et al. Low-level cadmium exposure and osteoporosis. J Bone Miner Res. 2000 Aug;15(8):1579-86. PMID: 10934657

127 Julin B, Wolk A, Johansson JE, et al. Dietary cadmium exposure and prostate cancer incidence: a population-based prospective cohort study. Br J Cancer. 2012 Aug 21;107(5):895-900. Epub 2012 Jul 31. PMID: 22850555

128 Julin B, Wolk A, Bergkvist L, et al. Dietary cadmium exposure and risk of postmenopausal breast cancer: a population-based prospective cohort study. Cancer Res. 2012 Mar 15;72(6):1459-66. CAN-11-0735. PMID: 22422990

129 Gallagher CM, Kovach JS, Meliker JR. Urinary cadmium and osteoporosis in U.S. Women >or= 50 years of age: NHANES 1988-1994 and 1999-2004. Environ Health Perspect. 2008 Oct;116(10):1338-43. Epub 2008 Jun 13. PMID: 18941575

130 Engström A, Michaëlsson K, Vahter M, et al. Associations between dietary cadmium exposure and bone miner-

al density and risk of osteoporosis and fractures among women. Bone. 2012 Jun;50(6):1372-8. Epub 2012 Mar 24. PMID: 22465267

131 Mann D, Can Heavy Metal in Foods, Cosmetics Spur Breast Cancer Spread? Yahoo News http://web.archive. org/web/20120426102047/http://news.yahoo.com/heavy-metal-foods-cosmetics-spur-breast-cancer-spread-200608223.html

132 Cadmium In Jewelry: Federal Regulators Failed To Protect Children From Cancer-Causing Metals, Huffington Post, 2012.10.14

133 FDA Consumer Updates, Mercury Poisoning Linked to Skin Products http://www.fda

134 Park JD, Zheng W. Human exposure and health effects of inorganic and elemental mercury. J Prev Med Public Health. 2012 Nov;45(6):344-52. Epub 2012 Nov 29. PMID: 23230464

135 Monika Mania 1, Maria Wojciechowska-Mazurek, Krystyna Starska, et al. Fish and seafood as a source of human exposure to methylmercury. PMID: 23173330

136 Bridges CC, Zalups RK. The aging kidney and the nephrotoxic effects of mercury. J Toxicol Environ Health B Crit Rev. 2017;20(2):55-80. Epub 2017 Feb 7. PMID: 28339347

137 Pizzorno J, The Path Ahead: Clinical Experience in Decreasing Mercury Load, IMCJ, Integrative Medicine • Vol. 10, No. 4 • Sept/Oct 2011

138 Pizzorno J. The Path Ahead: Is Mercury Toxicity an Epidemic? February, 2009,VOL. 8, NO. 1, p. 8-10

139 Houston MC. Role of mercury toxicity in hypertension, cardiovascular disease, and stroke.J Clin Hypertens (Greenwich). 2011 Aug;13(8):621-7. Epub 2011 Jul 11. PMID: 21806773

140 Monteiro CA, Cannon G, Levy RB, et al. Ultra-processed foods: what they are and how to identify them. Public Health Nutr. 2019 Apr;22(5):936-941. Epub 2019 Feb 12. PMID: 30744710

141 Zobel EH, Hansen TW, Rossing P, et al. Global Changes in Food Supply and the Obesity Epidemic. Curr Obes Rep. 2016 Dec;5(4):449-455. PMID: 27696237

142 Hall KD, Ayuketah A, Brychta R, et al. Ultra-Processed Diets Cause Excess Calorie Intake and Weight Gain: An Inpatient Randomized Controlled Trial of Ad Libitum Food Intake. Cell Metab. 2019 Jul 2;30(1):67-77.e3. Epub 2019 May 16. Erratum in: Cell Metab. 2019 Jul 2;30(1):226. Erratum in: Cell Metab. 2020 Oct 6;32(4):690. PMID: 31105044

143 Kim H, Hu EA, Rebholz CM. Ultra-processed food intake and mortality in the USA: results from the Third National Health and Nutrition Examination Survey (NHANES III, 1988-1994). Public Health Nutr. 2019 Jul;22(10):1777-1785. Epub 2019 Feb 21. PMID: 30789115; PMCID: PMC6554067

144 Schnabel L, Buscail C, Sabate JM, et al. Association Between Ultra-Processed Food Consumption and Functional Gastrointestinal Disorders: Results From the French NutriNet-Santé Cohort. Am J Gastroenterol. 2018 Aug;113(8):1217-1228. Epub 2018 Jun 15. PMID: 29904158.

145 Laster J, Frame LA. Beyond the Calories-Is the Problem in the Processing? Curr Treat Options Gastroenterol. 2019 Dec;17(4):577-586. PMID: 31786723

146 Mendonça RD, Lopes AC, Pimenta AM, et al. Ultra-Processed Food Consumption and the Incidence of Hypertension in a Mediterranean Cohort: The Seguimiento Universidad de Navarra Project. Am J Hypertens. 2017 Apr 1;30(4):358-366. PMID: 27927627.

147 Martínez Steele E, Popkin BM, Swinburn B, et al. The share of ultra-processed foods and the overall nutritional quality of diets in the US: evidence from a nationally representative cross-sectional study. Popul Health Metr. 2017 Feb 14;15(1):6. PMID: 28193285; PMCID: PMC5307821

148 Chen X, Zhang Z, Yang H, Qiu P, Wang H, Wang F, Zhao Q, Fang J, Nie J. Consumption of ultra-processed foods and health outcomes: a systematic review of epidemiological studies. Nutr J. 2020 Aug 20;19(1):86. PMID: 32819372; PMCID: PMC7441617

149 Tasić I, Popović M, Stojanović S, et al. Osteoporosis—a risk factor for cardiovascular diseases: a follow-up study. Srp Arh Celok Lek. Jan-Feb 2015;143(1-2):28-34. PMID: 25845249

150 Cirillo C, Bilancio G, Natale F, et al. Cardiovascular calcification and subcortical bone demineralization in hypertension. Hypertens Res. 2017 Sep;40(9):825-830. Epub 2017 Apr 6 PMID: 28381870

151 Baldini V, Mastropasqua M, Francucci C, et al. Cardiovascular disease and osteoporosis. Review J Endocrinol Invest. 2005;28(10 Suppl):69-72. PMID: 16550727

152 Chen J, Hogan C, Lyubomirsky G, et al. Women with cardiovascular disease have increased risk of osteoporotic fracture. Calcif Tissue Int. 2011 Jan;88(1):9-15. Epub 2010 Nov 4. PMID: 21046091

153 Bagger Y, Tankó L, Alexandersen P, et al. Radiographic measure of aorta calcification is a site-specific predictor of bone loss and fracture risk at the hip. J Intern Med. 2006 Jun;259(6):598-605. PMID: 16704561

154 Rajzbaum G, Bézie Y. Postmenopausal osteoporosis and atheroma. Joint Bone Spine. 2006 Dec;73(6):661-6. Epub 2006 Sep 5. PMID: 17064947

155 Vassalle C, Mazzone A. Bone loss and vascular calcification: A bi-directional interplay? Vascul Pharmacol. 2016 Nov;86:77-86. Epub 2016 Jul 4. PMID: 27389001

156 Tankó L, Christiansen C, Cox D, et al. Relationship between osteoporosis and cardiovascular disease in post-menopausal women. J Bone Miner Res. 2005 Nov;20(11):1912-20. Epub 2005 Jul 18. PMID: 16234963

157 Lee S, ChoY-Y, EunY-M, et al. Associations between osteoporosis and coronary artery disease in postmenopausal women. Climacteric . 2016 Oct;19(5):458-62. Epub 2016 Jul 9.PMID: 27397609

158 Ivanovic B, Tadic M. Hypercholesterolemia and Hypertension: Two Sides of the Same Coin. Am J Cardiovasc Drugs. 2015 Dec;15(6):403-14. PMID: 26062915

159 Borghi C, Urso R, Cicero AF. Renin-angiotensin system at the crossroad of hypertension and hypercholesterolemia. Nutr Metab Cardiovasc Dis. 2017 Feb;27(2):115-120. Epub 2016 Aug 6. PMID: 27745933

160 Ramasamy S, Kusumbe A, Schiller M, et al. Blood flow controls bone vascular function and osteogenesis. Nat Commun. 2016 Dec 6;7:13601. PMID: 27922003

161 Ilić K, Obradović N, Vujasinović-StuparN. The relationship among hypertension, antihypertensive medications, and osteoporosis: a narrative review. Calcif Tissue Int. 2013 Mar;92(3):217-27. Epub 2012 Nov 29. PMID: 23192372

162 Maria Pikilidou M, Yavropoulou M, Antoniou M, et al. The Contribution of Osteoprogenitor Cells to Arterial Stiffness and Hypertension. Review J Vasc Res. 2015;52(1):32-40. Epub 2015 Apr 23. PMID: 25925498

163 Vassalle C, Mazzone A. Bone loss and vascular calcification: A bi-directional interplay? Vascul Pharmacol. 2016 Nov;86:77-86. Epub 2016 Jul 4. PMID: 27389001

164 Leutner M, Matzhold C, Bellach L, et al. Diagnosis of osteoporosis in statin-treated patients is dose-dependent. Annals of the Rheumatic Diseases 2019;78:1706-1711. PMID: 31558481 https://ard.bmj.com/content/78/12/1706

165 Ilić K, Obradović N, Vujasinović-StuparN. The relationship among hypertension, antihypertensive medications, and osteoporosis: a narrative review. Calcif Tissue Int. 2013 Mar;92(3):217-27. Epub 2012 Nov 29. PMID: 23192372

166 Ghosh M, Majumdar S. Antihypertensive medications, bone mineral density, and fractures: a review of old cardiac drugs that provides new insights into osteoporosis. Review Endocrine. 2014 Aug;46(3):397-405. Epub 2014 Feb 7. PMID: 24504763

167 Suki W, Moore L. Phosphorus Regulation in Chronic Kidney Disease. Review Methodist Debakey Cardiovasc J. Oct-Dec 2016;12(4 Suppl):6-9. PMID: 28298956

168 McNerny E, Nickolas T. Bone Quality in Chronic Kidney Disease: Definitions and Diagnostics. Review Curr Osteoporos Rep. 2017 Jun;15(3):207-213. PMID: 28447312

169 Evenepoel P, Opdebeeck B, David K, et al. Bone-Vascular Axis in Chronic Kidney Disease. Review Adv Chronic Kidney Dis. 2019 Nov;26(6):472-483. PMID: 31831125 DOI: 10.1053/j.ackd.2019.09.006

170 Foster J. Update on Mineral and Bone Disorders in Chronic Kidney Disease. Review Vet Clin North Am Small Anim Pract.2016 Nov;46(6):1131-49. Epub 2016 Jul 16. PMID: 27436330

171 Evenepoel P, Opdebeeck B, David K, et al. Bone-Vascular Axis in Chronic Kidney Disease. Review Adv Chronic Kidney Dis. 2019 Nov;26(6):472-483. PMID: 31831125 DOI: 10.1053/j.ackd.2019.09.006

172 Bailey RL, Dodd KW, Goldman JA, et al. Estimation of total usual calcium and vitamin D intakes in the United States. J Nutr. 2010 Apr;140(4):817-22. PMID: 20181782

173 Evenepoel P, Claes K, Meijers B, et al. Poor Vitamin K Status Is Associated with Low Bone Mineral Density and Increased Fracture Risk in End-Stage Renal Disease. Clinical Trial J Bone Miner Res. 2019 Feb;34(2):262-269. Epub 2018 Nov 14. PMID: 30427544

174 Brandenburg VM, Reinartz S, Kaesler N, et al. Slower progress of aortic valve calcification with vitamin K supplementation: results from a prospective interventional proof-of-concept study. Circulation. 2017;135(21):2081–3. PMID: 28533322

175 Maurice Halder M, Petsophonsakul P, Akbulut A, Schurgers L, et al. Vitamin K: Double Bonds beyond Coagulation Insights into Differences between Vitamin K1 and K2 in Health and Disease. Review Int J Mol Sci. 2019 Feb 19;20(4):896. PMID: 30791399 PMCID: PMC6413124

176 Lau W, Savoj J, Nakata M, et al. Altered microbiome in chronic kidney disease: systemic effects of gut-derived uremic toxins Review Clin Sci (Lond) . 2018 Mar 9;132(5):509-522. Print 2018 Mar 15. PMID: 29523750

177 McNerny E, Nickolas T. Bone Quality in Chronic Kidney Disease: Definitions and Diagnostics. Review Curr Osteoporos Rep. 2017 Jun;15(3):207-213. PMID: 28447312

178 Lindeman R, Tobin J, Shock N. Longitudinal studies on the rate of decline in renal function with age. J Am Geriatr Soc. 1985 Apr;33(4):278-85. PMID: 3989190

179 Park Y, Choi JE, Hwang HS. Protein supplementation improves muscle mass and physical performance in undernourished prefrail and frail elderly subjects: a randomized, double-blind, placebo-controlled trial. Am J Clin Nutr. 2018 Nov 1;108(5):1026-1033. PMID: 30475969 https://academic.oup.com/ajcn/article/108/5/1026/5201551

180 Nunes E, Currier B, Lim C, et al. Nutrient-dense protein as a primary dietary strategy in healthy ageing: please sir, may we have more? Proc Nutr Soc. 2020 Oct 14;1-14. PMID: 33050965

181 Pizzorno, L., Canaries in the Phosphate-Toxicity Coal Mines. Integr Med (Encinitas), 2014. 13(6): p. 24-32. PMID: 26770122

182 Orr, S.E. and C.C. Bridges, Chronic Kidney Disease and Exposure to Nephrotoxic Metals. Int J Mol Sci, 2017.

18(5). PMID: 28498320

183 Liu, Q., et al., Arsenic Species in Chicken Breast: Temporal Variations of Metabolites, Elimination Kinetics, and Residual Concentrations. Environ Health Perspect, 2016. 124(8): p. 1174-81. PMID: 26992196

184 Wilson, D., Arsenic Consumption in the United States. J Environ Health, 2015. 78(3): p. 8-14; quiz 44. PMID: 26591332

185 Nachman, K.E., et al., Roxarsone, inorganic arsenic, and other arsenic species in chicken: a U.S.-based market basket sample. Environ Health Perspect, 2013. 121(7): p. 818-24. PMID: 23694900

186 Dobrakowski M, Pawlas N, Hudziec E, et al. Glutathione, glutathione-related enzymes, and oxidative stress in individuals with subacute occupational exposure to lead. Environ Toxicol Pharmacol. 2016 Jul;45:235-40. Epub 2016 Jun 7. PMID: 27331344

187 Bridges CC, Zalups RK.The aging kidney and the nephrotoxic effects of mercury. J Toxicol Environ Health B Crit Rev. 2017;20(2):55-80. Epub 2017 Feb 7. PMID: 28339347

188 Prezioso D, Strazzullo P, Lotti T, et al. Dietary treatment of urinary risk factors for renal stone formation. A review of CLU Working Group. Review Arch Ital Urol Androl . 2015 Jul 7;87(2):105-20. PMID: 26150027

189 Bailey DG, Dresser G, Arnold JM. Grapefruit-medication interactions: forbidden fruit or avoidable consequences? CMAJ. 2013 Mar 5;185(4):309-16. Epub 2012 Nov 26. PMID: 23184849; PMCID: PMC3589309

190 Prezioso D, Strazzullo P, Lotti T, et al. Dietary treatment of urinary risk factors for renal stone formation. A review of CLU Working Group. Review Arch Ital Urol Androl . 2015 Jul 7;87(2):105-20. PMID: 26150027

191 Liu W, Zhai Y, Heng X, et al. Oral bioavailability of curcumin: problems and advancements. Review J Drug Target . 2016 Sep;24(8):694-702. Epub 2016 Mar 17. PMID: 26942997

192 Chen C, Lin C, Kao C. Gastroesophageal reflux disease with proton pump inhibitor use is associated with an increased risk of osteoporosis: a nationwide population-based analysis. Osteoporos Int. 2016 Jun;27(6):2117-26. Epub 2016 Feb 10. PMID: 26860609

193 Poly TN, Islam MM, Yang HC, et al. Proton pump inhibitors and risk of hip fracture: a meta-analysis of observational studies. Osteoporos Int. 2019 Jan;30(1):103-114. Epub 2018 Dec 12. PMID: 30539272

194 Yu E, Bauer S, Bain P, et al. Proton pump inhibitors and risk of fractures: a meta-analysis of 11 international studies. Am J Med. 2011 Jun;124(6):519-26. PMID: 21605729

195 Fattahi M, Niknam R, Shams M, et al. The association between prolonged proton pump inhibitors use and bone mineral density. Risk Manag Healthc Policy. 2019 Dec 12;12:349-355. eCollection 2019. PMID: 31853206

196 Sipponen P, Härkönen M. Hypochlorhydric stomach: a risk condition for calcium malabsorption and osteoporosis? Scand J Gastroenterol. 2010;45(2):133-8. PMID: 19958055

197 Lee L, Ramos-Alvarez I, Ito T, et al. Insights into Effects/Risks of Chronic Hypergastrinemia and Lifelong PPI Treatment in Man Based on Studies of Patients with Zollinger-Ellison Syndrome. Review Int J Mol Sci. 2019 Oct 16;20(20):5128. PMID: 31623145

198 Saltzman JR, Russell RM. The aging gut. Nutritional issues. Review Gastroenterol Clin North Am. 1998 Jun;27(2):309-24. PMID: 9650019

199 Russell RM. The aging process as a modifier of metabolism. Review Am J Clin Nutr. 2000 Aug;72(2 Suppl):529S-32S. PMID: 10919955

200 Pilotto A, Franceschi M. Helicobacter pylori infection in older people. World J Gastroenterol. 2014 Jun 7; 20(21): 6364–6373. PMID: 24914358

201 Asaoka D, Nagahara A, Shimada, et al. Risk factors for osteoporosis in Japan: is it associated with Helicobacter pylori? Ther Clin Risk Manag. 2015 Mar 6;11:381-91. eCollection 2015. PMID: 25834453

202 Iki M. [Epidemiology of osteoporosis in Japan] Clin Calcium. 2012 Jun;22(6):797-803. PMID: 22653016

203 Wongtrakul W, Charoenngam N, Ungprasert P. The association between irritable bowel syndrome and osteoporosis: a systematic review and meta-analysis. Review Osteoporos Int. 2020 Jun;31(6):1049-1057. Epub 2020 Feb 1. PMID: 32008157

204 Brzozowski, B., Mazur-Bialy, A., Pajdo, R., Kwiecien, S., Bilski, J., Zwolinska-Wcislo, M., Mach, T., & Brzozowski, T. (2016). Mechanisms by which Stress Affects the Experimental and Clinical Inflammatory Bowel Disease (IBD): Role of Brain-Gut Axis. Current neuropharmacology, 14(8), 892–900. PMID: 27040468

205 Krela-Kaźmierczak I, Szymczak A, Lykowska-Szuber L, et al. Osteoporosis in Gastrointestinal Diseases. Adv Clin Exp Med. Jan-Feb 2016;25(1):185-90. PMID: 26935513

206 Chua C, Huang S, Cheng C, et al. Fatty acid components in Asian female patients with irritable bowel syndrome. Observational Study Medicine (Baltimore). 2017 Dec;96(49):e9094. PMID: 29245334

207 Fitzpatrick, L. R., & Jenabzadeh, P. (2020). IBD and Bile Acid Absorption: Focus on Pre-clinical and Clinical Observations. Frontiers in physiology, 11, 564. PMID: 32595517

208 Kojecký, V., Matouš, J., Zádorová, Z., Gřiva, M., Kianička, B., & Uher, M. (2019). Vitamin D supplementation dose needs to be higher in patients with inflammatory bowel disease: interventional study. U nemocných s idiopatickými střevními záněty je potřeba vitaminu D vyšší: intervenční studie. Vnitrni lekarstvi, 65(7-8), 470–474.

209 Oh H, Ryu K, Park B, et al. Osteoporosis and Osteoporotic Fractures in Gastrointestinal Disease. J Bone Metab.

2018 Nov;25(4):213-217. Epub 2018 Nov 30 PMID: 30574465

210 Krela-Kaźmierczak I, Szymczak A, Lykowska-Szuber L, et al. Osteoporosis in Gastrointestinal Diseases. Adv Clin Exp Med. Jan-Feb 2016;25(1):185-90. PMID: 26935513

211 Das U. Inflammatory bowel disease as a disorder of an imbalance between pro- and anti-inflammatory molecules and deficiency of resolution bioactive lipids. Lipids Health Dis. 2016 Jan 13;15:11. PMID: 26762544

212 Lavoie, B., Lian, J. B., & Mawe, G. M. (2017). Regulation of Bone Metabolism by Serotonin. Advances in experimental medicine and biology, 1033, 35–46. https://doi.org/10.1007/978-3-319-66653-2_3

213 Kumar, M., Jiloha, R. C., Kataria, D., Prasad, S., & Vohora, D. (2019). Effect of selective serotonin reuptake inhibitors on markers of bone loss. Psychiatry research, 276, 39–44. PMID: 31003023

214 Díez J, Molina I, Ibars M. Prevalence of thyroid dysfunction in adults over age 60 years from an urban community. Exp Clin Endocrinol Diabetes. 2003 Dec;111(8):480-5. PMID: 14714269

215 Gaitonde DY, Rowley KD, Sweeney LB. Hypothyroidism: an update. Am Fam Physician. 2012 Aug 1;86(3):244-51. PMID: 22962987

216 Konca Degertekin C, Turhan Iyidir O, Aktas Yılmaz B, et al. RANKL/Osteoprotegerin System and Bone Turnover in Hashimoto Thyroiditis. Calcif Tissue Int. 2016 Oct;99(4):365-72. Epub 2016 Jun 22. PMID: 27328677

217 Mazziotti G, Canalis E, Giustina A. Drug-induced osteoporosis: mechanisms and clinical implications. Am J Med. 2010 Oct;123(10):877-84. PMID: 20920685

218 Williams G, Bassett J. Thyroid diseases and bone health. J Endocrinol Invest. 2018 Jan;41(1):99-109. Epub 2017 Aug 29. PMID: 28853052

219 Fraser W. Hyperparathyroidism. Lancet . 2009 Jul 11;374(9684):145-58. PMID: 19595349

220 Yeh M, Ituarte P, Zhou H, et al. Incidence and prevalence of primary hyperparathyroidism in a racially mixed population. J Clin Endocrinol Metab. 2013 Mar;98(3):1122-9. Epub 2013 Feb 15. PMID: 23418315

221 https://www.niddk.nih.gov/health-information/endocrine-diseases/primary-hyperparathyroidism

222 J Clin Endocrinol Metab. 2013 Mar;98(3):1122-9. Epub 2013 Feb 15. PMID: 23418315

223 Lahner E, Zagari R, Zullo A, et al. Chronic atrophic gastritis: Natural history, diagnosis and therapeutic management. Practice Guideline Dig Liver Dis. 2019 Dec;51(12):1621-1632. Epub 2019 Oct 19. PMID: 31635944

224 Wright, J. V., & Lenard, L. (2001). Why stomach acid is good for you: natural relief from heartburn, indigestion, reflux, and GERD. New York: M. Evans. (pg. 20)

225 Wong, Chin K, Suhaimi F, et al. The Relationship between Metabolic Syndrome and Osteoporosis: A Review. Nutrients. 2016 Jun 7;8(6):347. PMID: 27338453

226 Raška Jr I, Rašková M, Zikán V, et al. Prevalence and Risk Factors of Osteoporosis in Postmenopausal Women with Type 2 Diabetes Mellitus Cent Eur J Public Health. 2017 Mar;25(1):3-10. PMID: 28399348

227 Walsh J, Vilaca T. Obesity, Type 2 Diabetes and Bone in Adults. Review Calcif Tissue Int. 2017 May;100(5):528-535. Epub 2017 Mar 9. PMID: 28280846

228 Vilaca, T., et al., The risk of hip and non-vertebral fractures in type 1 and type 2 diabetes: A systematic review and meta-analysis update. Bone, 2020. 137: p. 115457

229 Zhukouskaya V, Eller-Vainicher C, Gaudio A, et al. In postmenopausal female subjects with type 2 diabetes mellitus, vertebral fractures are independently associated with cortisol secretion and sensitivity. J Clin Endocrinol Metab. 2015 Apr;100(4):1417-25. Epub 2015 Jan 15. PMID: 25590217

230 Zhukouskaya V, Eller-Vainicher C, Gaudio A, et al. The utility of lumbar spine trabecular bone score and femoral neck bone mineral density for identifying asymptomatic vertebral fractures in well-compensated type 2 diabetic patients. Osteoporos Int. 2016 Jan;27(1):49-56. Epub 2015 Jul 3. PMID: 26138582

231 Vigevano F, Gregori G, Colleluori G, Chen R, Autemrongsawat V, Napoli N, Qualls C, Villareal DT, Armamento-Villareal R. In Men With Obesity, T2DM Is Associated With Poor Trabecular Microarchitecture and Bone Strength and Low Bone Turnover. J Clin Endocrinol Metab. 2021 Apr 23;106(5):1362-1376. PMID: 33537757

232 Jiajue R, Jiang Y, Wang O, et al. Suppressed bone turnover was associated with increased osteoporotic fracture risks in non-obese postmenopausal Chinese women with type 2 diabetes mellitus. Osteoporos Int. 2014 Aug;25(8):1999-2005. Epub 2014 Apr 24. PMID: 24760246

233 Raška Jr I, Rašková M, Zikán V, et al. Prevalence and Risk Factors of Osteoporosis in Postmenopausal Women with Type 2 Diabetes Mellitus Cent Eur J Public Health. 2017 Mar;25(1):3-10. PMID: 28399348

234 Walsh J, Vilaca T. Obesity, Type 2 Diabetes and Bone in Adults. Review Calcif Tissue Int. 2017 May;100(5):528-535. Epub 2017 Mar 9. PMID: 28280846

235 Abu-Samak MS, AbuRuz ME, Masa'Deh R, et al. Correlation of selected stress associated factors with vitamin D deficiency in Jordanian men and women. Int J Gen Med. 2019 Jun 28;12:225-233. eCollection 2019. PMID: 31303782

236 Muscogiuri G, Altieri B, Penna-Martinez M, et al. Focus on vitamin D and the adrenal gland. Horm Metab Res. 2015 Apr;47(4):239-46. Epub 2015 Feb 27.PMID: 25723858

237 Zhukouskaya V, Eller-Vainicher C, Gaudio A, et al. In postmenopausal female subjects with type 2 diabetes mellitus, vertebral fractures are independently associated with cortisol secretion and sensitivity. J Clin Endocrinol

Metab. 2015 Apr;100(4):1417-25. Epub 2015 Jan 15. PMID: 25590217

238 https://friedmanfellows.com/assets/pdfs/elibrary/Rosiglitazone%20associated%20fractures.ADOPT.PDF

239 Kumar R, Priyadarshi R, Anand U. Non-alcoholic Fatty Liver Disease: Growing Burden, Adverse Outcomes and Associations. Review J Clin Transl Hepatol. 2020 Mar 28;8(1):76-86. Epub 2019 Dec 28. PMID: 32274348

240 Poggiogalle E, Donini L, Lenzi A, et al. Non-alcoholic fatty liver disease connections with fat-free tissues: A focus on bone and skeletal muscle. Review World J Gastroenterol. 2017 Mar 14;23(10):1747-1757. PMID: 28348479

241 Eshraghian A. Bone metabolism in non-alcoholic fatty liver disease: vitamin D status and bone mineral density. Review Minerva Endocrinol. 2017 Jun;42(2):164-172. Epub 2016 Dec 14.PMID: 27973461

242 Dzoyem J, Kuete V, Eloff J. Chapter 23, Biochemical Parameters in Toxicological Studies in Africa: Significance, Principle of Methods, Data Interpretation, and Use in Plant Screenings,Toxicological Survey of African Medicinal Plants, Elsevier, 2014, Pages 659-715, https://doi.org/10.1016/B978-0-12-800018-2.00023-6 https://www.sciencedirect.com/science/article/pii/B9780128000182000236#s0015

243 Lee D, Low J, Chen J, et al. The Influence of Different Foods and Food Ingredients on Acute Postprandial Triglyceride Response: A Systematic Literature Review and Meta-Analysis of Randomized Controlled Trials. Adv Nutr. 2020 Nov 16;11(6):1529-1543. PMID: 32609800 PMCID: PMC7666897 (available on 2021-07-01)

244 Poggiogalle E, Donini L, Lenzi A, et al. Non-alcoholic fatty liver disease connections with fat-free tissues: A focus on bone and skeletal muscle. Review World J Gastroenterol. 2017 Mar 14;23(10):1747-1757. PMID: 28348479

245 Poggiogalle E, Donini L, Lenzi A, et al. Non-alcoholic fatty liver disease connections with fat-free tissues: A focus on bone and skeletal muscle. Review World J Gastroenterol. 2017 Mar 14;23(10):1747-1757. PMID: 28348479 https://www.ncbi.nlm.nih.gov/pmc/articles/PMC5352914/

246 Hales C, Carroll M, Fryar C, et al. Prevalence of Obesity and Severe Obesity Among Adults: United States, 2017–2018. NCHS Data Brief No. 360, February 2020. CDC Data Brief. https://www.cdc.gov/nchs/products/databriefs/db360.htm

247 Devlin M, Dosen C. The bone-fat interface: basic and clinical implications of marrow adiposity. Review Lancet Diabetes Endocrinol. 2015 Feb;3(2):141-7. Epub 2014 Feb 19. PMID: 24731667 PMCID: PMC4138282 DOI: 10.1016/S2213-8587(14)70007-5 https://www.ncbi.nlm.nih.gov/pmc/articles/PMC4138282/

248 Sadeghi O, Saneei P, Nasiri M, et al. Abdominal Obesity and Risk of Hip Fracture: A Systematic Review and Meta-Analysis of Prospective Studies. Review Adv Nutr. 2017 Sep 15;8(5):728-738. Print 2017 Sep. PMID: 28916573 PMCID: PMC5593104

249 Li X, Gong X, Jiang W. Abdominal obesity and risk of hip fracture: a meta-analysis of prospective studies. Meta-Analysis Osteoporos Int. 2017 Oct;28(10):2747-2757. Epub 2017 Jul 12. PMID: 28702682

250 Randa Saad R, Habli D, Sabbagh R, et al. Bone Health Following Bariatric Surgery: An Update. Review J Clin Densitom. Apr-Jun 2020;23(2):165-181. Epub 2019 Aug 9. PMID: 31519474

251 Scibora LM, Ikramuddin S, Buchwald H, et al. Examining the link between bariatric surgery, bone loss, and osteoporosis: a review of bone density studies. Obes Surg. 2012 Apr;22(4):654-67. PMID: 22271358

252 Fatimo Biobaku F, Ghanim H, Monte S, et al. Bariatric Surgery: Remission of Inflammation, Cardiometabolic Benefits, and Common Adverse Effects. Review J Endocr Soc. 2020 Aug 4;4(9):bvaa049. eCollection 2020 Sep 1. PMID: 32775937

253 http://bariatrics.stonybrookmedicine.edu/sleeve_gastrectomy

254 Gómez J, Rubió J, Curiel M, et al. Calcium citrate and vitamin D in the treatment of osteoporosis. Review Clin Drug Investg. 2011;31(5):285-98. PMID: 21405146

255 Biagioni M, Mendes A, Paiva S, et al. Use of Bone Biomarkers After Weight Loss:Example of Bariatric Surgery. V.R. Preedy (ed.), Biomarkers in Bone Disease, Biomarkers in Disease: Methods, Discoveries and Applications, DOI 10.1007/978-94-007-7745-3_8-1

256 Dupont J, Dedeyne L, Dalle S, et al. The role of omega-3 in the prevention and treatment of sarcopenia. 2019 Jun;31(6):825-836. Epub 2019 Feb 19. PMID: 30784011 PMCID: PMC6583677

257 Hirschfeld H, Kinsella R, Duque G. Osteosarcopenia: where bone, muscle, and fat collide. Review Osteoporos Int. 2017 Oct;28(10):2781-2790. Epub 2017 Jul 22. PMID: 28733716

258 Szlejf, C., Suemoto, C. K., Janovsky, C. C. P. S., Barreto, S. M., Diniz, M. de F. H. S., Lotufo, P. A., & Bensenor, I. M. (2020). Thyroid Function and Sarcopenia: Results from the ELSA-Brasil Study. Journal of the American Geriatrics Society. doi:10.1111/jgs.16416. PMID: 32167571

259 Cruz-Jentoft A, Sayer A. Sarcopenia. Review Lancet. 2019 Jun 29;393(10191):2636-2646. Epub 2019 Jun 3. PMID: 31171417

260 Mesinovic J, Zengin A, De Courten B, et al. Sarcopenia and type 2 diabetes mellitus: a bidirectional relationship. Diabetes Metab Syndr Obes. 2019 Jul 8;12:1057-1072. eCollection 2019. PMID: 31372016

261 Zhai Y, Xiao Q. The Common Mechanisms of Sarcopenia and NAFLD. Biomed Res Int. 2017;2017:6297651. Epub 2017 Dec 13. PMID: 29387723

262 Moorthi RN, Avin KG. Clinical relevance of sarcopenia in chronic kidney disease.Curr Opin Nephrol Hypertens. 2017 May;26(3):219-228. PMID: 28198733

263 Davis MP, Panikkar R. Sarcopenia associated with chemotherapy and targeted agents for cancer therapy. Ann

Palliat Med. 2019 Jan;8(1):86-101. Epub 2018 Sep 7. PMID: 30525762

264 Cetrone, M., Mele, A., & Tricarico, D. (2014). Effects of the Antidiabetic Drugs on the Age-Related Atrophy and Sarcopenia Associated with Diabetes Type II. Current Diabetes Reviews, 10(4), 231–237. PMID: 25245021

265 Cruz-Jentoft A, Sayer A. Sarcopenia. Review Lancet. 2019 Jun 29;393(10191):2636-2646. Epub 2019 Jun 3. PMID: 31171417

266 Woo J. Sarcopenia. Review Clin Geriatr Med. 2017 Aug;33(3):305-314. Epub 2017 May 13. PMID: 28689564

267 J. L. Krok-Schoen, A. Archdeacon Price, M. Luo, et al. Low Dietary Protein Intakes and Associated Dietary Patterns and Functional Limitations in an Aging Population: A NHANES Analysis. PMID: 30932132

268 Nunes E, Currier B, Lim C, et al. Nutrient-dense protein as a primary dietary strategy in healthy ageing: please sir, may we have more? Proc Nutr Soc. 2020 Oct 14;1-14. PMID: 33050965

269 Zhai Y, Xiao Q. The Common Mechanisms of Sarcopenia and NAFLD. Biomed Res Int. 2017;2017:6297651. Epub 2017 Dec 13. PMID: 29387723

270 Cruz-Jentoft A, Sayer A. Sarcopenia. Review Lancet. 2019 Jun 29;393(10191):2636-2646. Epub 2019 Jun 3. PMID: 31171417

271 Dupont J, Dedeyne L, Dalle S, et al. The role of omega-3 in the prevention and treatment of sarcopenia. 2019 Jun;31(6):825-836. Epub 2019 Feb 19. PMID: 30784011 PMCID: PMC6583677

272 Rondanelli M, Rigon C, Perna S, et al. Novel Insights on Intake of Fish and Prevention of Sarcopenia: All Reasons for an Adequate Consumption. Review Nutrients. 2020 Jan 24;12(2):307. PMID: 31991560 PMCID: PMC7071242

273 van Dronkelaar C, van Velzen A, Abdelrazek M, et al. Minerals and Sarcopenia; The Role of Calcium, Iron, Magnesium, Phosphorus, Potassium, Selenium, Sodium, and Zinc on Muscle Mass, Muscle Strength, and Physical Performance in Older Adults: A Systematic Review. J Am Med Dir Assoc. 2018 Jan;19(1):6-11.e3. Epub 2017 Jul 12. PMID: 28711425

274 Borack M, Volpi E. Efficacy and Safety of Leucine Supplementation in the Elderly. Review J Nutr. 2016 Dec;146(12):2625S-2629S. Epub 2016 Nov 9. PMID: 27934654

275 Oktaviana, J., Zanker, J., Vogrin, S., & Duque, G. (2018). The Effect of β-Hydroxy-β-Methylbutyrate (HMB) on Sarcopenia and Functional Frailty in Older Persons: A Systematic Review. The Journal of Nutrition, Health & Aging. PMID: 30697623

276 Pivonello R, Isidori AM, De Martino MC, et al. Complications of Cushing's syndrome: state of the art. Lancet Diabetes Endocrinol. 2016 Jul;4(7):611-29. Epub 2016 May 10. PMID: 27177728 Review.

277 S C Manolagas. Birth and death of bone cells: basic regulatory mechanisms and implications for the pathogenesis and treatment of osteoporosis. Endocr Rev. 2000 Apr;21(2):115-37. PMID: 10782361 https://www.sciencedirect.com/science/article/pii/B9780123705440500033

278 Morgan E, Barnes G, Einhorn, Osteoporosis, 3rd edition. Chapter 1—The Bone Organ System: Form and Function. https://www.sciencedirect.com/science/article/pii/B9780123705440500033

279 PMID: 30353360

280 Li D, Kaur RJ, Zhang CD, Ebbehoj A, Singh S, Atkinson EJ, Achenbach SJ, Rocca W, Khosla S, Bancos I. Risk of bone fractures after the diagnosis of adrenal adenomas: a population-based cohort study. Eur J Endocrinol. 2021 Apr;184(4):597-606. PMID: 33606665; PMCID: PMC7974392

281 Chiodini I, Morelli V, Masserini B, et al. Bone mineral density, prevalence of vertebral fractures, and bone quality in patients with adrenal incidentalomas with and without subclinical hypercortisolism: an Italian multicenter study. Clin Endocrinol Metab. 2009 Sep;94(9):3207-14. Epub 2009 Jun 23. PMID: 19549741

282 Goddard G, Ravikumar A, Levine A. Adrenal mild hypercortisolism. Endocrinol Metab Clin North Am. 2015 Jun;44(2):371-9. PMID: 26038206

283 Diacinti D, Guglielmi G. Vertebral morphometry.Radiol Clin North Am. 2010 May;48(3):561-75. PMID: 20609892

284 Chiodini I, Vainicher C, Morelli V, et al. MECHANISMS IN ENDOCRINOLOGY: Endogenous subclinical hypercortisolism and bone: a clinical review. Eur J Endocrinol. 2016 Dec;175(6):R265-R282. Epub 2016 Jul 13. PMID: 27412441

285 Hoy MK, Goldman JD. Calcium intake of the U.S. population, NHANES 2009-2010, USDA http://www.ars.usda.gov/SP2UserFiles/Place/80400530/pdf/DBrief/13_calcium_intake_0910.pdf

286 Chevalley T, Bonjour JP, van Rietbergen B, et al. Fractures during childhood and adolescence in healthy boys: relation with bone mass, microstructure, and strength. J Clin Endocrinol Metab. 2011 Oct;96(10):3134-42. Epub 2011 Jul 27. PMID: 21795454

287 Bonjour JP, Chevalley T. Pubertal timing, bone acquisition, and risk of fracture throughout life. Endocr Rev. 2014 Oct;35(5):820-47. Epub 2014 Aug 25. PMID: 25153348

288 Goulding A. Risk factors for fractures in normally active children and adolescents. Med Sport Sci. 2007;51:102-20. PMID: 17505122

289 Dodiuk-Gad RP, Rozen GS, Rennert G, et al. Sustained effect of short-term calcium supplementation on bone mass in adolescent girls with low calcium intake.Am J Clin Nutr. 2005 Jan;81(1):168-74. PMID: 15640477

290 Weaver CM. Age related calcium requirements due to changes in absorption and utilization. J Nutr. 1994

Aug;124(8 Suppl):1418S-1425S. PMID: 8064395

291   Heaney RP, Recker RR, Stegman MR, et al. Calcium absorption in women: relationships to calcium intake, estrogen status, and age. J Bone Miner Res. 1989 Aug;4(4):469-75. PMID: 2816496

292   Heaney RP, Gallagher JC, Johnston CC, et al. Calcium nutrition and bone health in the elderly. Am J Clin Nutr. 1982 Nov;36(5 Suppl):986-1013. PMID: 6765074

293   Weaver CM. Age related calcium requirements due to changes in absorption and utilization. J Nutr. 1994 Aug;124(8 Suppl):1418S-1425S. PMID: 8064395

294   Heaney RP, Recker RR, Stegman MR, Moy AJ. Calcium absorption in women: relationships to calcium intake, estrogen status, and age. J Bone Miner Res. 1989 Aug;4(4):469-75. PMID: 2816496

295   Gallagher JC, Riggs BL, DeLuca HF. Effect of estrogen on calcium absorption and serum vitamin D metabolites in postmenopausal osteoporosis. J Clin Endocrinol Metab. 1980 Dec;51(6):1359-64. PMID: 6255005

296   Tang BM, Eslick GD, Nowson C, et al. Use of calcium or calcium in combination with vitamin D supplementation to prevent fractures and bone loss in people age 50 years and older: a meta-analysis. Lancet. 2007 Aug 25;370(9588):657-66. PMID: 17720017

297   Adluri RS, Zhan L, Bagchi M, et al. Comparative effects of a novel plant-based calcium supplement with two common calcium salts on proliferation and mineralization in human osteoblast cells. Mol Cell Biochem. 2010 Jul;340(1-2):73-80. Epub 2010 Mar 7. PMID: 20213262

298   Michalek, J.E., Preuss, H.G., Croft, H.A. et al. Changes in total body bone mineral density following a common bone health plan with two versions of a unique bone health supplement: a comparative effectiveness research study. Nutr J 10, 32 (2011). PMID: 21492428

299   Kaats GR, Preuss HG, Stohs S, Perricone N. A 7-Year Longitudinal Trial of the Safety and Efficacy of a Vitamin/ Mineral Enhanced Plant-Sourced Calcium Supplement. J Am Coll Nutr. 2016;35(2):91-9. Epub 2016 Feb 17. Erratum in: J Am Coll Nutr. 2016 May-Jun;35(4):381. PMID: 26885697

300   Bolland MJ, Leung W, Reid IR, et al. Calcium intake and risk of fracture: systematic review BMJ September 2015;351:h4580. PMID: 26420387

301   Holick MF, Binkley NC, Bischoff-Ferrari HA, et al. Evaluation, treatment, and prevention of vitamin D deficiency: an Endocrine Society clinical practice guideline. J Clin Endocrinol Metab. 2011 Jul;96(7):1911-30. Epub 2011 Jun 6. PMID: 21646368

302   Pizzorno, L. Vitamin K2, but not vitamin K1, is helpful for bone density. Longevity Medicine Review 2009, http://www.lmreview.com/articles/view/vitamin-k2-but-not-vitamin-k1-is-helpfulfor-bone-density/.

303   Pizzorno, L. Vitamin D and Vitamin K team up to lower CVD risk: Part I, Longevity Medicine Review 2009, http://www.lmreview.com/articles/view/vitamin-d-and-vitamin-k-team-up-to-lower-cvdrisk-part-1/.

304   Pizzorno L. Vitamin K2: Optimal Levels Essential for the Prevention of Age-Associated Chronic Disease. Longevity Medicine Review 2011, http://www.lmreview.com/articles/view/Vitamin-K2-Essential-for-Prevention-of-Age-Associated-Chronic-Disease/

305   Wallace RB, Wactawski-Wende J, O'Sullivan MJ, et al. Urinary tract stone occurrence in the Women's Health Initiative randomized clinical trial of calcium and vitamin D supplements. Am J Clin Nutr. 2011 Apr 27. [Epub ahead of print] PMID: 21525191

306   Masterjohn C. Vitamin D toxicity redefined: vitamin K and the molecular mechanism. Med Hypotheses. 2007;68(5):1026-34. PMID: 17145139

307   Cowan A, Shinyoung J, Tooze J, et al. Total Usual Micronutrient Intakes Compared to the Dietary Reference Intakes among U.S. Adults by Food Security StatusNutrients. 2019 Dec 22;12(1):38. PMID: 31877853 PMCID: PMC7019721

308   Hoy MK, Goldman JD. Calcium intake of the U.S. population / What We Eat in America, NHANES 2009-2010, USDA http://www.ars.usda.gov/SP2UserFiles/Place/80400530/pdf/DBrief/13_calcium_intake_0910.pdf

309   Malmir H, Larijani B, Esmaillzadeh A. Consumption of milk and dairy products and risk of osteoporosis and hip fracture: a systematic review and Meta-analysis. Crit Rev Food Sci Nutr. 2020;60(10):1722-1737. Epub 2019 Mar 26. PMID: 30909722

310   Michaëlsson K, Wolk A, Langenskiöld S, et al. Milk intake and risk of mortality and fractures in women and men: cohort studies. BMJ. 2014 Oct 28;349:g6015. PMID: 25352269

311   Bian S, Hu J, Zhang K, Wang Y, Yu M, Ma J. Dairy product consumption and risk of hip fracture: a systematic review and meta-analysis. BMC Public Health. 2018 Jan 22;18(1):165. PMID: 29357845

312   Dekker P, Koenders D, Bruins M. Lactose-Free Dairy Products: Market Developments, Production, Nutrition and Health Benefits. Review Nutrients. 2019 Mar 5;11(3):551. PMID: 30841534. https://www.ncbi.nlm.nih.gov/pmc/articles/PMC6471712/

313   Straub DA. Calcium supplementation in clinical practice: a review of forms, doses, and indications. Nutr Clin Pract. 2007 Jun;22(3):286-96. PMID: 17507729

314   Bohmer H, Müller H, Resch KL. Calcium supplementation with calcium-rich mineral waters: a systematic review and meta-analysis of its bioavailability. Osteoporos Int. 2000;11(11):938-43. PMID: 11193246

315   Straub DA. Calcium supplementation in clinical practice: a review of forms, doses, and indications. Nutr Clin

Pract. 2007 Jun;22(3):286-96. PMID: 17507729

316 Pizzorno L. Canaries in the phosphate-toxicity coal mines. Review Integr Med (Encinitas). 2014 Dec;13(6):24-32. PMID: 26770122

317 Bristow SM, Gamble GD, Stewart A, et al. Acute and 3-month effects of microcrystalline hydroxyapatite, calcium citrate and calcium carbonate on serum calcium and markers of bone turnover: a randomised controlled trial in postmenopausal women. Br J Nutr. 2014 Nov 28;112(10):1611-20. Epub 2014 Oct 2. PMID: 25274192

318 Castelo-Branco C, Ciria-Recasens M, Cancelo-Hidalgo MJ, et al. Efficacy of ossein-hydroxyapatite complex compared with calcium carbonate to prevent bone loss: a meta-analysis. Menopause. 2009 Sep-Oct;16(5):984-91. PMID: 19407667

319 Castelo-Branco, C., & Dávila Guardia, J. (2014). Use of ossein–hydroxyapatite complex in the prevention of bone loss: a review. Review Climacteric. 2015 Feb;18(1):29-37. Epub 2014 Aug 17. PMID: 24893923

320 https://ods.od.nih.gov/factsheets/Calcium-HealthProfessional/

321 Straub DA. Calcium supplementation in clinical practice: a review of forms, doses, and indications. Nutr Clin Pract. 2007 Jun;22(3):286-96. PMID: 17507729

322 Reinwald S, Weaver CM, Kester JJ. The health benefits of calcium citrate malate: a review of the supporting science. Adv Food Nutr Res. 2008;54:219-346. PMID: 18291308

323 Recker RR. Calcium absorption and achlorhydria. N Engl J Med. 1985 Jul 11;313(2):70-3. PMID: 4000241

324 Tondapu P, Provost D, Adams-Huet B, et al. Comparison of the absorption of calcium carbonate and calcium citrate after Roux-en-Y gastric bypass. Obes Surg. 2009 Sep;19(9):1256-61. Epub 2009 May 13. PMID: 19437082

325 Adluri RS, Zhan L, Bagchi M, et al. Comparative effects of a novel plant-based calcium supplement with two common calcium salts on proliferation and mineralization in human osteoblast cells. Mol Cell Biochem. 2010 Jul;340(1-2):73-80. Epub 2010 Mar 7. PMID: 20213262

326 Michalek, J.E., Preuss, H.G., Croft, H.A. et al. Changes in total body bone mineral density following a common bone health plan with two versions of a unique bone health supplement: a comparative effectiveness research study. Nutr J 10, 32 (2011). PMID: 21492428

327 Kaats GR, Preuss HG, Croft HA, et al. A comparative effectiveness study of bone density changes in women over 40 following three bone health plans containing variations of the same novel plant-sourced calcium. Int J Med Sci. 2011 Mar 2;8(3):180-91. PMID: 21448303 Corrected chart: https://www.ncbi.nlm.nih.gov/pmc/articles/PMC3714389/

328 Kaats GR, Preuss HG, Stohs S, Perricone N. A 7-Year Longitudinal Trial of the Safety and Efficacy of a Vitamin/ Mineral Enhanced Plant-Sourced Calcium Supplement. J Am Coll Nutr. 2016;35(2):91-9. Epub 2016 Feb 17. Erratum in: J Am Coll Nutr. 2016 May-Jun;35(4):381. PMID: 26885697

329 Davis DR, Epp MD, Riordan HD. Changes in USDA food composition data for 43 garden crops, 1950 to 1999. J Am Coll Nutr. 2004 Dec;23(6):669-82. PMID: 15637215

330 Thomas D. The mineral depletion of foods available to us as a nation (1940-2002)-a review of the 6th Edition of McCance and Widdowson. Nutr Health. 2007;19(1-2):21-55. PMID: 18309763

331 Garvin DF, Welch RM, Finley JW. Historical shifts in the seed mineral micronutrient concentration of US hard red winter wheat germplasm. J. Sci. Food Agr. 2006;86:2213–20.

332 Recker RR. Calcium absorption and achlorhydria. N Engl J Med. 1985 Jul 11;313(2):70-3. PMID: 4000241

333 Martini L, Wood RJ. Relative bioavailability of calcium-rich dietary sources in the elderly. Am J Clin Nutr. 2002 Dec;76(6):1345-50.PMID: 12450902 in Straub DA. Calcium supplementation in clinical practice: a review of forms, doses, and indications. Nutr Clin Pract. 2007 Jun;22(3):286-96. PMID: 17507729

334 Heaney RP, Dowell MS, Bierman J, et al. Absorbability and cost effectiveness in calcium supplementation. J Am Coll Nutr. 2001 Jun;20(3):239-46. PMID: 11444420

335 Tondapu P, Provost D, Adams-Huet B, et al. Comparison of the absorption of calcium carbonate and calcium citrate after Roux-en-Y gastric bypass. Obes Surg. 2009 Sep;19(9):1256-61. Epub 2009 May 13. PMID: 19437082

336 Straub DA. Calcium supplementation in clinical practice: a review of forms, doses, and indications. Nutr Clin Pract. 2007 Jun;22(3):286-96. PMID: 17507729

337 Reinwald S, Weaver CM, Kester JJ. The health benefits of calcium citrate malate: a review of the supporting science. Adv Food Nutr Res. 2008;54:219-346. PMID: 18291308

338 Bronner F. Mechanisms of intestinal calcium absorption. J Cell Biochem. 2003 Feb 1;88(2):387-93. PMID: 12520541

339 Holick MF, Binkley NC, Bischoff-Ferrari HA, et al. Evaluation, treatment, and prevention of vitamin D deficiency: an Endocrine Society clinical practice guideline. J Clin Endocrinol Metab. 2011 Jul;96(7):1911-30. Epub 2011 Jun 6. PMID: 21646368

340 Heaney RP, Dowell MS, Hale CA, et al. Calcium absorption varies within the reference range for serum 25-hydroxyvitamin D. J Am Coll Nutr. 2003 Apr;22(2):142-6. PMID: 12672710, cited in Straub DA. Calcium supplementation in clinical practice: a review of forms, doses, and indications. Nutr Clin Pract. 2007 Jun;22(3):286-96. PMID: 17507729

341 Wacker M, Holick MF. Vitamin D - effects on skeletal and extraskeletal health and the need for supplementa-

tion. Nutrients. 2013 Jan 10;5(1):111-48. PMID: 23306192

342 Straub DA. Calcium supplementation in clinical practice: a review of forms, doses, and indications. Nutr Clin Pract. 2007 Jun;22(3):286-96. PMID: 17507729

343 Heaney RP. Factors influencing the measurement of bioavailability, taking calcium as a model. J Nutr. 2001 Apr;131(4 Suppl):1344S-8S. PMID: 11285351

344 Ju J, Kwak Y, Hao X, et al. Inhibitory effects of calcium against intestinal cancer in human colon cancer cells and Apc(Min/+) mice. Nutr Res Pract. 2012 Oct;6(5):396-404. Epub 2012 Oct 31. PMID: 23198018

345 Gonzalez J, Green B, Brown M. Calcium ingestion suppresses appetite and produces acute overcompensation of energy intake independent of protein in healthy adults. J Nutr. 2015 Mar;145(3):476-82. Epub 2015 Jan 14. PMID: 25733462

346 Ilich JZ, Kelly OJ, Liu PY, et al. Role of Calcium and Low-Fat Dairy Foods in Weight-Loss Outcomes Revisited: Results from the Randomized Trial of Effects on Bone and Body Composition in Overweight/Obese Postmenopausal Women.Nutrients. 2019 May 23;11(5):1157. PMID: 31126121

347 Gonzalez JT, Stevenson EJ. Calcium co-ingestion augments postprandial glucose-dependent insulinotropic peptide (1-42), glucagon-like peptide-1 and insulin concentrations in humans. Eur J Nutr. 2014;53(2):375-85. Epub 2013 May 21. PMID: 23689561

348 Chen YC, Smith HA, Hengist A, et al. Co-ingestion of whey protein hydrolysate with milk minerals rich in calcium potently stimulates glucagon-like peptide-1 secretion: an RCT in healthy adults. Eur J Nutr. 2020 Sep;59(6):2449-2462. Epub 2019 Sep 17.PMID: 31531707

349 Golic I, Velickovic K, Markelic M, et al. Calcium-induced alteration of mitochondrial morphology and mitochondrial-endoplasmic reticulum contacts in rat brown adipocytes. Eur J Histochem. 2014 Sep 9;58(3):2377. PMID: 25308841

350 Zhang F, Ye J, Zhu X, et al. Anti-Obesity Effects of Dietary Calcium: The Evidence and Possible Mechanisms. Int J Mol Sci. 2019 Jun 23;20(12):3072. PMID: 31234600

351 Loftus CJ, Volovetz J, Chaitoff A, et al. Effects of Calcium and Vitamin D Supplementation on Known Stone Formers. Abstract # FR-PO943, available at http://www.asn-online.org/abstracts

352 Nielsen FH, Lukaski HC. Update on the relationship between magnesium and exercise. Magnes Res. 2006 Sep;19(3):180-9. PMID: 17172008

353 Tarasov EA, Blinov DV, Zimovina UV, et al. [Magnesium deficiency and stress: Issues of their relationship, diagnostic tests, and approaches to therapy]. Ter Arkh. 2015;87(9):114-22. [Article in Russian] PMID: 26591563

354 Nechifor M. Magnesium in addiction - a general view. Magnes Res. 2018 Aug 1;31(3):90-98. PMID: 30714574.

355 Takase B, Akima T, Uehata A, et al. Effect of chronic stress and sleep deprivation on both flow-mediated dilation in the brachial artery and the intracellular magnesium level in humans. Clin Cardiol 2004;27(4): 223–227. PMID: 15119699

356 Dullo P, Vedi N. Changes in serum calcium, magnesium and inorganic phosphorus levels during different phases of the menstrual cycle. J Hum Reprod Sci. 2008 Jul;1(2):77-80. PMID: 19562050

357 Natural Medicines Comprehensive Database. Calcium [Natural Medicines Comprehensive Database website: http://www.naturaldatabase.com]

358 Pazianas M, Abrahamsen B, Ferrari S, et al. Eliminating the need for fasting with oral administration of bisphosphonates. Ther Clin Risk Manag. 2013;9:395-402. Epub 2013 Oct 18. PMID: 24204155

359 Shortt C, Madden A, Flynn A, et al. Influence of dietary sodium intake on urinary calcium excretion in selected Irish individuals. Eur J Clin Nutr. 1988 Jul;42(7):595-603. PMID: 3224603

360 Itoh R, Suyama Y, Oguma Y, et al. Dietary sodium, an independent determinant for urinary deoxypyridinoline in elderly women. A cross-sectional study on the effect of dietary factors on deoxypyridinoline excretion in 24-h urine specimens from 763 free-living healthy Japanese. Eur J Clin Nutr. 1999 Nov;53(11):886-90. PMID: 10557002

361 Park SM, Joung JY, Cho YY, et al. Effect of high dietary sodium on bone turnover markers and urinary calcium excretion in Korean postmenopausal women with low bone mass. Eur J Clin Nutr. 2015 Mar;69(3):361-6. Epub 2015 Feb 4. PMID: 25649239

362 López-González AA, Grases F, Monroy N, et al. Protective effect of myo-inositol hexaphosphate (phytate) on bone mass loss in postmenopausal women. Eur J Nutr. 2013 Mar;52(2):717-26. Epub 2012 May 22. PMID: 22614760

363 Heaney RP. Effects of caffeine on bone and the calcium economy. Food Chem Toxicol. 2002 Sep;40(9):1263-70. PMID: 12204390

364 Pizzorno L. Nothing Boring About Boron. Integr Med (Encinitas). 2015 Aug;14(4):35-48. PMID: 26770156

365 Pickering G, Mazur A, Trousselard M, Bienkowski P, Yaltsewa N, Amessou M, Noah L, Pouteau E. Magnesium Status and Stress: The Vicious Circle Concept Revisited. Nutrients. 2020; 12(12):3672. https://www.mdpi.com/2072-6643/12/12/3672

366 Tarasov EA, Blinov DV, Zimovina UV, et al. [Magnesium deficiency and stress: Issues of their relationship, diagnostic tests, and approaches to therapy].[Article in Russian] Ter Arkh. 2015;87(9):114-22. PMID: 26591563

367 Galland L. Magnesium, stress and neuropsychiatric disorders. Magnes Trace Elem. 1991-1992;10(2-4):287-301. PMID: 1844561

368 Lijnen P, Hespel P, Fagard R, et al. Erythrocyte, plasma and urinary magnesium in men before and after a marathon. Eur J Appl Physiol Occup Physiol. 1988;58(3):252-6. PMID: 3220063

369 Nielsen FH, Lukaski HC. Update on the relationship between magnesium and exercise. Magnes Res. 2006 Sep;19(3):180-9. PMID: 17172008

370 Takase B, Akima T, Uehata A, et al. Effect of chronic stress and sleep deprivation on both flow-mediated dilation in the brachial artery and the intracellular magnesium level in humans. Clin Cardiol 2004;27(4): 223–227. PMID: 15119699

371 Rude RK, Gruber HE. Magnesium deficiency and osteoporosis: animal and human observations. J Nutr Biochem. 2004 Dec;15(12):710-6. PMID: 15607643

372 Castiglioni S, Cazzaniga A, Albisetti W, et al. Magnesium and osteoporosis: current state of knowledge and future research directions. Nutrients. 2013 Jul 31;5(8):3022-33. PMID: 23912329

373 Hoorn EJ, Zietse R. Disorders of calcium and magnesium balance: a physiology-based approach. Pediatr Nephrol. 2013 Aug;28(8):1195-206. Epub 2012 Nov 10. PMID: 23142866

374 Kanazawa I, Yamamoto M, Yamaguchi T, et al. A case of magnesium deficiency associated with insufficient parathyroid hormone action and severe osteoporosis. Endocr J. 2007 Dec;54(6):935-40. Epub 2007 Nov 30. PMID: 18048993

375 Hoorn EJ, Zietse R. Disorders of calcium and magnesium balance: a physiology-based approach. Pediatr Nephrol. 2013 Aug;28(8):1195-206. Epub 2012 Nov 10. PMID: 23142866

376 Castiglioni S, Cazzaniga A, Albisetti W, et al. Magnesium and osteoporosis: current state of knowledge and future research directions. Nutrients. 2013 Jul 31;5(8):3022-33. PMID: 23912329

377 Rosanoff A, Weaver CM, Rude RK. Suboptimal magnesium status in the United States: are the health consequences underestimated? Nutr Rev. 2012 Mar;70(3):153-64. Epub 2012 Feb 15. PMID: 22364157

378 Hoorn EJ, Zietse R. Disorders of calcium and magnesium balance: a physiology-based approach. Pediatr Nephrol. 2013 Aug;28(8):1195-206. Epub 2012 Nov 10. PMID: 23142866

379 Rude RK, Singer FR, Gruber HE. Skeletal and hormonal effects of magnesium deficiency. J Am Coll Nutr. 2009 Apr;28(2):131-41. PMID: 19828898

380 Weglicki WB. Hypomagnesemia and inflammation: clinical and basic aspects. Annu Rev Nutr. 2012 Aug 21;32:55-71. Epub 2012 Mar 8. PMID: 22404119

381 Hoorn EJ, Zietse R. Disorders of calcium and magnesium balance: a physiology-based approach. Pediatr Nephrol. 2013 Aug;28(8):1195-206. Epub 2012 Nov 10. PMID: 23142866

382 Rosanoff A, Weaver CM, Rude RK. Suboptimal magnesium status in the United States: are the health consequences underestimated? Nutr Rev. 2012 Mar;70(3):153-64. Epub 2012 Feb 15. PMID: 22364157

383 Rosanoff A, Dai Q, Shapses S. Essential Nutrient Interactions: Does Low or Suboptimal Magnesium Status Interact with Vitamin D and/or Calcium Status? Advances in Nutrition, Volume 7, Issue 1, January 2016, Pages 25–43. PMID: 26773013

384 Shin HJ, Na HS, Do SH. Magnesium and Pain. Nutrients. 2020;12(8):2184. Published 2020 Jul 23. PMID: 32718032

385 Dullo P, Vedi N. Changes in serum calcium, magnesium and inorganic phosphorus levels during different phases of the menstrual cycle. J Hum Reprod Sci. 2008 Jul;1(2):77-80. PMID: 19562050

386 Nielsen FH, Lukaski HC. Update on the relationship between magnesium and exercise. Magnes Res. 2006 Sep;19(3):180-9. PMID: 17172008

387 Tarasov EA, Blinov DV, Zimovina UV, et al. [Magnesium deficiency and stress: Issues of their relationship, diagnostic tests, and approaches to therapy]. Ter Arkh. 2015;87(9):114-22. [Article in Russian] PMID: 26591563

388 Nechifor M. Magnesium in addiction - a general view. Magnes Res. 2018 Aug 1;31(3):90-98. PMID: 30714574.

389 Takase B, Akima T, Uehata A, et al. Effect of chronic stress and sleep deprivation on both flow-mediated dilation in the brachial artery and the intracellular magnesium level in humans. Clin Cardiol 2004;27(4): 223–227. PMID: 15119699

390 Dullo P, Vedi N. Changes in serum calcium, magnesium and inorganic phosphorus levels during different phases of the menstrual cycle. J Hum Reprod Sci. 2008 Jul;1(2):77-80. PMID: 19562050

391 Ranade VV, Somberg JC. Bioavailability and pharmacokinetics of magnesium after administration of magnesium salts to humans. Am J Ther. 2001 Sep-Oct;8(5):345-57. PMID: 11550076

392 Schuchardt J, Hahn A. Intestinal Absorption and Factors Influencing Bioavailability of Magnesium-An Update. Review Curr Nutr Food Sci. 2017 Nov;13(4):260-278. PMID: 29123461

393 Pizzorno L. Nothing boring about boron. Integr Med (Encinitas). 2015 Aug;14(4):35-48. PMID: 26770156

394 Pouteau E, Kabir-Ahmadi M, Noah L, et al. Superiority of magnesium and vitamin B6 over magnesium alone on severe stress in healthy adults with low magnesemia: A randomized, single-blind clinical trial.PLoS One. 2018 Dec 18;13(12):e0208454. eCollection 2018. PMID: 30562392

395 di Salvo ML, Safo MK, Contestabile R. Biomedical aspects of pyridoxal 5'-phosphate availability. Front Biosci (Elite Ed). 2012 Jan 1;4:897-913. PMID: 22201923

396 Spasov AA, Lezgitsa IN, Kharitonova MV, et al. [Effect of some organic and inorganic magnesium salts on lipoprotein state in rats fed with magnesium-deficient diet].Eksp Klin Farmakol. 2008 Jul-Aug;71(4):35-40. [Article in Russian] PMID: 18819439

397 Spasov AA, Petrov VI, Lezhitsa IN, et al. [Comparative study of magnesium salts bioavailability in rats fed a magnesium-deficient diet]. Vestn Ross Akad Med Nauk. 2010;(2):29-37. [Article in Russian] PMID: 20364677

398 Carter TC, Pangilinan F, Molloy AM, et al. Common Variants at Putative Regulatory Sites of the Tissue Nonspecific Alkaline Phosphatase Gene Influence Circulating Pyridoxal 5'-Phosphate Concentration in Healthy Adults. J Nutr. 2015 Jul;145(7):1386-93. Epub 2015 May 13. PMID: 25972531

399 Sakakeeny L, Roubenoff R, Obin M, et al. Plasma pyridoxal-5-phosphate is inversely associated with systemic markers of inflammation in a population of U.S. adults. J Nutr. 2012 Jul;142(7):1280-5. Epub 2012 May 23. PMID: 22623384

400 Elliott C, Newman N, Madan A. Gentamicin effects on urinary electrolyte excretion in healthy subjects. Clin Pharmacol Ther. 2000 Jan;67(1):16-21. PMID: 10668849

401 Sabra R, Branch RA. Amphotericin B nephrotoxicity. Drug Saf. 1990 Mar-Apr;5(2):94-108. PMID: 2182052

402 Romani AM. Cisplatin-induced renal toxicity magn...ified: role of magnesium deficiency in AKI onset. Am J Physiol Renal Physiol. 2015 Dec 15;309(12):F1005-6. Epub 2015 Oct 28. PMID: 26511648

403 Streb R, Püsküllüoğlu M, Glanowska I, et al. Assessment of frequency and severity of hypomagnesemia in patients with metastatic colorectal cancer treated with cetuximab, with a review of the literature. Oncol Lett. 2015 Dec;10(6):3749-3755. Epub 2015 Oct 12. PMID: 26788202

404 Ribeiro MC, Avila DS, Barbosa NB, et al. Hydrochlorothiazide and high-fat diets reduce plasma magnesium levels and increase hepatic oxidative stress in rats. Magnes Res. 2013 Jan-Feb;26(1):32-40. MID: 23657239

405 Spasov AA, Ozerov AA, Iezhitsa IN, et al. Correction of furosemide-induced magnesium deficiency with different stereoisomers of organic magnesium salts: a comparative study.Bull Exp Biol Med. 2011 Jul;151(3):333-5. PMID: 22451880

406 Palmery M, Saraceno A, Vaiarelli A, et al. Oral contraceptives and changes in nutritional requirements. Eur Rev Med Pharmacol Sci. 2013 Jul;17(13):1804-13. PMID: 23852908

407 Luk CP, Parsons R, Lee YP, et al. Proton pump inhibitor-associated hypomagnesemia: what do FDA data tell us? Ann Pharmacother. 2013 Jun;47(6):773-80. Epub 2013 Apr 30. PMID: 23632281

408 June CH, Thompson CB, Kennedy MS, et al. Profound hypomagnesemia and renal magnesium wasting associated with the use of cyclosporine for marrow transplantation. Transplantation. 1985 Jun;39(6):620-4. PMID: 3890292

409 Bronner F. Mechanisms of intestinal calcium absorption. J Cell Biochem. 2003 Feb 1;88(2):387-93. PMID: 12520541

410 Holick MF, Binkley NC, Bischoff-Ferrari HA, et al. Evaluation, treatment, and prevention of vitamin D deficiency: an Endocrine Society clinical practice guideline. J Clin Endocrinol Metab. 2011 Jul;96(7):1911-30. Epub 2011 Jun 6. PMID: 21646368

411 Tagliaferri C, Wittrant Y, Davicco MJ, et al. Muscle and bone, two interconnected tissues. Ageing Res Rev. 2015 May; 21:55-70. Epub 2015 Mar 21. PMID: 25804855

412 Bischoff-Ferrari HA, Dawson-Hughes B, Staehelin HB, et al. Fall prevention with supplemental and active forms of vitamin D: a meta-analysis of randomised controlled trials. BMJ. 2009 Oct 1;339:b3692. PMID: 19797342

413 Poole CD, Smith J, Davies JS. Cost-effectiveness and budget impact of Empirical vitamin D therapy on unintentional falls in older adults in the UK. BMJ Open. 2015 Sep 29;5(9):e007910. PMID: 26419680

414 Tagliaferri C, Wittrant Y, Davicco MJ, et al. Muscle and bone, two interconnected tissues. Ageing Res Rev. 2015 May;21:55-70. Epub 2015 Mar 21. PMID: 25804855

415 Gunton JE, Girgis CM, Baldock PA, et al. Bone muscle interactions and vitamin D. Bone. 2015 Nov;80:89-94. Epub 2015 Mar 6. PMID: 25745883

416 Girgis CM, Baldock PA, Downes M. Vitamin D, muscle and bone: Integrating effects in development, aging and injury. Mol Cell Endocrinol. 2015 Jul 15;410:3-10. Epub 2015 Mar 30. PMID: 25837735

417 Tagliaferri C, Wittrant Y, Davicco MJ, et al. Muscle and bone, two interconnected tissues. Ageing Res Rev. 2015 May;21:55-70. Epub 2015 Mar 21. PMID: 25804855

418 Dobnig H. A review of the health consequences of the vitamin D deficiency pandemic. J Neurol Sci. 2011 Dec 15;311(1-2):15-8. Epub 2011 Sep 22. PMID: 21939984

419 Ali N. Role of vitamin D in preventing of COVID-19 infection, progression and severity. J Infect Public Health. 2020 Oct;13(10):1373-1380. Epub 2020 Jun 20. PMID: 32605780; PMCID: PMC7305922

420 Correale J, Ysrraelit MC, Gaitán MI. Vitamin D-mediated immune regulation in multiple sclerosis. J Neurol Sci. 2011 Dec 15;311(1-2):23-31. Epub 2011 Jun 2. PMID: 21723567

421 Wahl, D.A., Cooper, C., Ebeling, P.R. et al. A global representation of vitamin D status in healthy populations. Arch Osteoporos 7, 155–172 (2012). PMID: 23225293

422 Mitchell PJ, Cooper C, Dawson-Hughes B, et al. Life-course approach to nutrition. Osteoporos Int. 2015 Dec;26(12):2723-42. Epub 2015 Sep 28. PMID: 26412214

423 Holick M, Binkley N, Bischoff-Ferrari H, et al. Guidelines for preventing and treating vitamin D deficiency and insufficiency revisited. J. Clin. Endocrinol. Metab. 2012, 97, 1153–1158

424 Sowah D, Fan X, Dennett L, Hagtvedt R, Straube S. Vitamin D levels and deficiency with different occupations: a systematic review. BMC Public Health. 2017 Jun 22;17(1):519. PMID: 28637448; PMCID: PMC5480134.

425 Mazahery H, von Hurst PR. Factors Affecting 25-Hydroxyvitamin D Concentration in Response to Vitamin D Supplementation. Nutrients. 2015 Jun 25;7(7):5111-42. Review. PMID: 26121531

426 Webb AR, Kline L, Holick MF. Influence of season and latitude on the cutaneous synthesis of vitamin D3: exposure to winter sunlight in Boston and Edmonton will not promote vitamin D3 synthesis in human skin. J Clin Endocrinol Metab. 1988 Aug;67(2):373-8. PMID: 2839537

427 Holick MF. Environmental factors that influence the cutaneous production of vitamin D. Am J Clin Nutr. 1995 Mar;61(3 Suppl):638S-645S. PMID: 7879731

428 Holick MF, Chen TC, Lu Z, Sauter E. Vitamin D and skin physiology: a D-lightful story. J Bone Miner Res. 2007 Dec;22 Suppl 2:V28-33. PMID: 18290718

429 Binkley N, Novotny R, Krueger D, et al. Low vitamin D status despite abundant sun exposure. J Clin Endocrinol Metab. 2007 Jun;92(6):2130-5. Epub 2007 Apr 10. PMID: 17426097

430 Frith J, Day CP, Henderson E. Non-alcoholic fatty liver disease in older people. Gerontology. 2009;55(6):607-13. Epub 2009 Aug 19. PMID: 19690397

431 Frassetto LA, Morris RC Jr, Sebastian A. Effect of age on blood acid-base composition in adult humans: role of age-related renal functional decline. Am J Physiol. 1996 Dec;271(6 Pt 2):F1114-22. PMID: 8997384

432 Whiting SJ, Calvo MS. Correcting poor vitamin D status: do older adults need higher repletion doses of vitamin D3 than younger adults? Mol Nutr Food Res. 2010 Aug;54(8):1077-84. PMID: 20440693

433 Kohlmeier M. Nutrient Metabolism, Structures, Functions and Genes, 2nd edition. Elsevier: San Diego, 2015, p. 507

434 Zittermann A, Ernst JB, Gummert JF, et al. Vitamin D supplementation, body weight and human serum 25-hydroxyvitamin D response: a systematic review. Eur J Nutr. 2014;53(2):367-74. Epub 2013 Dec 1. Review. PMID: 24292820

435 Pereira-Santos M, Costa PR, Assis AM, et al. Obesity and vitamin D deficiency: a systematic review and meta-analysis. Obes Rev. 2015 Apr;16(4):341-9. Epub 2015 Feb 17. PMID: 25688659

436 Adachi JD, Brown JP, Ioannidis G. Characterizing the assessment and management of vitamin d levels in patients with osteoporosis in clinical practice: a chart review initiative. J Osteoporos. 2015;2015:312952. Epub 2015 Jan 29. PMID: 25709852

437 Yao Y, Zhu L, He L, et al. A meta-analysis of the relationship between vitamin D deficiency and obesity. Int J Clin Exp Med. 2015 Sep 15;8(9):14977-84. eCollection 2015. PMID: 26628980

438 Ekwaru JP, Zwicker JD, Holick MF, et al. The importance of body weight for the dose response relationship of oral vitamin D supplementation and serum 25-hydroxyvitamin D in healthy volunteers. PLoS One. 2014 Nov 5;9(11):e111265. eCollection 2014. PMID: 25372709

439 Mazahery H, von Hurst PR. Factors Affecting 25-Hydroxyvitamin D Concentration in Response to Vitamin D Supplementation. Nutrients. 2015 Jun 25;7(7):5111-42. Review. PMID: 26121531

440 Casella A, Long C, Zhou J. Differential Frequency of CYP2R1 Variants Across Populations Reveals Pathway Selection for Vitamin D Homeostasis. J Clin Endocrinol Metab. 2020 May 1;105(5):1302–15. PMID: 32115644; PMCID: PMC7096315

441 Aloia J, Mikhail M, Dhaliwal R, et al. Free 25(OH)D and the Vitamin D Paradox in African Americans. J Clin Endocrinol Metab. 2015 Sep;100(9):3356-3363. Epub 2015 Jul 10. PMID: 26161453

442 Powe CE, Evans MK, Wenger J, et al. Vitamin D-binding protein and vitamin D status of black Americans and white Americans. N Engl J Med. 2013 Nov 21;369(21):1991-2000. PMID: 24256378

443 Aloia J, Mikhail M, Dhaliwal R, et al. Free 25(OH)D and the Vitamin D Paradox in African Americans. J Clin Endocrinol Metab. 2015 Sep;100(9):3356-3363. Epub 2015 Jul 10. PMID: 26161453

444 Holick MF. Bioavailability of vitamin D and its metabolites in black and white adults. N Engl J Med. 2013 Nov 21;369(21):2047-8. PMID: 24256384

445 Wacker M, Holick MF. Vitamin D - effects on skeletal and extraskeletal health and the need for supplementation. Nutrients. 2013 Jan 10;5(1):111-48. PMID: 23306192

446 Holick MF. Bioavailability of vitamin D and its metabolites in black and white adults. N Engl J Med. 2013 Nov 21;369(21):2047-8. PMID: 24256384

447 Afzal S, Brøndum-Jacobsen P, Bojesen SE, et al. Genetically low vitamin D concentrations and increased mortality: Mendelian randomisation analysis in three large cohorts. BMJ. 2014 Nov 18;349:g6330. PMID: 25406188

448 Wang TJ, Zhang F, Richards JB, et al. Common genetic determinants of vitamin D insufficiency: A genome-wide association study. Lancet. 2010 Jul 17;376(9736):180-8. Epub 2010 Jun 10. PMID: 20541252

449 Boroń D, Kamiński A, Kotrych D, et al. Polymorphism of vitamin D3 receptor and its relation to mineral bone density in perimenopausal women. Osteoporos Int. 2015 Mar;26(3):1045-52. Epub 2014 Nov 19. PMID: 25407264

450 Mohammadi Z, Fayyazbakhsh F, Ebrahimi M, et al. Association between vitamin D receptor gene polymorphisms (Fok1 and Bsm1) and osteoporosis: a systematic review. J Diabetes Metab Disord. 2014 Oct 17;13(1):98. eCollection 2014. PMID: 25364703

451 Al-Daghri NM, Al-Attas OS, Alkharfy KM, et al. Association of VDR-gene variants with factors related to the metabolic syndrome, type 2 diabetes and vitamin D deficiency. Gene. 2014 Jun 1;542(2):129-33. Epub 2014 Mar 25. PMID: 24680778

452 Holick MF. Evidence-based D-bate on health benefits of vitamin D revisited. Dermatoendocrinol. 2012 Apr 1;4(2):183-90. PMID: 22928075

453 Veugelers PJ, Pham TM, Ekwaru JP. Optimal Vitamin D Supplementation Doses that Minimize the Risk for Both Low and High Serum 25-Hydroxyvitamin D Concentrations in the General Population. Nutrients. 2015 Dec 4;7(12):10189-208. PMID: 26690210

454 Garland CF, French CB, Baggerly LL, Heaney RP. Vitamin D supplement doses and serum 25-hydroxyvitamin D in the range associated with cancer prevention. Anticancer Res. 2011 Feb;31(2):607-11. PMID: 21378345

455 Balvers MG, Brouwer-Brolsma EM, Endenburg S, et al. Recommended intakes of vitamin D to optimise health, associated circulating 25-hydroxyvitamin D concentrations, and dosing regimens to treat deficiency: workshop report and overview of current literature. J Nutr Sci. 2015 May 25;4:e23. eCollection 2015. PMID: 26090099

456 Dudenkov DV, Yawn BP, Oberhelman SS, et al. Changing Incidence of Serum 25-Hydroxyvitamin D Values Above 50 ng/mL: A 10-Year Population-Based Study. Mayo Clin Proc. 2015 May;90(5):577-86. PMID: 25939935

457 Houghton LA, Vieth R. The case against ergocalciferol (vitamin D2) as a vitamin supplement. Am J Clin Nutr. 2006 Oct;84(4):694-7. PMID: 17023693

458 Heaney RP, Recker RR, Grote J, Horst RL, Armas LA. Vitamin D3 Is More Potent Than Vitamin D2 in Humans. J Clin Endocrinol Metab. 2010 Dec 22. [Epub ahead of print] PMID: 21177785

459 Logan VF, Gray AR, Peddie MC, et al. Long term vitamin D3 supplementation is more effective than vitamin D2 in maintaining serum 25-hydroxyvitamin D status over the winter months. Br J Nutr. 2013 Mar 28;109(6):1082-8. Epub 2012 Jul 11. PMID: 23168298

460 Trang HM, Cole DE, Rubin LA, et al. Evidence that vitamin D3 increases serum 25-hydroxyvitamin D more efficiently than does vitamin D2. Am J Clin Nutr. 1998 Oct;68(4):854-8. PMID: 9771862

461 Tripkovic L, Lambert H, Hart K, et al. Comparison of vitamin D2 and vitamin D3 supplementation in raising serum 25-hydroxyvitamin D status: a systematic review and meta-analysis. Am J Clin Nutr. 2012 Jun;95(6):1357-64. Epub 2012 May 2. PMID: 22552031

462 Chowdhury R, Kunutsor S, Vitezova A, et al. Vitamin D and risk of cause specific death: systematic review and meta-analysis of observational cohort and randomised intervention studies. BMJ. 2014 Apr 1;348:g1903. PMID: 24690623

463 Bjelakovic G, Gluud LL, Nikolova D, et al. Vitamin D supplementation for prevention of mortality in adults. Cochrane Database Syst Rev. 2014 Jan 10;1:CD007470. PMID: 24414552

464 Mazahery H, von Hurst PR. Factors Affecting 25-Hydroxyvitamin D Concentration in Response to Vitamin D Supplementation. Nutrients. 2015 Jun 25;7(7):5111-42. Review. PMID: 26121531

465 McDuffie JR, Calis KA, Booth SL, et al. Effects of orlistat on fat-soluble vitamins in obese adolescents. Pharmacotherapy. 2002 Jul;22(7):814-22. PMID: 12126214

466 Gotfredsen A, Westergren Hendel H, Andersen T. Influence of orlistat on bone turnover and body composition. Int J Obes Relat Metab Disord. 2001 Aug;25(8):1154-60. PMID: 11486790

467 Glueck CJ, Budhani SB, Masineni SS, et al. Vitamin D deficiency, myositis-myalgia, and rev#ersible statin intolerance. Curr Med Res Opin. 2011 Sep;27(9):1683-90. Epub 2011 Jul 6. PMID: 21728907

468 Bhattacharyya S, Bhattacharyya K, Maitra A. Possible mechanisms of interaction between statins and vitamin D. QJM. 2012 May;105(5):487-91. Epub 2012 Feb 9. PMID: 22323613

469 Shea MK, Dallal GE, Dawson-Hughes B, et al. Vitamin K, circulating cytokines, and bone mineral density in older men and women. Am J Clin Nutr. 2008 Aug;88(2):356-63. PMID: 18689371

470 McCann JC, Ames BN. Vitamin K, an example of triage theory: is micronutrient inadequacy linked to diseases of aging? Am J Clin Nutr. 2009 Oct;90(4):889-907. Epub 2009 Aug 19. PMID: 19692494

471 Mundy GR. Osteoporosis and inflammation. Nutr Rev. 2007 Dec;65(12 Pt 2):S147-51. PMID: 18240539

472 Shea MK, Dallal GE, Dawson-Hughes B, et al. Vitamin K, circulating cytokines, and bone mineral density in older men and women. Am J Clin Nutr. 2008 Aug;88(2):356-63. PMID: 18689371

473 Hart JP, Catterall A, Dodds RA, et al. Circulating vitamin K1 levels in fractured neck of femur. Lancet. 1984 Aug 4;2(8397):283. PMID: 6146829

474 Booth SL, Tucker KL, Chen H, et al. Dietary vitamin K intakes are associated with hip fracture but not with bone mineral density in elderly men and women. Am J Clin Nutr 2000 May;71(5):1201-8. PMID: 10799384

475 Iwamoto J, Sato Y, Takeda T, et al. High-dose vitamin K supplementation reduces fracture incidence in post-

menopausal women: a review of the literature. Nutr Res. 2009 Apr;29(4):221-8. PMID: 19410972

476 Rosillo MÁ, Alcaraz MJ, Sánchez-Hidalgo M, et al. Anti-inflammatory and joint protective effects of extra-virgin olive-oil polyphenol extract in experimental arthritis. J Nutr Biochem. 2014 Dec;25(12):1275-81. Epub 2014 Sep 16. PMID: 25294776

477 Liu H, Huang H, Li B, et al. Olive oil in the prevention and treatment of osteoporosis after artificial menopause. Clin Interv Aging. 2014 Dec 2;9:2087-95. eCollection 2014. PMID: 25506212

478 Troy LM, Jacques PF, Hannan MT, et al. Dihydrophylloquinone intake is associated with low bone mineral density in men and women. Am J Clin Nutr. 2007 Aug;86(2):504-8. PMID: 17684225

479 Fu X, Harshman SG, Shen X, Haytowitz DB, Karl JP, Wolfe BE, Booth SL. Multiple Vitamin K Forms Exist in Dairy Foods. Curr Dev Nutr. 2017 Jun 1;1(6):e000638. PMID: 29955705; PMCID: PMC5998353

480 Schurgers LJ, Vermeer C. Differential lipoprotein transport pathways of K-vitamins in healthy subjects. Biochim Biophys Acta. 2002 Feb 15;1570(1):27-32. PMID: 11960685

481 Flore R, Ponziani FR, Di Rienzo TA, Zocco MA, Flex A, Gerardino L, Lupascu A, Santoro L, Santoliquido A, Di Stasio E, Chierici E, Lanti A, Tondi P, Gasbarrini A. Something more to say about calcium homeostasis: the role of vitamin K2 in vascular calcification and osteoporosis. Eur Rev Med Pharmacol Sci. 2013 Sep;17(18):2433-40. PMID: 24089220.

482 Flore R, Ponziani FR, Di Rienzo TA, et al. Something more to say about calcium homeostasis: the role of vitamin K2 in vascular calcification and osteoporosis. Eur Rev Med Pharmacol Sci. 2013 Sep;17(18):2433-40. PMID: 24089220

483 Geleijnse JM, Vermeer C, Grobbee DE, et al. Dietary intake of menaquinone is associated with a reduced risk of coronary heart disease: the Rotterdam Study. J Nutr. 2004 Nov;134(11):3100-5. PMID: 15514282

484 Fujita Y, Iki M, Tamaki J, et al. Association between vitamin K intake from fermented soybeans, natto, and bone mineral density in elderly Japanese men: the Fujiwara-kyo Osteoporosis Risk in Men (FORMEN) study. Osteoporos Int. 2012 Feb;23(2):705-14. Epub 2011 Mar 11. PMID: 21394493

485 Manoury E, Jourdon K, Boyaval P, Fourcassié P. Quantitative measurement of vitamin K2 (menaquinones) in various fermented dairy products using a reliable high-performance liquid chromatography method. J Dairy Sci. 2013 Mar;96(3):1335-46. Epub 2013 Jan 17. PMID: 23332840

486 Schurgers LJ, Vermeer C. Determination of phylloquinone and menaquinones in food. Effect of food matrix on circulating vitamin K concentrations. Haemostasis. 2000 Nov-Dec;30(6):298-307. PMID: 11356998

487 Elder SJ, Haytowitz DB, Howe J, Peterson JW, Booth SL. Vitamin k contents of meat, dairy, and fast food in the U.S. Diet. J Agric Food Chem. 2006 Jan 25;54(2):463-7. PMID: 16417305

488 Vermeer C, Raes J, van 't Hoofd C, Knapen MHJ, Xanthoulea S. Menaquinone Content of Cheese. Nutrients. 2018;10(4):446. Published 2018 Apr 4. PMID: 29617314

489 Vermeer C, Raes J, van 't Hoofd C, Knapen MHJ, Xanthoulea S. Menaquinone Content of Cheese. Nutrients. 2018;10(4):446. Published 2018 Apr 4. PMID: 29617314

490 Manoury E, Jourdon K, Boyaval P, Fourcassié P. Quantitative measurement of vitamin K2 (menaquinones) in various fermented dairy products using a reliable high-performance liquid chromatography method. J Dairy Sci. 2013 Mar;96(3):1335-46. Epub 2013 Jan 17. PMID: 23332840

491 Hojo K, Watanabe R, Mori T, Taketomo N. Quantitative measurement of tetrahydromenaquinone-9 in cheese fermented by propionibacteria. J Dairy Sci. 2007 Sep;90(9):4078-83. PMID: 17699024

492 Elder SJ, Haytowitz DB, Howe J, Peterson JW, Booth SL. Vitamin k contents of meat, dairy, and fast food in the u.S. Diet. J Agric Food Chem. 2006 Jan 25;54(2):463-7. PMID: 16417305

493 Schurgers LJ, Geleijnse JM, Grobbee DE, et al. "Nutritional intake of vitamins K1 (phylloquinone) and K2 (menaquinone) in the Netherlands." Journal of nutritional & environmental medicine 9.2 (1999): 115-122

494 Sato T, Schurgers LJ, Uenishi K. Comparison of menaquinone-4 and menaquinone-7 bioavailability in healthy women. Nutr J. 2012 Nov 12;11:93. PMID: 23140417; PMCID: PMC3502319.

495 Geleijnse JM, Vermeer C, Grobbee DE, et al. Dietary intake of menaquinone is associated with a reduced risk of coronary heart disease: the Rotterdam Study. J Nutr. 2004 Nov;134(11):3100-5. PMID: 15514282

496 Schurgers LJ, Teunissen KJ, Hamulyák K, et al. Vitamin K-containing dietary supplements: comparison of synthetic vitamin K1 and natto-derived menaquinone-7. Blood. 2007 Apr 15;109(8):3279-83. Epub 2006 Dec 7. PMID: 17158229

497 Sato T, Schurgers LJ, Uenishi K. Comparison of menaquinone-4 and menaquinone-7 bioavailability in healthy women. Nutr J. 2012 Nov 12;11:93. PMID: 23140417

498 Schurgers LJ, Vermeer C. Differential lipoprotein transport pathways of K-vitamins in healthy subjects. Biochim Biophys Acta. 2002 Feb 15;1570(1):27-32. PMID: 11960685

499 Schurgers LJ, Vermeer C. Differential lipoprotein transport pathways of K-vitamins in healthy subjects. Biochim Biophys Acta. 2002 Feb 15;1570(1):27-32. PMID: 11960685

500 Bhalerao S, Clandinin TR. Cell biology. Vitamin K2 takes charge. Science. 2012 Jun 8;336(6086):1241-2. PMID: 22679087

501 Lovern D, Marbois B. Does menaquinone participate in brain astrocyte electron transport? Med Hypotheses.

2013 Oct;81(4):587-91. Epub 2013 Jul 30. PMID: 23910074

502 Phillips MC. Apolipoprotein E isoforms and lipoprotein metabolism. IUBMB Life. 2014 Sep;66(9):616-23. PMID: 25328986

503 Shearer MJ, Fu X, Booth SL. Vitamin K nutrition, metabolism, and requirements: current concepts and future research. Adv Nutr. 2012 Mar 1;3(2):182-95. PMID: 22516726

504 Pilkey RM, Morton AR, Boffa MB, et al. Subclinical vitamin K deficiency in hemodialysis patients. Am J Kidney Dis. 2007 Mar;49(3):432-9. PMID: 17336705

505 Kaneki M. [Genomic approaches to bone and joint diseases. New insights into molecular mechanisms underlying protective effects of vitamin K on bone health].[Article in Japanese]Clin Calcium. 2008 Feb;18(2):224-32. PMID: 18245893

506 Jeenduang N, Porntadavity S, Wanmasae S. Combined PCSK9 and APOE Polymorphisms are Genetic Risk Factors Associated with Elevated Plasma Lipid Levels in a Thai Population. Lipids. 2015 Jun;50(6):543-53. Epub 2015 Apr 22. PMID: 25899039

507 Kohnke H, Sörlin K, Granath G, Wadelius M. Warfarin dose related to apolipoprotein E (APOE) genotype. Eur J Clin Pharmacol. 2005 Jul;61(5-6):381-8. Epub 2005 Jun 11. PMID: 15952022

508 Haraikawa M, Tsugawa N, Sogabe N, et al. Effects of gamma-glutamyl carboxylase gene polymorphism (R325Q) on the association between dietary vitamin K intake and gamma-carboxylation of osteocalcin in young adults. Asia Pac J Clin Nutr. 2013;22(4):646-54. PMID: 24231026

509 Sogabe N, Tsugawa N, Maruyama R, et al. Nutritional effects of gamma-glutamyl carboxylase gene polymorphism on the correlation between the vitamin K status and gamma-carboxylation of osteocalcin in young males. J Nutr Sci Vitaminol (Tokyo). 2007 Oct;53(5):419-25. PMID: 18079608

510 Vossen LM, Schurgers LJ, van Varik BJ, et al. Menaquinone-7 Supplementation to Reduce Vascular Calcification in Patients with Coronary Artery Disease: Rationale and Study Protocol (VitaK-CAC Trial). Nutrients. 2015 Oct 28;7(11):8905-15. PMID: 26516910

511 Holden RM, Booth SL, Day AG, et al. Inhibiting the progression of arterial calcification with vitamin K in HemoDialysis patients (iPACK-HD) trial: rationale and study design for a randomized trial of vitamin K in patients with end stage kidney disease. Can J Kidney Health Dis. 2015 May 1;2:17. eCollection 2015. PMID: 26075081

512 Guralp O, Erel CT. Effects of vitamin K in postmenopausal women: mini review. Maturitas. 2014 Mar;77(3):294-9. Epub 2013 Nov 27. PMID: 24342502

513 Caluwé R, Vandecasteele S, Van Vlem B, et al. Vitamin K2 supplementation in haemodialysis patients: a randomized dose-finding study. Nephrol Dial Transplant. 2014 Jul;29(7):1385-90. Epub 2013 Nov 26. PMID: 24285428

514 Yamaguchi M. Regulatory mechanism of food factors in bone metabolism and prevention of osteoporosis. Yakugaku Zasshi. 2006 Nov;126(11):1117-37. PMID: 17077614

515 Hamidi MS, Gajic-Veljanoski O, Cheung AM. Vitamin K and bone health. J Clin Densitom. 2013 Oct-Dec;16(4):409-13. Epub 2013 Oct 3. PMID: 24090644

516 Knapen MH, Drummen NE, Smit E, Vermeer C, Theuwissen E. Three-year low-dose menaquinone-7 supplementation helps decrease bone loss in healthy postmenopausal women. Osteoporos Int. 2013 Sep;24(9):2499-507. Epub 2013 Mar 23. PMID: 23525894

517 El Asmar MS, Naoum JJ, Arbid EJ. Vitamin k dependent proteins and the role of vitamin k2 in the modulation of vascular calcification: a review. Oman Med J. 2014 May;29(3):172-7. PMID: 24936265

518 Flore R, Ponziani FR, Di Rienzo TA, et al. Something more to say about calcium homeostasis: the role of vitamin K2 in vascular calcification and osteoporosis. Eur Rev Med Pharmacol Sci. 2013 Sep;17(18):2433-40. PMID: 24089220

519 Schurgers LJ, Uitto J, Reutelingsperger CP. Vitamin K-dependent carboxylation of matrix Gla-protein: a crucial switch to control ectopic mineralization. Trends Mol Med. 2013 Apr;19(4):217-26. Epub 2013 Jan 30. PMID: 23375872

520 Dalmeijer GW, van der Schouw YT, Vermeer C, et al. Circulating matrix Gla protein is associated with coronary artery calcification and vitamin K status in healthy women. J Nutr Biochem. 2013 Apr;24(4):624-8. Epub 2012 Jul 20. PMID: 22819559

521 van den Heuvel EG, van Schoor NM, Lips P, et al. Circulating uncarboxylated matrix Gla protein, a marker of vitamin K status, as a risk factor of cardiovascular disease. Maturitas. 2014 Feb;77(2):137-41. Epub 2013 Oct 24. PMID: 24210635

522 Tsukamoto Y, Ichise H, Kakuda H, et al. Intake of fermented soybean (natto) increases circulating vitamin K2 (menaquinone-7) and gamma-carboxylated osteocalcin concentration in normal individuals. J Bone Miner Metab. 2000;18(4):216-22. PMID: 10874601

523 Knapen MH, Drummen NE, Smit E, et al. Three-year low-dose menaquinone-7 supplementation helps decrease bone loss in healthy postmenopausal women. Osteoporos Int. 2013 Sep;24(9):2499-507. Epub 2013 Mar 23. PMID: 23525894

524 Caluwé R, Vandecasteele S, Van Vlem B, et al. Vitamin K2 supplementation in haemodialysis patients: a

randomized dose-finding study. Nephrol Dial Transplant. 2014 Jul;29(7):1385-90. Epub 2013 Nov 26. PMID: 24285428

525 Tsukamoto Y, Ichise H, Kakuda H, et al. Intake of fermented soybean (natto) increases circulating vitamin K2 (menaquinone-7) and gamma-carboxylated osteocalcin concentration in normal individuals. J Bone Miner Metab. 2000;18(4):216-22. PMID: 10874601

526 Fujita Y, Iki M, Tamaki J, et al. Association between vitamin K intake from fermented soybeans, natto, and bone mineral density in elderly Japanese men: the Fujiwara-kyo Osteoporosis Risk in Men (FORMEN) study. Osteoporos Int. 2012 Feb;23(2):705-14. Epub 2011 Mar 11. PMID: 21394493

527 IOM recommendations: https://www.ncbi.nlm.nih.gov/books/NBK56068/table/summarytables.t7/?report=objectonly accessed 1-23-21

528 Poterucha TJ, Goldhaber SZ. Warfarin and Vascular Calcification. Am J Med. 2015 Dec 20. pii: S0002-9343(15)30031-0. [Epub ahead of print] PMID: 26714212

529 Tantisattamo E, Han KH, O'Neill WC. Increased vascular calcification in patients receiving warfarin. Arterioscler Thromb Vasc Biol. 2015 Jan;35(1):237-42. Epub 2014 Oct 16. PMID: 25324574

530 Namba S, Yamaoka-Tojo M, Hashikata T, et al. Long-term warfarin therapy and biomarkers for osteoporosis and atherosclerosis. BBA Clin. 2015 Aug 12;4:76-80. eCollection 2015. PMID: 26674156

531 Suárez-Pinilla M, Fernández-Rodríguez Á, Benavente-Fernández L, et al. Vitamin K antagonist-associated intracerebral hemorrhage: lessons from a devastating disease in the dawn of the new oral anticoagulants. J Stroke Cerebrovasc Dis. 2014 Apr;23(4):732-42. Epub 2013 Aug 15. PMID: 23954605

532 Zapata-Wainberg G, Ximénez-Carrillo Rico Á, Benavente Fernández L, et al. Epidemiology of Intracranial Haemorrhages Associated with Vitamin K Antagonist Oral Anticoagulants in Spain: TAC Registry. Interv Neurol. 2015 Oct;4(1-2):52-8. Epub 2015 Sep 18. PMID: 26600798

533 Mazziotti G, Canalis E, Giustina A. Drug-induced osteoporosis: mechanisms and clinical implications. Am J Med. 2010 Oct;123(10):877-84. PMID: 20920685

534 Pearson DA. Bone health and osteoporosis: the role of vitamin K and potential antagonism by anticoagulants. Nutr Clin Pract. 2007 Oct;22(5):517-44. PMID: 17906277

535 Sugiyama T, Kugimiya F, Kono S, Kim YT, et al. Warfarin use and fracture risk: an evidence-based mechanistic insight. Osteoporos Int. 2015 Mar;26(3):1231-2. Epub 2014 Oct 10. PMID: 25300528

536 Danziger J. Vitamin K-dependent proteins, warfarin, and vascular calcification. Clin J Am Soc Nephrol. 2008 Sep;3(5):1504-10. Epub 2008 May 21. PMID: 18495950

537 Cozzolino M, Brandenburg V. Warfarin: to use or not to use in chronic kidney disease patients? J Nephrol. 2010 Nov-Dec;23(6):648-52. PMID: 20349408

538 Theuwissen E, Teunissen K, Spronk H, et al. Effect of low-dose supplements of menaquinone-7 [vitamin K2(35)] on the stability of oral anticoagulant treatment: dose-response relationship in healthy volunteers. J Thromb Haemost. 2013 Mar 26. [Epub ahead of print] PMID: 23530987

539 Tufano A, Coppola A, Contaldi P, et al. Oral anticoagulant drugs and the risk of osteoporosis: new anticoagulants better than old? Semin Thromb Hemost. 2015 Jun;41(4):382-8. Epub 2015 Feb 19. PMID: 25703521

540 Cranenburg EC, Schurgers LJ, Vermeer C. Vitamin K: the coagulation vitamin that became omnipotent. PMID: 17598002 Thromb Haemost. 2007 Jul;98(1):120-5

541 Theuwissen E, Teunissen K, Spronk H, et al. Effect of low-dose supplements of menaquinone-7 [vitamin K2(35)] on the stability of oral anticoagulant treatment: dose-response relationship in healthy volunteers. J Thromb Haemost. 2013 Mar 26. [Epub ahead of print] PMID: 23530987

542 Roca B, Roca M. The new oral anticoagulants: Reasonable alternatives to warfarin. Cleve Clin J Med. 2015 Dec;82(12):847-54. PMID: 26651894

543 Siegal DM, Curnutte JT, Connolly SJ, et al. Andexanet Alfa for the Reversal of Factor Xa Inhibitor Activity. N Engl J Med. 2015 Dec 17;373(25):2413-24. Epub 2015 Nov 11. PMID: 26559317

544 O'Malley PA.The Antidote Is Finally Here! Idarucizumab, A Specific Reversal Agent for the Anticoagulant Effects of Dabigatran. Clin Nurse Spec. 2016 Mar-Apr;30(2):81-3. PMID: 26848896

545 Casado-Díaz A, Santiago-Mora R, Dorado G, et al. The omega-6 arachidonic fatty acid, but not the omega-3 fatty acids, inhibits osteoblastogenesis and induces adipogenesis of human mesenchymal stem cells: potential implication in osteoporosis. Osteoporos Int. 2013 May;24(5):1647-61. Epub 2012 Oct 27. PMID: 23104199

546 Kelly OJ, Gilman JC, Kim Y, et al. Long-chain polyunsaturated fatty acids may mutually benefit both obesity and osteoporosis. Nutr Res. 2013 Jul;33(7):521-33. Epub 2013 Jun 10. PMID: 23827126

547 Thanabalasundaram G, Arumalla N, Tailor HD, et al. Regulation of differentiation of mesenchymal stem cells into musculoskeletal cells. Curr Stem Cell Res Ther. 2012 Mar;7(2):95-102. PMID: 22023628

548 Kelly OJ, Gilman JC, Kim Y, et al. Long-chain polyunsaturated fatty acids may mutually benefit both obesity and osteoporosis. Nutr Res. 2013 Jul;33(7):521-33. Epub 2013 Jun 10. PMID: 23827126

549 Chen C. COX-2's new role in inflammation. Nat Chem Biol. 2010 Jun;6(6):401-2. PMID: 20479749

550 http://appliedresearch.cancer.gov/diet/foodsources/fatty_acids/table4.htm

551 Komprda T, Zelenka J, Fajmonová E, et al. Arachidonic acid and long-chain n-3 polyunsaturated fatty acid contents in meat of selected poultry and fish species in relation to dietary fat sources. J Agric Food Chem. 2005 Aug 24;53(17):6804-12. PMID: 16104803

552 Kouba M, Mourot J. A review of nutritional effects on fat composition of animal products with special emphasis on n-3 polyunsaturated fatty acids. Biochimie. 2011 Jan;93(1):13-7. Epub 2010 Feb 25. PMID: 20188790

553 Viladomiu M, Hontecillas R, Bassaganya-Riera J. Modulation of inflammation and immunity by dietary conjugated linoleic acid. Eur J Pharmacol. 2015 May 15. pii: S0014-2999(15)00459-8. [Epub ahead of print] PMID: 25987426

554 Kraft J, Collomb M, Möckel P, et al. Differences in CLA isomer distribution of cow's milk lipids. Lipids. 2003 Jun;38(6):657-64. PMID: 12934676

555 https://cronometer.com/#foods

556 Poulsen RC, Moughan PJ, Kruger MC. Long-chain polyunsaturated fatty acids and the regulation of bone metabolism. Exp Biol Med (Maywood). 2007 Nov;232(10):1275-88. PMID: 17959840

557 Claassen N, Coetzer H, Steinmann CM, Kruger MC. The effect of different n-6/n-3 essential fatty acid ratios on calcium balance and bone in rats. Prostaglandins Leukot Essent Fatty Acids. 1995 Jul;53(1):13-9. PMID: 7675819

558 Brenna JT, Salem N Jr, Sinclair AJ,et al. alpha-Linolenic acid supplementation and conversion to n-3 long-chain polyunsaturated fatty acids in humans. Prostaglandins Leukot Essent Fatty Acids. 2009 Feb-Mar;80(2-3):85-91. Epub 2009 Mar 9. PMID: 19269799

559 Plourde M, Cunnane SC. Extremely limited synthesis of long chain polyunsaturates in adults: implications for their dietary essentiality and use as supplements. Appl Physiol Nutr Metab. 2007 Aug;32(4):619-34. PMID: 17622276

560 Burdge G. Alpha-linolenic acid metabolism in men and women: nutritional and biological implications. Curr Opin Clin Nutr Metab Care. 2004 Mar;7(2):137-44. PMID: 15075703

561 Linus Pauling Institute Essential Fatty Acids http://lpi.oregonstate.edu/mic/other-nutrients/essential-fatty-acids#reference6

562 http://media.grubhub.com/files/doc_downloads/GrubHub-Inc-Men-vs-Women-Eating-Preferences-White-Paper_v001_b3cw14.pdf

563 Giltay EJ, Gooren LJ, Toorians AW, et al. Docosahexaenoic acid concentrations are higher in women than in men because of estrogenic effects. Am J Clin Nutr. 2004 Nov;80(5):1167-74. PMID: 15531662

564 Poulsen RC, Moughan PJ, Kruger MC. Long-chain polyunsaturated fatty acids and the regulation of bone metabolism. Exp Biol Med (Maywood). 2007 Nov;232(10):1275-88. PMID: 17959840

565 Claassen N, Coetzer H, Steinmann CM, Kruger MC. The effect of different n-6/n-3 essential fatty acid ratios on calcium balance and bone in rats. Prostaglandins Leukot Essent Fatty Acids. 1995 Jul;53(1):13-9. PMID: 7675819

566 Park JD, Zheng W. Human exposure and health effects of inorganic and elemental mercury. J Prev Med Public Health. 2012 Nov;45(6):344-52. Epub 2012 Nov 29. PMID: 23230464

567 Judd N, Griffith WC, Faustman EM. Contribution of PCB exposure from fish consumption to total dioxin-like dietary exposure. Regul Toxicol Pharmacol. 2004 Oct;40(2):125-35. PMID: 15450716

568 Moffat CF, McGill AS. Variability of the composition of fish oils: significance for the diet. Proc Nutr Soc. 1993 Oct;52(3):441-56. PMID: 8302886

569 Lawson LD, Hughes BG. Absorption of eicosapentaenoic acid and docosahexaenoic acid from fish oil triacylglycerols or fish oil ethyl esters co-ingested with a high-fat meal. Biochem Biophys Res Commun. 1988 Oct 31;156(2):960-3.PMID: 2847723

570 Offman E, Davidson M, Abu-Rashid M, et al. Systemic Bioavailability and Dose Proportionality of Omega-3 Administered in Free Fatty Acid Form Compared With Ethyl Ester Form: Results of a Phase 1 Study in Healthy Volunteers. Eur J Drug Metab Pharmacokinet. 2017 Jan 23. [Epub ahead of print] PMID: 28116646

571 Opperman M, Benade S. Analysis of the omega-3 fatty acid content of South African fish oil supplements: a follow-up study. Cardiovasc J Afr. 2013 Sep;24(8):297-302. PMID: 24240381

572 Dyerberg J, Madsen P, Møller JM, et al. Bioavailability of marine n-3 fatty acid formulations. Prostaglandins Leukot Essent Fatty Acids. 2010 Sep;83(3):137-41. PMID: 20638827

573 Marze S. Bioaccessibility of lipophilic micro-constituents from a lipid emulsion. Food Funct. 2015 Oct 7;6(10):3218-27. PMID: 26327276

574 Walker R, Decker EA, McClements DJ. Development of food-grade nanoemulsions and emulsions for delivery of omega-3 fatty acids: opportunities and obstacles in the food industry. Food Funct. 2015 Jan;6(1):42-55. doi: 10.1039/c4fo00723a. Epub 2014 Nov 11.

575 Albert B, Derraik J, Cameron-Smith D, et al. Fish oil supplements in New Zealand are highly oxidized and do not meet label content of n-3 PUFA, Nature.com, Scientific Reports, January 21, 2015, http://www.nature.com/articles/srep07928

576 Ruyter B, Grimmer S, Thorkildsen T, Todorcevic M, Lalic M. Vol. 196. Trondheim: Rubin; 2010. Lite Oksiderte

Omega-3 Oljer og Potensielle Helsefordeler. pp. 1–60 cited in Rupp H, Rupp KG. Adverse effects of ethyl esters or oxidation products in omega-3 preparations? Cardiovasc J Afr. 2014 Mar-Apr;25(2):86-7. PMID: 24844555

577 Opperman M, Benade S. Analysis of the omega-3 fatty acid content of South African fish oil supplements: a follow-up study. Cardiovasc J Afr. 2013 Sep;24(8):297-302. PMID: 24240381

578 Hoogenboom R, Traag W, Fernandes A, et al. European developments following incidents with dioxins and PCBs in the food and feed chain, Food Control 50(2015) 670-683

579 Jacobs MN, Covaci A, Schepens P. Investigation of selected persistent organic pollutants in farmed Atlantic salmon (Salmo salar), salmon aquaculture feed, and fish oil components of the feed. Environ Sci Technol. 2002 Jul 1;36(13):2797-805. PMID: 12144249

580 Montory M, Habit E, Fernandez P, et al. Polybrominated diphenyl ether levels in wild and farmed Chilean salmon and preliminary flow data for commercial transport. J Environ Sci (China). 2012;24(2):221-7. PMID: 22655380

581 Yogui GT, Sericano JL. Polybrominated diphenyl ether flame retardants in the U.S. marine environment: a review. Environ Int. 2009 Apr;35(3):655-66. Epub 2008 Dec 18. PMID: 19100622

582 de Wit CA, Herzke D, Vorkamp K. Brominated flame retardants in the Arctic environment--trends and new candidates. Sci Total Environ. 2010 Jul 1;408(15):2885-918. Epub 2009 Oct 7. PMID: 19815253

583 Ikeda I, Sasaki E, Yasunami H, et al. Digestion and lymphatic transport of eicosapentaenoic and docosahexae-noic acids given in the form of triacylglycerol, free acid and ethyl ester in rats. Biochim Biophys Acta. 1995 Dec 7;1259(3):297-304. PMID: 8541338

584 Hong DD, Takahashi Y, Kushiro M, Ide T. Divergent effects of eicosapentaenoic and docosahexaenoic acid ethyl esters, and fish oil on hepatic fatty acid oxidation in the rat. Biochim Biophys Acta. 2003 Nov 30;1635(1):29-36. PMID: 14642774

585 Albert B, Derraik J, Cameron-Smith D, et al. Fish oil supplements in New Zealand are highly oxidized and do not meet label content of n-3 PUFA, Nature.com, Scientific Reports, January 21, 2015, http://www.nature.com/articles/srep07928

586 Borra SK, Mahendra J, Gurumurthy P, et al. Effect of curcumin against oxidation of biomolecules by hydroxyl radicals. J Clin Diagn Res. 2014 Oct;8(10):CC01-5. Epub 2014 Oct 20. PMID: 25478334

587 Prasad S, Gupta SC, Tyagi AK, et al. Curcumin, a component of golden spice: from bedside to bench and back. Biotechnol Adv. 2014 Nov 1;32(6):1053-64. Epub 2014 Apr 30. PMID: 24793420

588 (https://pubmed.ncbi.nlm.nih.gov/?term=curcumin&filter=datesearch.y_5&filter=hum_ani.humans)

589 French DL, Muir JM, Webber CE.The ovariectomized, mature rat model of postmenopausal osteoporosis: an assessment of the bone sparing effects of curcumin. Phytomedicine. 2008 Dec;15(12):1069-78. Epub 2008 Aug 6. PMID: 18693096

590 Yang MW, Wang TH, Yan PP, et al. Curcumin improves bone microarchitecture and enhances mineral density in APP/PS1 transgenic mice. Phytomedicine. 2011 Jan 15;18(2-3):205-13. Epub 2010 Jul 16. PMID: 20637579

591 Gammone MA, Riccioni G,, D'Orazio N. Marine Carotenoids against Oxidative Stress: Effects on Human Health. Mar Drugs. 2015 Sep 30;13(10):6226-46. PMID: 26437420

592 Saw CL, Yang AY, Guo Y, Kong AN. Astaxanthin and omega-3 fatty acids individually and in combination protect against oxidative stress via the Nrf2-ARE pathway. Food Chem Toxicol. 2013 Dec;62:869-75. Epub 2013 Oct 21. PMID: 24157545

593 Dong H, Hutchins-Wiese H, Kleppinger A, et al. Effects of Omega-3 Polyunsaturated Fatty Acid Supplementa-tion on Bone Turnover in Older Women. Int J Vitam Nutr Res. 2014;84(3-4):124-32. PMID: 26098476

594 Hutchins-Wiese HL, Picho K, Watkins BA, et al. High-dose eicosapentaenoic acid and docosahexaenoic acid supplementation reduces bone resorption in postmenopausal breast cancer survivors on aromatase inhibi-tors: a pilot study. Nutr Cancer. 2014;66(1):68-76. Epub 2013 Nov 25. PMID: 24274259

595 Phillips MC. Apolipoprotein E isoforms and lipoprotein metabolism. IUBMB Life. 2014 Sep;66(9):616-23. PMID: 25328986

596 Chouinard-Watkins R, Plourde M. Fatty acid metabolism in carriers of apolipoprotein E epsilon 4 allele: is it contributing to higher risk of cognitive decline and coronary heart disease? Nutrients. 2014 Oct 20;6(10):4452-71. PMID: 25333200

597 Peter I, Crosier MD, Yoshida M, et al. Associations of APOE gene polymorphisms with bone mineral density and fracture risk: a meta-analysis. Osteoporos Int. 2011 Apr;22(4):1199-209. Epub 2010 Jun 9. PMID: 20533025

598 Chouinard-Watkins R, Plourde M. Fatty acid metabolism in carriers of apolipoprotein E epsilon 4 allele: is it contributing to higher risk of cognitive decline and coronary heart disease? Nutrients. 2014 Oct 20;6(10):4452-71. PMID: 25333200

599 Simopoulos AP. Evolutionary aspects of the dietary omega-6:omega-3 fatty acid ratio: medical implications. World Rev Nutr Diet. 2009;100:1-21. Epub 2009 Aug 17. PMID: 19696523

600 Kruger MC, Coetzer H, de Winter R, et al. Eicosapentaenoic acid and docosahexaenoic acid supplementation increases calcium balance. Nutrition Research, Volume 15, Issue 2, February 1995, Pages 211–219, http://www.sciencedirect.com/science/article/pii/027153179592587A?np=y

601 Kelly OJ, Gilman JC, Kim Y, et al. Long-chain polyunsaturated fatty acids may mutually benefit both obesity and osteoporosis. Nutr Res. 2013 Jul;33(7):521-33. Epub 2013 Jun 10. PMID: 23827126

602 Järvinen R, Tuppurainen M, Erkkilä AT, et al. Associations of dietary polyunsaturated fatty acids with bone mineral density in elderly women. Eur J Clin Nutr. 2012 Apr;66(4):496-503. Epub 2011 Nov 23. PMID: 22113249

603 Farina EK, Kiel DP, Roubenoff R, et al. Protective effects of fish intake and interactive effects of long-chain polyunsaturated fatty acid intakes on hip bone mineral density in older adults: the Framingham Osteoporosis Study. Am J Clin Nutr. 2011 May;93(5):1142-51. Epub 2011 Mar 2. PMID: 21367955

604 Gómez Candela C, Bermejo López LM, Loria Kohen V. Importance of a balanced omega 6/omega 3 ratio for the maintenance of health: nutritional recommendations. Nutr Hosp. 2011 Mar-Apr;26(2):323-9. PMID: 21666970

605 Whelan J. The health implications of changing linoleic acid intakes. Prostaglandins Leukot Essent Fatty Acids. 2008 Sep-Nov;79(3-5):165-7. Epub 2008 Nov 5. PMID: 18990554

606 Abedi E, Sahari MA. Long-chain polyunsaturated fatty acid sources and evaluation of their nutritional and functional properties. Food Sci Nutr. 2014 Sep;2(5):443-63. Epub 2014 Jun 29. PMID: 25473503

607 Adam O, Tesche A, Wolfram G. Impact of linoleic acid intake on arachidonic acid formation and eicosanoid biosynthesis in humans. Prostaglandins Leukot Essent Fatty Acids. 2008 Sep-Nov;79(3-5):177-81. Epub 2008 Oct 29. PMID: 18973995

608 Plourde M, Cunnane SC. Extremely limited synthesis of long-chain polyunsaturates in adults: implications for their dietary essentiality and use as supplements. Appl Physiol Nutr Metab. 2007 Aug;32(4):619-34. PMID: 17622276

609 Simopoulos AP. Evolutionary aspects of the dietary omega-6:omega-3 fatty acid ratio: medical implications. World Rev Nutr Diet. 2009;100:1-21. Epub 2009 Aug 17. PMID: 19696523

610 Strobel C, Jahreis G, Kuhnt K. Survey of n-3 and n-6 polyunsaturated fatty acids in fish and fish products. Lipids Health Dis. 2012 Oct 30;11:144. PMID: 23110317

611 Weaver KL, Ivester P, Chilton JA, et al. The content of favorable and unfavorable polyunsaturated fatty acids found in commonly eaten fish. J Am Diet Assoc. 2008 Jul;108(7):1178-85. PMID: 18589026

612 Weaver KL, Ivester P, Chilton JA, et al. The content of favorable and unfavorable polyunsaturated fatty acids found in commonly eaten fish. J Am Diet Assoc. 2008 Jul;108(7):1178-85. PMID: 18589026

613 PMID: 26210791. https://www.ncbi.nlm.nih.gov/pmc/articles/PMC4514959/

614 Pizzorno L. Nothing Boring About Boron. Integr Med (Encinitas). 2015 Aug;14(4):35-48. PMID: 26770156

615 Rosen V, Wozney JM. Bone morphogenetic proteins. In: Bilezikian JP, Raisz LG, Rodan GA, editors. Principles of bone biology, vol. 2, second edition 2002. p. 919–28 [Chapter 50].

616 Chen D, Zhao M, Mundy GR. Bone morphogenetic proteins. Growth Factors. 2004 Dec;22(4):233-41. Review. PMID: 15621726

617 Lavery K, Swain P, Falb D, et al. BMP-2/4 and BMP-6/7 differentially utilize cell surface receptors to induce osteoblastic differentiation of human bone marrow-derived mesenchymal stem cells. J Biol Chem. 2008 Jul 25;283(30):20948-58. Epub 2008 Apr 24. PMID: 18436533.

618 Phimphilai M, Zhao Z, Boules H, et al. BMP signaling is required for RunX2-dependent induction of the osteoblast phenotype. J Bone Miner Res. 2006 Apr;21(4):637-46. Epub 2006 Apr 5. PMID: 16598384

619 Nielsen F, Hunt C, Mullen L, et al. 1987. Effect of dietary boron on mineral, estrogen, and testosterone metabolism in postmenopausal women. FASEB J Nov;1(5):394–7. PMID: 3678698

620 Jones G, Prosser DE, Kaufmann M. 25-Hydroxyvitamin D-24-hydroxylase (CYP24A1): its important role in the degradation of vitamin D. Arch Biochem Biophys. 2012 Jul 1;523(1):9-18. Epub 2011 Nov 12. PMID: 22100522

621 Nielsen FH, Mullen LM, Gallegher SK. Effect of boron depletion and repletion on blood indicators of calcium status in humans fed a magnesium-low diet. J Trace Elem Exp Med 1990;3:45–54. http://handle.nal.usda.gov/10113/49316

622 Miljkovic D, Scorei RI, Cimpoiaşu VM, et al. Calcium fructoborate: plant-based dietary boron for human nutrition. J Diet Suppl. 2009;6(3):211-26. PMID: 22435474

623 Nielsen FH, Hunt CD, Mullen LM, et al. Effect of dietary boron on mineral, estrogen, and testosterone metabolism in postmenopausal women. FASEB J. 1987 Nov;1(5):394-7. PMID: 3678698

624 Beattie JH, Peace HS. The influence of a low-boron diet and boron supplementation on bone, major mineral and sex steroid metabolism in postmenopausal women. Br J Nutr. 1993 May;69(3):871-84. PMID: 8329361

625 Naghii MR, Mofid M, Asgari AR, et al. Comparative effects of daily and weekly boron supplementation on plasma steroid hormones and proinflammatory cytokines. J Trace Elem Med Biol. 2011 Jan;25(1):54-8. Epub 2010 Dec 3. PMID: 21129941

626 Nielsen F, Hunt C, Mullen L, et al. 1987. Effect of dietary boron on mineral, estrogen, and testosterone metabolism in postmenopausal women. FASEB J Nov;1(5):394–7. PMID: 3678698

627 Naghii MR, Mofid M, Asgari AR, et al. Comparative effects of daily and weekly boron supplementation on plasma steroid hormones and proinflammatory cytokines. J Trace Elem Med Biol. 2011 Jan;25(1):54-8. Epub 2010 Dec 3. PMID: 21129941

628 Pizzorno L. Nothing Boring About Boron. Integr Med (Encinitas). 2015 Aug;14(4):35-48. PMID: 26770156

629 Başaran N, Duydu Y, Bolt HM. J Reproductive toxicity in boron exposed workers in Bandirma, Turkey. Trace Elem Med Biol. 2012 Jun;26(2-3):165-7. Epub 2012 May 8. PMID: 22575543

630 Rainey C, Nyquist L. Multicountry estimation of dietary boron intake. Biol Trace Elem Res. 1998 Winter;66(1-3):79-86. PMID: 10050910

631 Food and Nutrition Board. Standing Committee on the Scientific Evaluation of Dietary Reference Intake, Institute of Medicine, Dietary reference intakes for vitamin A, vitamin K, arsenic, boron, chromium, copper, iodine, iron, manganese, molybdenum, nickel, silicon, vanadium, and zinc. Washington, DC: National Academy Press; 2002.

632 Landete-Castillejos T, Currey JD, Estevez JA, et al. Do drastic weather effects on diet influence changes in chemical composition, mechanical properties and structure in deer antlers? Bone 47, 815-825 (2010) PMID: 20673821

633 Landete-Castillejos T, Molina-Quilez I, Estevez JA, et al. Alternative hypothesis for the origin of osteoporosis: the role of Mn. Front Biosci (Elite Ed). 2012 Jan 1;4:1385-90. PMID: 22201963

634 Keen CL, Zidenberg-Cherr S. Manganese, Encyclopedia of Food Sciences and Nutrition, Academic Press, 2003, p. 3686-3691, https://doi.org/10.1016/B0-12-227055-X/00732-X

635 Samsel A, Seneff S. Glyphosate, pathways to modern diseases III: Manganese, neurological diseases, and associated pathologies. Surg Neurol Int. 2015 Mar 24;6:45. eCollection 2015. PMID: 25883837 PMCID: PMC4392553

636 Jing Y, Jing J, Ye L, et al. Chondrogenesis and osteogenesis are one continuous developmental and lineage defined biological process. Sci Rep. 2017 Aug 30;7(1):10020. PMID: 28855706

637 Keen CL, Zidenberg-Cherr S. Manganese, Encyclopedia of Food Sciences and Nutrition, Academic Press, 2003, p. 3686-3691, https://doi.org/10.1016/B0-12-227055-X/00732-X

638 Saltman PD, Strause LG. The role of trace minerals in osteoporosis. J Am Coll Nutr. 1993 Aug;12(4):384-9. PMID: 8409100

639 Watts DL. The nutritional relationships of manganese. Journal of Orthomolecular Medicine. Vol. 5, No. 4, 1990. http://orthomolecular.org/library/jom/1990/toc4.shtml

640 Li Y, Yu C, Shen G, et al. Sirt3-MnSOD axis represses nicotine-induced mitochondrial oxidative stress and mtDNA damage in osteoblasts. Acta Biochim Biophys Sin (Shanghai). 2015 Apr;47(4):306-12. Epub 2015 Mar 10. PMID: 25757953

641 Zou X, Santa-Maria CA, O'Brien J, et al. Manganese Superoxide Dismutase Acetylation and Dysregulation, Due to Loss of SIRT3 Activity, Promote a Luminal B-Like Breast Carcinogenic-Permissive Phenotype. Antioxid Redox Signal. 2016 Aug 20;25(6):326-36. Epub 2016 Apr 15. PMID: 26935174

642 Saltman PD, Strause LG. The role of trace minerals in osteoporosis. J Am Coll Nutr. 1993 Aug;12(4):384-9. PMID: 8409100

643 Saltman PD, Strause LG. The role of trace minerals in osteoporosis. J Am Coll Nutr. 1993 Aug;12(4):384-9. PMID: 8409100

644 Freeland-Graves J, Mousa T, Sanjeevi N, Chapter 2, Nutritional requirements for manganese, in Manganese in health and disease, ed. Costa LG, Aschner M. Royal Society of Chemistry, Nov 27, 2014.

645 SNPedia, rs 4880, https://www.snpedia.com/index.php/Rs4880

646 Bresciani G, da Cruz IB, González-Gallego J. Manganese superoxide dismutase and oxidative stress modulation. Adv Clin Chem. 2015;68:87-130. Epub 2015 Jan 7. PMID: 25858870

647 Freeland-Graves J, Mousa T, Sanjeevi N, Chapter 2, Nutritional requirements for manganese, in Manganese in health and disease, ed. Costa LG, Aschner M. Royal Society of Chemistry, Nov 27, 2014. https://books.google.com/books?hl=en&lr=&id=zGooDwAAQBAJ&oi=fnd&pg=PR9&dq=Manganese+in+health+and+disease,+ed.+Costa+LG,+Aschner+M&ots=a5gtgoVC1c&sig=7L4hKLc1-_g0dy8-7mSRCRYu_b8#v=onepage&q=Manganese%20in%20health%20and%20disease%2C%20ed.%20Costa%20LG%2C%20Aschner%20M&f=false

648 Spungen JH, Pouillot R, Hoffman-Pennesi D, et al. Current Data on Manganese in Foods and in U.S. Diets from the U.S. Food and Drug Administration's Total Diet Study, Published Online:1 Apr 2016Abstract Number:677.18.

649 Ekholm P, Reinivuo H, Mattila P, et al. Changes in the mineral and trace element contents of cereals: fruits and vegetables in Finland. J. Food Compost. Anal. Volume 20, Issue 6, September 2007, Pages 487-495

650 Ficco DB, Riefolo C, Nicastro G, et al. 2009. Phytate and mineral elements concentration in a collection of Italian durum wheat cultivars. Field Crops Res. 111, 235–242.

651 Marles RJ. Mineral nutrient composition of vegetables, fruits and grains: The context of reports of apparent historical declines. Journal of Food Composition and Analysis. Volume 56, March 2017, Pages 93-103. https://doi.org/10.1016/j.jfca.2016.11.012,

652 Oghbaei M, Prakash J, Yildiz F. Effect of primary processing of cereals and legumes on its nutritional quality A comprehensive review. Cogent Food & Agriculture, Vol. 2, Issue 1, 2016. http://www.tandfonline.com/doi/full/10.1080/23311932.2015.1136015

653 Samsel A, Seneff S. Glyphosate, pathways to modern diseases III: Manganese, neurological diseases, and asso-

ciated pathologies. Surg Neurol Int. 2015 Mar 24;6:45. eCollection 2015. PMID: 25883837 PMCID: PMC4392553

654 Benbrook CM. Trends in glyphosate herbicide use in the United States and globally. Environmental Sciences Europe. 2016;28(1):3. PMID: 27752438

655 Pastoriza S, Mesías M, Cabrera C, et al. Healthy properties of green and white teas: an update. Food Funct. 2017 Aug 1;8(8):2650-2662. Epub 2017 Jun 22. PMID: 28640307

656 BioMinerals, Take Back Your Farm, Effects of Glyphosate on Soils and Plants, http://www.biomineralstechnologies.com/farm-solutions/reduce-chemicals/effects-of-glyphosate-on-soils-and-plants

657 Barrett KA, McBride MB. Oxidative degradation of glyphosate and aminomethylphosphonate by manganese oxide. Environ Sci Technol. 2005 Dec 1;39(23):9223-8. PMID: 16382946

658 Manganese - Nutrient Management Spear Program, nmsp.cals.cornell.edu/publications/factsheets/factsheet49.pdf

659 Samsel A, Seneff S. Glyphosate, pathways to modern diseases III: Manganese, neurological diseases, and associated pathologies. Surg Neurol Int. 2015 Mar 24;6:45. eCollection 2015. PMID: 25883837 PMCID: PMC4392553

660 Gaby A. "Manganese," Chapter 35 in Nutritional Medicine, 2nd edition, Fritz Perlberg Publishing, Concord, NH, p.181.

661 Samsel A, Seneff S. Glyphosate, pathways to modern diseases III: Manganese, neurological diseases, and associated pathologies. Surg Neurol Int. 2015 Mar 24;6:45. eCollection 2015. PMID: 25883837 PMCID: PMC4392553

662 Agency for Toxic Substances & Disease Registry: Public Health Statement for Manganese https://www.atsdr.cdc.gov/phs/phs.asp?id=100&tid=23

663 Oulhote Y, Mergler D, Bouchard MF. Sex- and age-differences in blood manganese levels in the U.S. general population: national health and nutrition examination survey 2011-2012. Environ Health. 2014 Oct 24;13:87. PMID: 25342305

664 Jakob F, Becker K, Paar E, et al. Expression and regulation of thioredoxin reductases and other selenoproteins in bone. Methods Enzymol. 2002;347:168-79. PMID: 11898403

665 Ebert R, Ulmer M, Zeck S, et al. Selenium supplementation restores the antioxidative capacity and prevents cell damage in bone marrow stromal cells in vitro.Stem Cells. 2006 May;24(5):1226-35. Epub 2006 Jan 19. PMID: 16424399

666 Zhang Z, Zhang J, Xiao J. Selenoproteins and selenium status in bone physiology and pathology. Biochim Biophys Acta. 2014 Nov;1840(11):3246-3256. Epub 2014 Aug 10. PMID: 25116856

667 McCarty MF, DiNicolantonio JJ. An increased need for dietary cysteine in support of glutathione synthesis may underlie the increased risk for mortality associated with low protein intake in the elderly. Age (Dordr). 2015 Oct;37(5):96. Epub 2015 Sep 11. PMID: 26362762 PMCID: PMC5005830

668 Zhang Z, Zhang J, Xiao J. Selenoproteins and selenium status in bone physiology and pathology. Biochim Biophys Acta. 2014 Nov;1840(11):3246-3256. Epub 2014 Aug 10. PMID: 25116856

669 Zeng H, Cao JJ, Combs GF Jr. Selenium in bone health: roles in antioxidant protection and cell proliferation. Nutrients. 2013 Jan 10;5(1):97-110. PMID: 23306191

670 Zhang Z, Zhang J, Xiao J. Selenoproteins and selenium status in bone physiology and pathology. Biochim Biophys Acta. 2014 Nov;1840(11):3246-3256. Epub 2014 Aug 10. PMID: 25116856

671 Beukhof CM, Medici M, van den Beld AW, et al. Selenium Status Is Positively Associated with Bone Mineral Density in Healthy Aging European Men. PLoS One. 2016 Apr 7;11(4):e0152748. eCollection 2016. PMID: 27055238

672 Jakob F, Becker K, Paar E, et al. Expression and regulation of thioredoxin reductases and other selenoproteins in bone. Methods Enzymol. 2002;347:168-79. PMID: 11898403

673 Zhang Z, Zhang J, Xiao J. Selenoproteins and selenium status in bone physiology and pathology. Biochim Biophys Acta. 2014 Nov;1840(11):3246-3256. Epub 2014 Aug 10. PMID: 25116856

674 Beukhof CM, Medici M, van den Beld AW, et al. Selenium Status Is Positively Associated with Bone Mineral Density in Healthy Aging European Men. PLoS One. 2016 Apr 7;11(4):e0152748. eCollection 2016. PMID: 27055238

675 Hoeg A, Gogakos A, Murphy E, et al. Bone turnover and bone mineral density are independently related to selenium status in healthy euthyroid postmenopausal women. J Clin Endocrinol Metab. 2012 Nov;97(11):4061-70. Epub 2012 Aug 17. 22904175

676 Beukhof CM, Medici M, van den Beld AW, et al. Selenium Status Is Positively Associated with Bone Mineral Density in Healthy Aging European Men. PLoS One. 2016 Apr 7;11(4):e0152748. eCollection 2016. PMID: 27055238

677 Williams, G. R. Actions of thyroid hormones in bone. Endokrynol Pol 2009 Sep-Oct;60(5):380–8. PMID: 19885809

678 Zaidi, M., T. F. Davies, A. Zallone, H. C. Blair, et al. Thyroid-stimulating hormone, thyroid hormones, and bone loss. Curr Osteoporos Rep 2009 Jul;7(2):47–52. PMID: 19631028

679 Hoeg A, Gogakos A, Murphy E, et al. Bone turnover and bone mineral density are independently related to selenium status in healthy euthyroid postmenopausal women. J Clin Endocrinol Metab. 2012 Nov;97(11):4061-70. Epub 2012 Aug 17. 22904175

680 Yoshihara A, Yoshimura Noh J, Mukasa K, et al. The characteristics of osteoporotic patients in Graves'

disease patients newly diagnosed after menopause: a prospective observational study. Endocr J. 2016 Dec 30;63(12):1113-1122. Epub 2016 Sep 7. PMID: 27600197

681 Pawlas N, Dobrakowski M, Kasperczyk A, et al. The Level of Selenium and Oxidative Stress in Workers Chronically Exposed to Lead. Biol Trace Elem Res. 2016 Mar;170(1):1-8. Epub 2015 Jul 17. PMID: 26179085

682 Zwolak I, Zaporowska H. Selenium interactions and toxicity: a review. Selenium interactions and toxicity. Cell Biol Toxicol. 2012 Feb;28(1):31-46. Epub 2011 Sep 14. PMID: 21913064

683 How You Can Avoid Low-Level Arsenic in Rice and Chicken, Cleveland Clinic, February 2018, https://health.clevelandclinic.org/2015/02/how-you-can-avoid-low-level-arsenic-in-rice-and-chicken/, accessed 1-19-21

684 Pizzorno JE, The Toxin Solution, Harper One, NY, 2018, p. 207

685 Ralston NV, Raymond LJ. Dietary selenium's protective effects against methylmercury toxicity. Toxicology. 2010 Nov 28;278(1):112-23. Epub 2010 Jun 16. PMID: 20561558

686 Yamashita Y, Yabu T, Yamashita M. Discovery of the strong antioxidant selenoneine in tuna and selenium redox metabolism. World J Biol Chem. 2010 May 26;1(5):144-50. PMID: 21540999

687 Yamashita M, Yamashita Y, Suzuki T, et al. Selenoneine, a novel selenium-containing compound, mediates detoxification mechanisms against methylmercury accumulation and toxicity in zebrafish embryo. Mar Biotechnol (NY). 2013 Oct;15(5):559-70. Epub 2013 May 25. PMID: 23709046

688 Hoeg A, Gogakos A, Murphy E, et al. Bone turnover and bone mineral density are independently related to selenium status in healthy euthyroid postmenopausal women. J Clin Endocrinol Metab. 2012 Nov;97(11):4061-70. Epub 2012 Aug 17. 22904175

689 Zhang Z, Zhang J, Xiao J. Selenoproteins and selenium status in bone physiology and pathology. Biochim Biophys Acta. 2014 Nov;1840(11):3246-3256. Epub 2014 Aug 10. PMID: 25116856

690 Wrobel JK, Power R, Toborek M. Biological activity of selenium: Revisited. IUBMB Life. 2016 Feb;68(2):97-105. Epub 2015 Dec 30. PMID: 26714931

691 Zeng H, Cao JJ, Combs GF Jr. Selenium in bone health: roles in antioxidant protection and cell proliferation. Nutrients. 2013 Jan 10;5(1):97-110. PMID: 23306191

692 National Institutes of Health. Office of Dietary Supplements. Selenium, dietary supplement fact sheet for Health Professionals, https://ods.od.nih.gov/factsheets/Selenium-HealthProfessional/ accessed 8-3-17

693 Gaby A. "Selenium" in Nutritional Medicine, 2nd edition, Fritz Perlburg Publishing: Concord, NH, April 2017, pgs. 176-179.

694 Pedrera-Zamorano JD, Calderon-García JF, Roncero-Martin R, et al. The protective effect of calcium on bone mass in postmenopausal women with high selenium intake. J Nutr Health Aging. 2012;16(9):743-8. PMID: 23131814

695 Price CT, Koval KJ, Langford JR. Silicon: a review of its potential role in the prevention and treatment of postmenopausal osteoporosis. Int J Endocrinol. 2013;2013:316783. Epub 2013 May 15. PMID: 23762049

696 Jugdaohsingh R. Silicon and bone health. J Nutr Health Aging. 2007 Mar-Apr;11(2):99-110. PMID: 17435952

697 Charnot Y, Pérès G. [Study of the endocrine control of silicon metabolism]. [Article in French] Ann Endocrinol (Paris). 1971 May-Jun;32(3):397-402. PMID: 5114904

698 Jugdaohsingh R. Silicon and bone health. J Nutr Health Aging. 2007 Mar-Apr;11(2):99-110. PMID: 17435952

699 Wang W, Li J, Liu H, Ge S. Advancing Versatile Ferroelectric Materials Toward Biomedical Applications. Adv Sci (Weinh). 2020 Dec 3;8(1):2003074. PMID: 33437585; PMCID: PMC7788502.

700 Price CT, Koval KJ, Langford JR. Silicon: a review of its potential role in the prevention and treatment of postmenopausal osteoporosis. Int J Endocrinol. 2013; 2013:316783. Epub 2013 May 15. PMID: 23762049

701 Jugdaohsingh R, Tucker KL, Qiao N, et al. Dietary silicon intake is positively associated with bone mineral density in men and premenopausal women of the Framingham Offspring cohort. J Bone Miner Res. 2004 Feb;19(2):297-307. Epub 2003 Dec 16. PMID: 14969400

702 Schiano A, Eisinger F, Detolle P, et al. [Article in French] [Silicon, bone tissue and immunity]. Rev Rhum Mal Osteoartic. 1979 Jul-Sep;46(7-9):483-6. PMID: 504950

703 discussed in Jugdaohsingh R. Silicon and bone health. J Nutr Health Aging. 2007 Mar-Apr;11(2):99-110. Review. PMID: 17435952 https://europepmc.org/article/med/504950

704 Spector TD, Calomme MR, Anderson SH, et al. Choline-stabilized orthosilicic acid supplementation as an adjunct to calcium/vitamin D3 stimulates markers of bone formation in osteopenic females: a randomized, placebo-controlled trial. BMC Musculoskelet Disord. 2008 Jun 11;9:85. PMID: 18547426

705 Macdonald HM, Hardcastle AC, Jugdaohsingh R, et al. Dietary silicon interacts with oestrogen to influence bone health: evidence from the Aberdeen Prospective Osteoporosis Screening Study. Bone. 2012 Mar;50(3):681-7. Epub 2011 Dec 7. PMID: 22173054

706 Price CT, Koval KJ, Langford JR. Silicon: a review of its potential role in the prevention and treatment of postmenopausal osteoporosis. Int J Endocrinol. 2013;2013:316783. Epub 2013 May 15. PMID: 23762049

707 Jugdaohsingh R. Silicon and bone health. J Nutr Health Aging. 2007 Mar-Apr;11(2):99-110. PMID: 17435952 https://www.ncbi.nlm.nih.gov/pmc/articles/PMC2658806/

708   Rodella LF, Bonazza V, Labanca M, et al. A review of the effects of dietary silicon intake on bone homeostasis and regeneration. J Nutr Health Aging. 2014;18(9):820-6. PMID: 25389960

709   Jugdaohsingh R, Anderson S, Tucker K, et al. Dietary silicon intake and absorption, The American Journal of Clinical Nutrition, Volume 75, Issue 5, May 2002, Pages 887–893, https://doi.org/10.1093/ajcn/75.5.887

710   Prescha A, Zabłocka-Słowińska K, Grajeta H. Dietary Silicon and Its Impact on Plasma Silicon Levels in the Polish Population. Nutrients. 2019;11(5):980. Published 2019 Apr 29. PMID: 31035649

711   Langman M, Expert Group on Vitamins and Minerals, https://cot.food.gov.uk/sites/default/files/vitmin2003.pdf

712   Sigel A, Sigel H, Siegel R, eds. Interrelations between Essential Metal Ions and Human Diseases in Metal Ions in Life Sciences, Book 13, Springer, 2014, p. 455, ISBN 978-94-007-7500-8

713   Jugdaohsingh R. Silicon and bone health. J Nutr Health Aging. 2007 Mar-Apr;11(2):99-110. PMID: 17435952 https://www.ncbi.nlm.nih.gov/pmc/articles/PMC2658806/

714   Casey TR, Bamforth CW. Silicon in beer and brewing. J Sci Food Agric. 2010 Apr 15;90(5):784-8. PMID: 20355113 https://www.sciencedaily.com/releases/2010/02/100208091922.htm

715   http://www.derma.ee/files/Biosil%20monograaf.pdf

716   Jugdaohsingh R, Hui M, Anderson SH, et al. The silicon supplement 'Monomethylsilanetriol' is safe and increases the body pool of silicon in healthy Pre-menopausal women. Nutr Metab (Lond). 2013 Apr 26;10(1):37. PMID: 23622499

717   Vanden Berghe DA. There are not enough data to conclude that Monomethylsilanetriol is safe. Nutr Metab (Lond). 2013 Oct 25;10(1):66. PMID: 24499245 PMCID: PMC4029377

718   Jugdaohsingh R. Silicon and bone health. J Nutr Health Aging. 2007 Mar-Apr;11(2):99-110. PMID: 17435952 https://www.ncbi.nlm.nih.gov/pmc/articles/PMC2658806/

719   Sripanyakorn S, Jugdaohsingh R, Dissayabutr W, et al. The comparative absorption of silicon from different foods and food supplements. Br J Nutr. 2009 Sep;102(6):825-34. Epub 2009 Apr 9. PMID: 19356271

720   Casey TR, Bamforth CW. Silicon in beer and brewing. J Sci Food Agric. 2010 Apr 15;90(5):784-8. PMID: 20355113 https://www.sciencedaily.com/releases/2010/02/100208091922.htm

721   Pors Nielsen S. The biological role of strontium. Bone. 2004 Sep;35(3):583-8. PMID: 15336592

722   Genuis SJ, Schwalfenberg GK. Picking a bone with contemporary osteoporosis management: nutrient strategies to enhance skeletal integrity. Clin Nutr. 2007 Apr;26(2):193-207. Epub 2006 Oct 13. PMID: 17046114

723   https://en.wikipedia.org/wiki/Mineral_(nutrient)#Essential_chemical_elements_for_humans

724   Pors Nielsen S. The biological role of strontium. Bone. 2004 Sep;35(3):583-8. PMID: 15336592

725   ATSDR (Agency for Toxic Substances & Disease Registry) https://www.atsdr.cdc.gov/substances/toxsubstance. asp?toxid=25

726   The Toxin and Toxin-Target Database: http://www.t3db.ca/toxins/T3D1709

727   ToxNO: https://www.toxno.com.au/toxins/substance_id_7907.html

728   Marie PJ, Ammann P, Boivin G, et al. Mechanisms of action and therapeutic potential of strontium in bone. Calcif Tissue Int. 2001 Sep;69(3):121-9. PMID: 11683526

729   Pors Nielsen S. The biological role of strontium. Bone. 2004 Sep;35(3):583-8. PMID: 15336592 DOI: 10.1016/j.bone.2004.04.

730   Blake G, Fogelman I. The correction of BMD measurements for bone strontium content. J Clin Densitom. Jul-Sep 2007;10(3):259-65. Epub 2007 Jun 1. PMID: 17543560

731   Liao J, Blake G, McGregor A, et al. The effect of bone strontium on BMD is different for different manufacturers' DXA Systems. Bone. 2010 Nov;47(5):882-7. Epub 2010 Aug 10. PMID: 20699129

732   Dahl SG, crystal surface of the bone matrix Allain P, Marie PJ, et al. Incorporation and distribution of strontium in bone. Bone. 2001 Apr;28(4):446-53. PMID: 11336927

733   Marie PJ, Ammann P, Boivin G, et al. Mechanisms of action and therapeutic potential of strontium in bone. Calcif Tissue Int. 2001 Sep;69(3):121-9. PMID: 11683526

734   Cianferotti L, Gomes AR, Fabbri S, et al. The calcium-sensing receptor in bone metabolism: from bench to bedside and back. Osteoporos Int. 2015 Aug;26(8):2055-71. Epub 2015 Jun 23. PMID: 26100412

735   Shorr E, Carter AC. The usefulness of strontium as an adjuvant to calcium in the mineralization of the skeleton in man. Bull Hosp Joint Dis. 1952 Apr;13(1):59-66. PMID: 14935450

736   Saidak Z, Marie PJ. Strontium signaling: molecular mechanisms and therapeutic implications in osteoporosis. Pharmacol Ther. 2012 Nov;136(2):216-26. Epub 2012 Jul 20. PMID: 22820094

737   Bovijn J, Krebs K, Chen C, et al. Evaluating the cardiovascular safety of sclerostin inhibition using evidence from meta-analysis of clinical trials and human genetics. Sci Transl Med. 2020 Jun 24;12(549):eaay6570. PMID: 32581134

738   Marie PJ, Ammann P, Boivin G, et al. Mechanisms of action and therapeutic potential of strontium in bone. Calcif Tissue Int. 2001 Sep;69(3):121-9. PMID: 11683526

739   Riedel C, Zimmermann EA, Zustin J, et al. The incorporation of fluoride and strontium in hydroxyapatite affects the composition, structure, and mechanical properties of human cortical bone. J Biomed Mater Res A. 2017

Feb;105(2):433-442. Epub 2016 Oct 21. PMID: 27684387

740   Moise H, Chettle DR, Pejović-Milić A. Monitoring bone strontium intake in osteoporotic females self-supple-menting with strontium citrate with a novel in-vivo X-ray fluorescence based diagnostic tool. Bone. 2014 Apr;61:48-54. Epub 2014 Jan 14. PMID: 24434614

741   Moise H, Chettle DR, Pejović-Milić A. Modeling elemental strontium in human bone based on in vivo x-ray fluorescence measurements in osteoporotic females self-supplementing with strontium citrate. Physiol Meas. 2016 Mar;37(3):429-41. Epub 2016 Feb 24. PMID: 26910208

742   Calvo MS, Moshfegh AJ, Tucker KL. Assessing the health impact of phosphorus in the food supply: issues and considerations. Adv Nutr. 2014 Jan 1;5(1):104-13. PMID: 24425729

743   Pizzorno L. Canaries in the Phosphate-Toxicity Coal Mines. Integr Med (Encinitas). 2014 Dec;13(6):24-32. PMID: 26770122 PMCID: PMC4566440

744   Marie PJ, Ammann P, Boivin G, et al. Mechanisms of action and therapeutic potential of strontium in bone. Calcif Tissue Int. 2001 Sep;69(3):121-9. PMID: 11683526

745   Ozgür S, Sümer H, Koçoğlu G. Rickets and soil strontium. Arch Dis Child. 1996 Dec;75(6):524-6. PMID: 9014608 This is why you should err on the side of safety and always consume twice as much calcium as strontium.

746   https://pubmed.ncbi.nlm.nih.gov/?term=zinc+and+the+immune+system

747   King JC, Brown KH, Gibson RS, et al. Biomarkers of Nutrition for Development (BOND)-Zinc Review. J Nutr. 2016 Mar 9. pii: jn220079. [Epub ahead of print] PMID: 26962190

748   Zofkova I, Davis M, Blahos J. Trace elements have beneficial, as well as detrimental effects on bone homeosta-sis. Physiol Res. 2017 Jul 18;66(3):391-402. Epub 2017 Feb 28. PMID: 28248532

749   Meunier N, O'Connor JM, Maiani G, et al. Importance of zinc in the elderly: the ZENITH study. Eur J Clin Nutr. 2005 Nov;59 Suppl 2:S1-4. PMID: 16254574

750   Prasad A. Impact of discovery of human zinc deficiency on health. Journal of Trace Elements in Medicine and Biology 28 (2014) 357–363. http://dx.doi.org/10.1016/j.jtemb.2014.09.002.

751   Mahdavi-Roshan M, Ebrahimi M, Ebrahimi A. Copper, magnesium, zinc and calcium status in osteopenic and osteoporotic post-menopausal women. Clin Cases Miner Bone Metab. 2015 Jan-Apr;12(1):18-21. doi: 10.11138/ccmbm/2015.12.1.018. PMID: 26136790

752   Lowe NM, Lowe NM, Fraser WD, et al. Is there a potential therapeutic value of copper and zinc for osteoporosis? Proc Nutr Soc. 2002 May;61(2):181-5. Proc Nutr Soc. 2002 May;61(2):181-5. PMID: 12133199

753   https://www.sciencedirect.com/topics/neuroscience/alkaline-phosphatase

754   Hosea HJ, Taylor CG, Wood T, et al. Zinc-deficient rats have more limited bone recovery during repletion than diet-restricted rats. Exp Biol Med (Maywood). 2004 Apr;229(4):303-11. PMID: 15044713

755   Ryz NR, Weiler HA, Taylor CG. Zinc deficiency reduces bone mineral density in the spine of young adult rats: a pilot study. Ann Nutr Metab. 2009;54(3):218-26. Epub 2009 Jun 9. PMID: 19506366

756   Ferreira ECS, Bortolin RH, Freire-Neto FP, et al. Zinc supplementation reduces RANKL/OPG ratio and prevents bone architecture alterations in ovariectomized and type 1 diabetic rats.Nutr Res. 2017 Apr;40:48-56. Epub 2017 Mar 14. PMID: 28473060

757   Dermience M, Lognay G, Mathieu F, et al. Effects of thirty elements on bone metabolism. J Trace Elem Med Biol. 2015 Oct;32:86-106. Epub 2015 Jun 26. PMID: 26302917

758   Seo HJ, Cho YE, Kim T, Shin HI, Kwun IS. Zinc may increase bone formation through stimulating cell prolifera-tion, alkaline phosphatase activity and collagen synthesis in osteoblastic MC3T3-E1 cells. Nutr Res Pract. 2010 Oct;4(5):356-61. Epub 2010 Oct 26. PMID: 21103080

759   Dermience M, Lognay G, Mathieu F, et al. Effects of thirty elements on bone metabolism. J Trace Elem Med Biol. 2015 Oct;32:86-106. Epub 2015 Jun 26. PMID: 26302917

760   Zofkova I, Davis M, Blahos J. Trace elements have beneficial, as well as detrimental effects on bone homeosta-sis. Physiol Res. 2017 Jul 18;66(3):391-402. Epub 2017 Feb 28. PMID: 28248532

761   Dermience M, Lognay G, Mathieu F, et al. Effects of thirty elements on bone metabolism. J Trace Elem Med Biol. 2015 Oct;32:86-106. Epub 2015 Jun 26. PMID: 26302917

762   Prasad A. Impact of discovery of human zinc deficiency on health. Journal of Trace Elements in Medicine and Biology 28 (2014) 357–363. http://dx.doi.org/10.1016/j.jtemb.2014.09.002.

763   Jamieson JA, Taylor CG, Weiler HA. Marginal zinc deficiency exacerbates bone lead accumulation and high dietary zinc attenuates lead accumulation at the expense of bone density in growing rats. Toxicol Sci. 2006 Jul;92(1):286-94. Epub 2006 Apr 19. PMID: 16624848

764   Haase H, Rink L. Multiple impacts of zinc on immune function. Metallomics. 2014 Jul;6(7)-80. PMID: 24531756

765   Hojyo S, Fukada T. Roles of Zinc Signaling in the Immune System. J Immunol Res. 2016:6762343. Epub 2016 Oct 31. PMID: 27872866

766   Prasad A. Zinc: An antioxidant and anti-inflammatory agent: Role of zinc in degenerative disorders of aging. Journal of Trace Elements in Medicine and Biology 28 (2014) 364–371. PMID: 25200490

767   King JC, Brown KH, Gibson RS, et al. Biomarkers of Nutrition for Development (BOND)-Zinc Review. J Nutr.

2016 Mar 9. pii: jn220079. [Epub ahead of print] PMID: 26962190

768 Lowe NM, Lowe NM, Fraser WD, et al. Is there a potential therapeutic value of copper and zinc for osteoporosis? Proc Nutr Soc. 2002 May;61(2):181-5. Proc Nutr Soc. 2002 May;61(2):181-5. PMID: 12133199

769 Prasad A. Zinc: An antioxidant and anti-inflammatory agent: Role of zinc in degenerative disorders of aging. Journal of Trace Elements in Medicine and Biology 28 (2014) 364–371. PMID: 25200490

770 Kohlmeier M, ed. Nutrient Metabolism, Structures, Functions and Genes, 2nd ed. Chapter 11, Minerals and Trace Elements, Elsevier, NY, 2015, p. 732

771 Maret W, Sandstead HH. Zinc requirements and the risks and benefits of zinc supplementation. J Trace Elem Med Biol. 2006;20(1):3-18. Epub 2006 Feb 21. PMID: 16632171

772 http://www.chemistry.wustl.edu/~edudev/LabTutorials/CourseTutorials/Tutorials/Vitamins/calcium.htm#:~:-text=Our%20bodies%20contain%20a%20staggering,%2C%20and%20the%20cellular%20fluid)

773 King JC, Brown KH, Gibson RS, et al. Biomarkers of Nutrition for Development (BOND)-Zinc Review. J Nutr. 2016 Mar 9. pii: jn220079. [Epub ahead of print] PMID: 26962190

774 Wessells KR, Singh GM, Brown KH. Estimating the global prevalence of inadequate zinc intake from national food balance sheets: effects of methodological assumptions. PLoS One. 2012;7(11):e50565. Epub 2012 Nov 29. PMID: 23209781

775 Maret W, Sandstead HH. Zinc requirements and the risks and benefits of zinc supplementation. J Trace Elem Med Biol. 2006;20(1):3-18. Epub 2006 Feb 21. PMID: 16632171

776 King JC, Brown KH, Gibson RS, et al. Biomarkers of Nutrition for Development (BOND)-Zinc Review. J Nutr. 2016 Mar 9. pii: jn220079. [Epub ahead of print] PMID: 26962190

777 Sandstead HH, Freeland-Graves JH. Dietary phytate, zinc and hidden zinc deficiency. Journal of Trace Elements in Medicine and Biology. 28 (2014) 414–417. PMID: 25439135

778 King JC, Brown KH, Gibson RS, et al. Biomarkers of Nutrition for Development (BOND)-Zinc Review. J Nutr. 2016 Mar 9. pii: jn220079. [Epub ahead of print] PMID: 26962190

779 Lowe NM, Lowe NM, Fraser WD, et al. Is there a potential therapeutic value of copper and zinc for osteoporosis? Proc Nutr Soc. 2002 May;61(2):181-5. Proc Nutr Soc. 2002 May;61(2):181-5. PMID: 12133199

780 Dermience M, Lognay G, Mathieu F, et al. Effects of thirty elements on bone metabolism. J Trace Elem Med Biol. 2015 Oct;32:86-106. Epub 2015 Jun 26. PMID: 26302917

781 King JC, Brown KH, Gibson RS, et al. Biomarkers of Nutrition for Development (BOND)-Zinc Review. J Nutr. 2016 Mar 9. pii: jn220079. [Epub ahead of print] PMID: 26962190

782 Sandstead HH, Freeland-Graves JH. Dietary phytate, zinc and hidden zinc deficiency. Journal of Trace Elements in Medicine and Biology. 28 (2014) 414–417. PMID: 25439135

783 Institute of Medicine, Food and Nutrition Board. Dietary Reference Intakes for Vitamin A, Vitamin K, Arsenic, Boron, Chromium, Copper, Iodine, Iron, Manganese, Molybdenum, Nickel, Silicon, Vanadium, and Zinc. Washington, DC: National Academy Press, 2001

784 https://www.westonaprice.org/health-topics/vegetarianism-and-plant-foods/living-with-phytic-acid/

785 Gustafsson EL, Sandberg AS. (1995), Phytate Reduction in Brown Beans (Phaseolus vulgaris L.). Journal of Food Science, 60: 149–152. doi:10.1111/j.1365-2621.1995.tb05626.x-- http://onlinelibrary.wiley.com/doi/10.1111/j.1365-2621.1995.tb05626.x/abstract

786 Luo Y, Xie W, Luo F. Effect of several germination treatments on phosphatases activities and degradation of phytate in faba bean (Vicia faba L.) and azuki bean (Vigna angularis L.). J Food Sci. 2012 Oct;77(10):C1023-9. Epub 2012 Aug 31. PMID: 22938099

787 Leenhardt F, Levrat-Verny MA, Chanliaud E, et al. Moderate decrease of pH by sourdough fermentation is sufficient to reduce phytate content of whole wheat flour through endogenous phytase activity. J Agric Food Chem. 2005 Jan 12;53(1):98-102. PMID: 15631515

788 King JC, Brown KH, Gibson RS, et al. Biomarkers of Nutrition for Development (BOND)-Zinc Review. J Nutr. 2016 Mar 9. pii: jn220079. [Epub ahead of print] PMID: 26962190

789 Bhardwaj A, Swe KM, Sinha NK, et al. Treatment for osteoporosis in people with ß-thalassaemia. Cochrane Database Syst Rev. 2016 Mar 10;3:CD010429. PMID: 26964506

790 Nidumuru S, Boddula V, Vadakedath S, et al. Evaluating the Role of Zinc in Beta Thalassemia Major: A Prospective Case-Control Study from a Tertiary Care Teaching Hospital in India. Cureus. 2017 Jul 20;9(7):e1495. PMID: 28948115

791 Claro da Silva T, Hiller C, Gai Z, et al. Vitamin D3 transactivates the zinc and manganese transporter SLC30A10 via the Vitamin D receptor. J Steroid Biochem Mol Biol. 2016 Oct;163:77-87. Epub 2016 Apr 20. PMID: 27107558

792 Lazarte C, Carlsson N, Almgren A, et al. Phytate, zinc, iron and calcium content of common Bolivian food, and implications for mineral bioavailability, J Food Comp & Analysis, Vol 39, May 2015, pgs. 111-119, www.sciencedirect.com/science/article/pii/S0889157515000162#bib0015

793 Knez M, Graham RD, Welch RM, et al. New perspectives on the regulation of iron absorption via cellular zinc concentrations in humans. Crit Rev Food Sci Nutr. 2017 Jul 3;57(10):2128-2143. PMID: 26177050

794 Bjørklund G, Aaseth J, Skalny AV, et al. Interactions of iron with manganese, zinc, chromium, and selenium as related to prophylaxis and treatment of iron deficiency. J Trace Elem Med Biol. 2017 May;41:41-53. Epub 2017 Feb 12. PMID: 28347462

795 Mónica A, Lautaro B, Fernando P, et al. Calcium and zinc decrease intracellular iron by decreasing transport during iron repletion in an in vitro model. Eur J Nutr. 2017 Sep 7. [Epub ahead of print] PMID: 28884360

796 Chen Y, Zhang Z, Yang K, et al. Myeloid zinc-finger 1 (MZF-1) suppresses prostate tumor growth through enforcing ferroportin-conducted iron egress. Oncogene. 2015 Jul;34(29):3839-47. Epub 2014 Oct 6. PMID: 25284586

797 Anderson GJ, Frazer DM. Current understanding of iron homeostasis. Am J Clin Nutr. 2017 Oct 25. pii: ajcn155804. [Epub ahead of print] PMID: 29070551

798 Shamshirsaz AA, Bekheirnia MR, Kamgar M, et al. Bone mineral density in Iranian adolescents and young adults with beta-thalassemia major. Pediatr Hematol Oncol. 2007 Oct-Nov;24(7):469-79. PMID: 17786783

799 Mashhadi MA, Sepehri Z, Heidari Z, et al. The prevalence of zinc deficiency in patients with thalassemia in South East of iran, sistan and baluchistan province. Iran Red Crescent Med J. 2014 Aug;16(8):e6243. Epub 2014 Aug 5. PMID: 25389495 PMCID: PMC4222021

800 Ozturk Z, Genc GE, Gumuslu S. Minerals in thalassaemia major patients: An overview. J Trace Elem Med Biol. 2017 May;41:1-9. Epub 2017 Jan 16. PMID: 28347454

801 Barrie S, Wright J, Pizzorno J, et al. Comparative Absorption of Zinc Picolinate, Zinc Citrate and Zinc Gluconate in Humans. Agents Actions 21, no. 1-2 (Jun 1987): 223–8. PMID: 3630857

802 Wegmüller R, Tay F, Zeder C, et al. Zinc absorption by young adults from supplemental zinc citrate is comparable with that from zinc gluconate and higher than from zinc oxide. J Nutr. 2014 Feb;144(2):132-6. Epub 2013 Nov 20. PMID: 24259556

803 Saper R, Rash R. Zinc: An Essential Micronutrient. Am Fam Physician. 2009 May 1;79(9):768-772. www.aafp.org/afp/2009/0501/p768.html

804 Barrie S, Wright J, Pizzorno J, et al. Comparative Absorption of Zinc Picolinate, Zinc Citrate and Zinc Gluconate in Humans. Agents Actions 21, no. 1-2 (Jun 1987): 223–8. PMID: 3630857

805 King JC, Brown KH, Gibson RS, et al. Biomarkers of Nutrition for Development (BOND)-Zinc Review. J Nutr. 2016 Mar 9. pii: jn220079. [Epub ahead of print] PMID: 26962190

806 Zofková I, Nemcikova P, Matucha P.Trace elements and bone health. Clin Chem Lab Med. 2013 Aug;51(8):1555-61. PMID: 23509220

807 Gaby A. Nutritional Medicine, 2nd edition, Fritz Perlberg Publishing, 2017, p. 164

808 Claro da Silva T, Hiller C, Gai Z, et al. Vitamin D3 transactivates the zinc and manganese transporter SLC30A10 via the Vitamin D receptor. J Steroid Biochem Mol Biol. 2016 Oct;163:77-87. Epub 2016 Apr 20. PMID: 27107558

809 Mezzetti A, Pierdomenico SD, Costantini F, et al. Copper/zinc ratio and systemic oxidant load: effect of aging and aging-related degenerative diseases. Free Radic Biol Med. 1998 Oct;25(6):676-81. PMID: 9801067

810 Lowe NM, Lowe NM, Fraser WD, et al. Is there a potential therapeutic value of copper and zinc for osteoporosis? Proc Nutr Soc. 2002 May;61(2):181-5. Proc Nutr Soc. 2002 May;61(2):181-5. PMID: 12133199

811 Gaier ED, Kleppinger A, Ralle M, et al.High serum Cu and Cu/Zn ratios correlate with impairments in bone density, physical performance and overall health in a population of elderly men with frailty characteristics. Exp Gerontol. 2012 Jul;47(7):491-6. Epub 2012 Mar 29. PMID: 22484083

812 Mezzetti A, Pierdomenico SD, Costantini F, et al. Copper/zinc ratio and systemic oxidant load: effect of aging and aging-related degenerative diseases. Free Radic Biol Med. 1998 Oct;25(6):676-81. PMID: 9801067

813 Malavolta M, Piacenza F, Basso A, et al. Serum copper to zinc ratio: Relationship with aging and health status. Mech Ageing Dev. 2015 Nov;151:93-100. Epub 2015 Feb 7. PMID: 25660061

814 Medeiros DM, Ilich J, Ireton J, Matkovic V, et al. Femurs from rats fed diets deficient in copper or iron have decreased mechanical strength and altered mineral composition. J Trace Elem Exp Med. 1997;10:197–203. doi: 10.1002/(SICI)1520-670X(1997)10:3<197::AID-JTRA7>3.0.CO;2-8.

815 Mahdavi-Roshan M, Ebrahimi M, Ebrahimi A. Copper, magnesium, zinc and calcium status in osteopenic and osteoporotic post-menopausal women. Clin Cases Miner Bone Metab. 2015 Jan-Apr;12(1):18-21. PMID: 26136790; PMCID: PMC4469220.

816 Sierpinska T, Konstantynowicz J, Orywal K, et al. Copper deficit as a potential pathogenic factor of reduced bone mineral density and severe tooth wear. Osteoporos Int. 2014 Feb;25(2):447-54. PMID: 23797848

817 Brookes SJ, Shore RC, Robinson C, Wood SR, Kirham J. Copper ions inhibit the demineralization of human enamel. Arch Oral Biol. 2003;48:25–30. PMID: 12615138

818 Dermience M, Lognay G, Mathieu F, et al. Effects of thirty elements on bone metabolism. J Trace Elem Med Biol. 2015 Oct;32:86-106. Epub 2015 Jun 26. PMID: 26302917

819 Zofková I, Nemcikova P, Matucha P. Trace elements and bone health. Clin Chem Lab Med. 2013 Aug;51(8):1555-61. PMID: 23509220

820 Zofkova I, Davis M, Blahos J. Trace elements have beneficial, as well as detrimental effects on bone homeostasis. Physiol Res. 2017 Jul 18;66(3):391-402. Epub 2017 Feb 28. PMID: 28248532

821 Gaby A. Nutritional Medicine, 2nd edition, Fritz Perlberg Publishing, 2017, p. 164.

822 Food and Nutrition Board, Institute of Medicine. Copper. Dietary reference intakes for vitamin A, vitamin K, boron, chromium, copper, iodine, iron, manganese, molybdenum, nickel, silicon, vanadium, and zinc. Washington, D.C.: National Academy Press; 2001:224-257.

823 Joo NS, Yang SW, Song BC, et al. Vitamin A intake, serum vitamin D and bone mineral density: analysis of the Korea National Health and Nutrition Examination Survey (KNHANES, 2008-2011). Nutrients. 2015 Mar 10;7(3):1716-27. PMID: 25763530

824 Michaëlsson K, Lithell H, Vessby B, et al. Serum retinol levels and the risk of fracture. N Engl J Med. 2003 Jan 23;348(4):287-94. PMID: 12540641

825 Boucher BJ. Serum retinol levels and fracture risk. N Engl J Med. 2003 May 8;348(19):1927-8; author reply 1927-8. Comment on Hypervitaminosis A and fractures. [N Engl J Med. 2003] PMID: 12736290

826 Mata-Granados JM, Cuenca-Acevedo JR, Luque de Castro MD, et al. Vitamin D insufficiency together with high serum levels of vitamin A increases the risk for osteoporosis in postmenopausal women. Arch Osteoporos. 2013;8:124. Epub 2013 Feb 16. PMID: 23417776

827 Caire-Juvera G, Ritenbaugh C, Wactawski-Wende J, et al. Vitamin A and retinol intakes and the risk of fractures among participants of the Women's Health Initiative Observational Study. Am J Clin Nutr. 2009 Jan;89(1):323-30. Epub 2008 Dec 3. PMID: 19056568

828 Conaway HH, Henning P, Lerner UH. Vitamin A metabolism, action, and role in skeletal homeostasis. Endocr Rev. 2013 Dec;34(6):766-97. Epub 2013 May 29. PMID: 23720297

829 Uitterlinden AG, Fang Y, Van Meurs JB, et al. Genetics and biology of vitamin D receptor polymorphisms. Gene. 2004 Sep 1;338(2):143-56. PMID: 15315818

830 Sanchez-Martinez R, Castillo A, Steinmeyer A, et al. The retinoid X receptor ligand restores defective signaling by the vitamin D receptor. EMBO Rep. 2006 Oct;7(10):1030-4. PMID: 16936639

831 Bettoun DJ, Burris TP, Houck KA, et al. Retinoid X receptor is a nonsilent major contributor to vitamin D receptor-mediated transcriptional activation. Mol Endocrinol. 2003 Nov;17(11):2320-8. PMID: 12893883

832 Kohlmeier M, ed. Nutrient Metabolism, 2nd edition, Chapter 9, Fat soluble vitamins and nonnutrients, Elsevier, NY, 2015 p. 497

833 Conaway HH, Henning P, Lerner UH. Vitamin a metabolism, action, and role in skeletal homeostasis. Endocr Rev. 2013 Dec;34(6):766-97. Epub 2013 May 29. PMID: 23720297

834 Henning P, Conaway HH, Lerner UH. Retinoid receptors in bone and their role in bone remodeling. Front Endocrinol (Lausanne). 2015 Mar 11;6:31. eCollection 2015. PMID: 25814978

835 Caire-Juvera G, Ritenbaugh C, Wactawski-Wende J, et al. Vitamin A and retinol intakes and the risk of fractures among participants of the Women's Health Initiative Observational Study. Am J Clin Nutr. 2009 Jan;89(1):323-30. Epub 2008 Dec 3. PMID: 19056568

836 Pizzorno L. Vitamin A: tolerance extends longevity. Longevity Medicine Review. 2009 http://www.lmreview.com/articles/view/vitamin-a-tolerance-extends-longevity/

837 Ertesvåg A, Naderi S, Blomhoff HK. Regulation B cell proliferation and differentiation by retinoic acid. Semin Immunol. 2009 Feb;21(1):36-41. PMID: 18703353

838 Pino-Lagos K, Benson MJ, Noelle RJ. Retinoic acid in the immune system. Ann N Y Acad Sci. 2008 Nov;1143:170-87. PMID: 19076350

839 Lu LF, Rudensky A. Molecular orchestration of differentiation and function of regulatory T cells. Genes Dev. 2009 Jun 1;23(11):1270-82. PMID: 19487568

840 Strober W. Vitamin A rewrites the ABCs of oral tolerance. Mucosal Immunol. 2008 Mar;1(2):92-5. PMID: 19079166

841 Pizzorno JE, Murray JT, eds., Textbook of Natural Medicine, 5th edition, Vitamin A, Chapter 125, p. 910-918, Elsevier: St. Louis, MO, 2020.

842 Chiu H, Fischman D, Hammerling U. Vitamin A depletion causes oxidative stress, mitochondrial dysfunction, and PARP-1-dependent energy deprivation. FASEB J. 22, 3878–3887 (2008). PMID: 18676402

843 Rhéume-Bleue K. Vitamin K and the Calcium Paradox, John Wiley & Sons: Mississauga, Ontario, 2012, p. 201

844 Fu X, Wang XD, Mernitz H, et al. 9-Cis retinoic acid reduces 1alpha,25-dihydroxycholecalciferol-induced renal calcification by altering vitamin K-dependent gamma-carboxylation of matrix gamma-carboxyglutamic acid protein in A/J male mice. J Nutr. 2008 Dec;138(12):2337-41. PMID: 19022954

845 Farzaneh-Far A, Weissberg PL, Proudfoot D, et al. Transcriptional regulation of matrix gla protein. Z Kardiol. 2001;90 Suppl 3:38-42. PMID: 11374031

846 Proudfoot D, Shanahan CM. Molecular mechanisms mediating vascular calcification: role of matrix Gla protein. Nephrology (Carlton). 2006 Oct;11(5):455-61. PMID: 17014561

847 Morgan, A. F. Kimmel, L. Hawkins, N. C. "A comparison of the hypervitaminoses induced by irradiated ergosterol and fish liver oil concentrates," The Journal of Biological Chemistry, 1937; 120(1): 85-102

848 Clark, I. Bassett, C. A. L. "The amelioration of hypervitaminosis D in rats with vitamin A," J Exp Med., 1962; 115:

147-156.

849 Callari, D. Garra, M. L. Billitteri, A. "Retinoic acid action on D3 hypervitaminosis," Boll. Soc. It. Biol. Sper., 1986; LXII (6): 835-841.

850 Westenfeld R, Krueger T, Schlieper G, et al. Effect of vitamin K2 supplementation on functional vitamin K deficiency in hemodialysis patients: a randomized trial. Am J Kidney Dis. 2012;59(2):186-195. PMID: 22169620

851 Fusaro M, D'Angelo A, Gallieni M. Consequences of vitamin K2 deficiency in hemodialysis patients. Am J Kidney Dis. 2012 Jul;60(1):169. PMID: 22709599

852 Price, P. A. Faus, S. A. Williamson, M. K. "Warfarin-Induced Artery Calcification Is Accelerated by Growth and Vitamin D," Arterioscler Thromb Vasc Biol., 2000; 20: 317-327

853 Rhéume-Bleue K. Vitamin K and the Calcium Paradox, John Wiley & Sons: Mississauga, Ontario, 2012, p. 201

854 Masterjohn C. From Seafood to Sunshine: A New Understanding of Vitamin D Safety. Wise Traditions, December 17, 2006, http://www.westonaprice.org/health-topics/abcs-of-nutrition/from-seafood-to-sunshine-a-new-understanding-of-vitamin-d-safety/#2v3

855 Bardaoui M, Sakly R, Neffati F, et al. Effect of vitamin A supplemented diet on calcium oxalate renal stone formation in rats. Exp Toxicol Pathol. 2010 Sep;62(5):573-6. Epub 2009 Sep 18. PMID: 19766470

856 Wagner J. Potential role of retinoids in the therapy of renal disease. Nephrol Dial Transplant. 2001 Mar;16(3):441-4. PMID: 11239012

857 Sakly R, Fekih M, Ben Amor A, et al. [Possible role of vitamin A and E deficiency in human idiopathic lithiasis]. [Article in French] Ann Urol (Paris). 2003 Aug;37(4):217-9. PMID: 12951718

858 Barber T, Esteban-Pretel G, Marín MP, et al. Vitamin A deficiency and alterations in the extracellular matrix. Nutrients. 2014 Nov 10;6(11):4984-5017. PMID: 25389900

859 Favus, M. J. "Intestinal Absorption of Calcium, Magnesium and Phosphorus," in Coe, F. L. Favus, M. J. eds., Disorders of Bone and Mineral Metabolism, 2nd Edition, Baltimore, MD: Lippincott Williams and Wilkins, 2002

860 Aburto, A. Edwards, H. M. Britton, W. M. "The Influence of Vitamin A on the Utilization and Amelioration of Toxicity of Cholecalciferol, 25- Masterjohn C. From Seafood to Sunshine: A New Understanding of Vitamin D Safety. Wise Traditions, December 17, 2006, http://www.westonaprice.org/health-topics/abcs-of-nutrition/from-seafood-to-sunshine-a-new-understanding-of-vitamin-d-safety/#2v3.

861 Hydroxycholecalciferol, and 1,25 Dihydroxycholecalciferol in Young Broiler Chickens," Poultry Science, 1998; 77: 585-593

862 Oliva A, Della Ragione F, Fratta M, et al. Effect of retinoic acidon osteocalcin gene expression in human osteoblasts. Biochem Biophys Res Commun. 1993 Mar 31;191(3):908-14. PMID: 8466530

863 Jääskeläinen T, Ryhänen S, Mäenpää PH. 9-cis retinoic acid accelerates calcitriol-induced osteocalcin production and promotes degradation of both vitamin D receptor and retinoid X receptor in human osteoblastic cells. J Cell Biochem. 2003 Aug 15;89(6):1164-76. PMID: 12898515

864 Shiraki M, Yamazaki Y, Shiraki Y, et al. High level of serum undercarboxylated osteocalcin in patients with incident fractures during bisphosphonate treatment. J Bone Miner Metab. 2010 Sep;28(5):578-84. Epub 2010 Mar 11. PMID: 20221651

865 Arunakul M, Niempoog S, Arunakul P, et al. Level of undercarboxylated osteocalcin in hip fracture Thai female patients. J Med Assoc Thai. 2009 Sep;92 Suppl5:S7-11. PMID: 19891375

866 Inaba N, Sato T, Yamashita T. Low-Dose Daily Intake of Vitamin K(2) (Menaquinone-7) Improves Osteocalcin γ-Carboxylation: A Double-Blind, Randomized Controlled Trials. J Nutr Sci Vitaminol (Tokyo). 2015;61(6):471-80. PMID: 26875489

867 Villa JK, Diaz MA, Pizziolo VR. Effect of vitamin K in bone metabolism and vascular calcification: a review of mechanisms of action and evidences. Crit Rev Food Sci Nutr. 2016 Jul 20:0. [Epub ahead of print] PMID: 27437760

868 Nozière P, Grolier P, Durand D, et al. Variations in carotenoids, fat-soluble micronutrients, and color in cows' plasma and milk following changes in forage and feeding level. J Dairy Sci. 2006 Jul;89(7):2634-48. PMID: 16772583

869 Hulshof PJM, van Roekel-Jansen T, van de Bovenkamp P, et al. Variation in retinol and carotenoid content of milk and milk products in The Netherlands. Journal of Food Composition and Analysis 19(1):67-75 · February 2006, DOI: 10.1016/j.jfca.2005.04.005

870 Leung WC, Hessel S, Méplan C, Flint J, Oberhauser V, Tourniaire F, Hesketh JE, von Lintig J, Lietz G. Two common single nucleotide polymorphisms in the gene encoding beta-carotene 15,15'-monoxygenase alter beta-carotene metabolism in female volunteers. FASEB J. 2009 Apr;23(4):1041-53. PMID: 19103647

871 Lietz G, Oxley A, Leung W, et al. Single nucleotide polymorphisms upstream from the β-carotene 15,15'-monoxygenase gene influence provitamin A conversion efficiency in female volunteers. J Nutr. 2012 Jan;142(1):161S-5S. Epub 2011 Nov 23. PMID: 22113863

872 Pizzorno L, Common genetic variants and other host-related factors greatly increase susceptibility to vitamin A deficiency, Longevity Medicine Review, 2009, https://lmreview.com/common-genetic-variants-and-other-host-related-factors-greatly-increase-susceptibility-to-vitamin-a-deficiency/

873 Tang G. Bioconversion of dietary provitamin A carotenoids to vitamin A in humans. Am J Clin Nutr. 2010 May;91(5):1468S-1473S. Epub 2010 Mar 3. PMID: 20200262

874 Scott KJ, Rodriquez-Amaya D. Pro-vitamin A carotenoid conversion factors: retinol equivalents – fact or fiction? Food Chemistry 69 (2000) 127-127. http://dx.doi.org/10.1016/S0308-8146(99)00256-3

875 Kohlmeier RH. "Vitamin A," in "Fat soluble vitamins and non-nutrients," Nutrient Metabolism, Elsevier: London, p. 464-478

876 Green MH, Ford JL, Green JB. Development of a Compartmental Model to Investigate the Influence of Inflammation on Predictions of Vitamin A Total Body Stores by Retinol Isotope Dilution in Theoretical Humans. J Nutr. 2021 Jan 20:nxaa407. Epub ahead of print. PMID: 33484140.

877 Patrick L, Beta-carotene: the controversy continues. Altern Med Rev. 2000 Dec;5(6):530-45. PMID: 11134976

878 Mitra S, De A, Chowdhury A. Epidemiology of non-alcoholic and alcoholic fatty liver diseases. Transl Gastroenterol Hepatol. 2020;5:16. Published 2020 Apr 5. PMID: 32258520

879 Wang XD. Alcohol, vitamin A, and cancer. Alcohol. 2005 Apr;35(3):251-8. PMID: 16054987

880 Stargrove M, Treasure J, McKee D. Herb, Nutrient, and Drug Interactions: Clinical Implications and Therapeutic Strategies. Mosby:Elsevier: St Louis, MO, 2008, pp. 235-236

881 Odabasi M. Halogenated volatile organic compounds from the use of chlorine-bleach-containing household products. Environ Sci Technol. 2008 Mar 1;42(5):1445-51. PMID: 18441786

882 https://ods.od.nih.gov/factsheets/VitaminA-HealthProfessional/#h2

883 Knapen MH, Braam LA, Drummen NE, et al. Menaquinone-7 supplementation improves arterial stiffness in healthy postmenopausal women. A double-blind randomised clinical trial. Thromb Haemost. 2015 May;113(5):1135-44. Epub 2015 Feb 19. PMID: 25694037

884 Knapen MH, Drummen NE, Smit E, Vermeer C, Theuwissen E. Three-year low-dose menaquinone-7 supplementation helps decrease bone loss in healthy postmenopausal women. Osteoporos Int. 2013 Sep;24(9):2499-507. Epub 2013 Mar 23. PMID: 23525894

885 Vossen LM, Schurgers LJ, van Varik BJ, et al. Menaquinone-7 Supplementation to Reduce Vascular Calcification in Patients with Coronary Artery Disease: Rationale and Study Protocol (VitaK-CAC Trial). Nutrients. 2015 Oct 28;7(11):8905-15. PMID: 26516910

886 Caluwé R, Vandecasteele S, Van Vlem B, Vermeer C, De Vriese AS. Vitamin K2 supplementation in haemodialysis patients: a randomized dose-finding study. Nephrol Dial Transplant. 2014 Jul;29(7):1385-90. Epub 2013 Nov 26. PMID: 24285428

887 Westenfeld R, Krueger T, Schlieper G, et al. Effect of vitamin K2 supplementation on functional vitamin K deficiency in hemodialysis patients: a randomized trial. Am J Kidney Dis. 2012;59(2):186-195.PMID: 22169620

888 https://ods.od.nih.gov/factsheets/VitaminA-HealthProfessional/#h2

889 Whitney E, Rolfes S. Chapter 11, "The Fat-Soluble Vitamins," in Understanding Nutrition, Wadsworth: Belmont, CA, 2008, p. 369-389

890 Kohlmeier M. Chapter 9, Fat-soluble vitamins and nonnutrients, Vitamin A, in Nutrient Metabolism, 2nd edition. Elsevier: London, 2015, p. 486-500

891 Rutkowski M, Grzegorczyk K. Adverse effects of antioxidative vitamins. Int J Occup Med Environ Health. 2012 Jun;25(2):105-21. Epub 2012 Apr 19. PMID: 22528540

892 Penniston KL, Tanumihardjo SA. The acute and chronic toxic effects of vitamin A. Am J Clin Nutr. 2006 Feb;83(2):191-201. PMID: 16469975

893 Klutstein M, Nejman D, Greenfield R, et al. DNA Methylation in Cancer and Aging. Cancer Res. 2016 Jun 15;76(12):3446-50. Epub 2016 Jun 2. Review. PMID: 27256564

894 Gomes MV, Pelosi GG. Epigenetic vulnerability and the environmental influence on health. Exp Biol Med (Maywood). 2013 Aug 1;238(8):859-65. Epub 2013 Jul 4. PMID: 23828586

895 Loenen WA. S-adenosylmethionine: jack of all trades and master of everything? Biochem Soc Trans. 2006 Apr;34(Pt 2):330-3. PMID: 16545107

896 Lu SC, Mato JM. S-adenosylmethionine in liver health, injury, and cancer. Physiol Rev. 2012 Oct;92(4):1515-42. PMID: 23073625

897 Saito M, Fujii K, Marumo K. Degree of mineralization-related collagen crosslinking in the femoral neck cancellous bone in cases of hip fracture and controls. Calcif Tissue Int. 2006 Sep;79(3):160-8. Epub 2006 Sep 11. PMID: 16969591

898 Saito M, Marumo K. Collagen cross-links as a determinant of bone quality: a possible explanation for bone fragility in aging, osteoporosis, and diabetes mellitus. Osteoporos Int. 2010 Feb;21(2):195-214. PMID: 19760059

899 Vaes BL, Lute C, Blom HJ, et al. Vitamin B(12) deficiency stimulates osteoclastogenesis via increased homocysteine and methylmalonic acid. Calcif Tissue Int. 2009 May;84(5):413-22. Epub 2009 Apr 12. PMID: 19363664

900 Herrmann M, Tami A, Wildemann B, et al. Hyperhomocysteinemia induces a tissue specific accumulation of homocysteine in bone by collagen binding and adversely affects bone. Bone. 2009 Mar;44(3):467-75. Epub 2008 Nov 12. PMID: 19056526

901 Petramala L, Acca M, Francucci CM, et al. Hyperhomocysteinemia: a biochemical link between bone and cardiovascular system diseases? J Endocrinol Invest. 2009;32(4 Suppl):10-4. PMID: 19724160

902 Yang J, Hu X, Zhang Q, et al. Homocysteine level and risk of fracture: A meta-analysis and systematic review. Bone. 2012 Sep;51(3):376-82. Epub 2012 Jun 26. PMID: 22749888

903 Gjesdal CG, Vollset SE, Ueland PM, et al. Plasma total homocysteine level and bone mineral density: the Horda-land Homocysteine Study. Arch Intern Med. 2006 Jan 9;166(1):88-94. PMID: 16401815

904 McLean RR, Jacques PF, Selhub J, et al. Homocysteine as a predictive factor for hip fracture in older persons. N Engl J Med. 2004 May 13;350(20):2042-9. PMID: 15141042

905 Feigerlova E, Demarquet L, Guéant JL. One carbon metabolism and bone homeostasis and remodeling: A review of experimental research and population studies. Biochimie. 2016 Jul;126:115-23. Epub 2016 Apr 13. PMID: 27086080

906 Yang J, Hu X, Zhang Q, et al. Homocysteine level and risk of fracture: A meta-analysis and systematic review. Bone. 2012 Sep;51(3):376-82. Epub 2012 Jun 26. PMID: 22749888

907 van Wijngaarden JP, Doets EL, Szczecińska A, et al. Vitamin B12, folate, homocysteine, and bone health in adults and elderly people: a systematic review with meta-analyses. J Nutr Metab. 2013;2013:486186. Epub 2013 Feb 20. PMID: 23509616

908 Pizzorno J. Homocysteine: Friend or Foe? Integr Med (Encinitas). 2014 Aug;13(4):8-14. PMID: 26770102 PMCID: PMC4566450

909 Pizzorno J. Homocysteine: Friend or Foe? Integr Med (Encinitas). 2014 Aug;13(4):8-14. PMID: 26770102 PMCID: PMC4566450

910 Yadav U, Kumar P, Gupta S, Rai V. Distribution of MTHFR C677T Gene Polymorphism in Healthy North Indian Population and an Updated Meta-analysis. Indian J Clin Biochem. 2017 Oct;32(4):399-410. Epub 2016 Oct 11. PMID: 29062171; PMCID: PMC5634971

911 Dalto DB, Matte JJ. Pyridoxine (Vitamin B_6) and the Glutathione Peroxidase System; a Link between One-Car-bon Metabolism and Antioxidation. Nutrients. 2017 Feb 24;9(3). pii: E189. PMID: 28245568 PMCID: PMC5372852 https://www.ncbi.nlm.nih.gov/pubmed/28245568

912 Boylan LM, Spallholz JE. In vitro evidence for a relationship between magnesium and vitamin B-6. Magnes Res. 1990 Jun;3(2):79-85. PMID: 2133627

913 Gaby A. "Vitamin B6," Chapter 18, Nutritional Medicine, 2nd edition, 2017 p. 89 https://www.amazon.com/Nutritional-Medicine-Second-Alan-Gaby/dp/1532322097

914 Dodds RA, Catterall A, Bitensky L, Chayen J. Abnormalities in fracture healing induced by vitamin B6-deficiency in rats. Bone. 1986;7(6):489-95. PMID: 3801238

915 Reynolds TM. Vitamin B6 deficiency may also be important. Clin Chem. 1998 Dec;44(12):2555-6. PMID: 9836732

916 Lienhart WD, Gudipati V, Macheroux P. The human flavoproteome. Arch Biochem Biophys. 2013 Jul 15;535(2):150-62. Epub 2013 Mar 15. PMID: 23500531

917 Katsyuba E, Auwerx J. Modulating NAD+ metabolism, from bench to bedside. MBO J. 2017 Aug 7. pii: e201797135. [Epub ahead of print] PMID: 28784597

918 Stein LR, Imai S. The dynamic regulation of NAD metabolism in mitochondria. Trends in endocrinology and metabolism: TEM. 2012;23(9):420-428. PMID: 22819213

919 Lienhart WD, Gudipati V, Macheroux P. The human flavoproteome. Arch Biochem Biophys. 2013 Jul 15;535(2):150-62. Epub 2013 Mar 15. PMID: 23500531

920 Williams GR, Bassett JHD. Thyroid diseases and bone health. J Endocrinol Invest. 2017 Aug 29. [Epub ahead of print] PMID: 28853052

921 Gietka-Czernel M. The thyroid gland in postmenopausal women: physiology and diseases. Prz Menopauzalny. 2017 Jun;16(2):33-37. Epub 2017 Jun 30. PMID: 28721126

922 Marenzana M, Arnett TR. The Key Role of the Blood Supply to Bone. Bone Res. 2013 Sep 25;1(3):203-15. eCol-lection 2013 Sep. PMID: 26273504

923 Evans DM, Ralston SH. Nitric oxide and bone. J Bone Miner Res. 1996 Mar;11(3):300-5. PMID: 8852940

924 Griffith JF, Yeung DK, Tsang PH, et al. Compromised bone marrow perfusion in osteoporosis. .J Bone Miner Res. 2008 Jul;23(7):1068-75. PMID: 18302498

925 Vestergaard P, Rejnmark L, Mosekilde L. Hypertension is a risk factor for fractures. Calcif Tissue Int. 2009 Feb;84(2):103-11. Epub 2008 Dec 5. PMID: 19067019

926 Marenzana M, Arnett TR. The Key Role of the Blood Supply to Bone. Bone Res. 2013 Sep 25;1(3):203-15. eCol-lection 2013 Sep. PMID: 26273504

927 Kaplon RE, Gano LB, Seals DR. Vascular endothelial function and oxidative stress are related to dietary niacin intake among healthy middle-aged and older adults. J Appl Physiol (1985). 2014 Jan 15;116(2):156-63. Epub 2013 Dec 5. PMID: 24311750

928 Mudryj AN, de Groh M, Aukema HM, et al. Folate intakes from diet and supplements may place certain Canadi-ans at risk for folic acid toxicity. Br J Nutr. 2016 Oct;116(7):1236-1245. Epub 2016 Sep 9. PMID: 27609220

929 https://www.ncbi.nlm.nih.gov/books/NBK45182/#:~:text=Estimated%20Average%20Requirement%20 (EAR)%3A,healthy%20individuals%20in%20a%20group

930 Sovianne ter Borg S, Verlaan S, Hemsworth J, et al. Micronutrient intakes and potential inadequacies of community-dwelling older adults: a systematic review. Br J Nutr. 2015 Apr 28;113(8):1195-206. Epub 2015 Mar 30. PMID: 25822905

931 http://www.mayoclinic.org/diseases-conditions/anemia/symptoms-causes/dxc-20183157

932 Bird JK, Murphy RA, Ciappio ED, et al. Risk of Deficiency in Multiple Concurrent Micronutrients in Children and Adults in the United States. Nutrients. 2017 Jun 24;9(7). pii: E655. PMID: 28672791

933 Guralnik JM, Eisenstaedt RS, Ferrucci L, et al. Prevalence of anemia in persons 65 years and older in the United States: evidence for a high rate of unexplained anemia. Blood. 2004 Oct 15;104(8):2263-8. Epub 2004 Jul 6. PMID: 15238427

934 Gaby A. "Vitamin B6," Chapter 18, Nutritional Medicine, 2nd edition, 2017, p. 86.

935 Porter K, Hoey L, Hughes CF, et al. Causes, Consequences and Public Health Implications of Low B-Vitamin Status in Ageing. Nutrients. 2016 Nov 16;8(11). pii: E725. PMID: 27854316

936 https://ods.od.nih.gov/factsheets/Riboflavin-HealthProfessional/

937 Bates B, Cox L, Page S, National Diet and Nutrition Survey: Results from Years 5 and 6 (Combined) of the Rolling Programme (2012/2013–2013/2014); Public Health England: London, UK, 2016

938 Powers HJ. Riboflavin (vitamin B-2) and health. Am J Clin Nutr. 2003 Jun;77(6):1352-60. PMID: 12791609

939 https://www.snpedia.com/index.php/Rs70991108

940 Scaglione F, Panzavolta G. Folate, folic acid and 5-methyltetrahydrofolate are not the same thing. Xenobiotica. 2014 May;44(5):480-8. Epub 2014 Feb 4. PMID: 24494987

941 Selhub J, Rosenberg IH. Excessive folic acid intake and relation to adverse health outcome. Biochimie. 2016 Jul;126:71-8. Epub 2016 Apr 27. PMID: 27131640

942 Kim YI. Does a high folate [folic acid] intake increase the risk of breast cancer? Nutr Rev. 2006 Oct;64(10 Pt 1):468-75. PMID: 17063929

943 Mudryj AN, de Groh M, Aukema HM, et al. Folate intakes from diet and supplements may place certain Canadi- ans at risk for folic acid toxicity. Br J Nutr. 2016 Oct;116(7):1236-1245. Epub 2016 Sep 9. PMID: 27609220

944 Troen AM, Mitchell B, Sorensen B, et al. Unmetabolized folic acid in plasma is associated with reduced natural killer cell cytotoxicity among postmenopausal women. J Nutr. 2006 Jan;136(1):189-94. PMID: 16365081

945 Morris MS, Jacques PF, Rosenberg IH, et al. Circulating unmetabolized folic acid and 5-methyltetrahydrofolate in relation to anemia, macrocytosis, and cognitive test performance in American seniors. Am J Clin Nutr. 2010 Jun;91(6):1733-44. Epub 2010 Mar 31. PMID: 20357042

946 Li Z, Wu C, Li L, et al. Effect of long-term proton pump inhibitor administration on gastric mucosal atrophy: A meta-analysis. Saudi J Gastroenterol. 2017 Jul-Aug;23(4):222-228. PMID: 28721975

947 Lam JR, Schneider JL, Zhao W, et al. Proton pump inhibitor and histamine 2 receptor antagonist use and vitamin B12 deficiency. JAMA. 2013 Dec 11;310(22):2435-42. PMID: 24327038

948 Valuck RJ, Ruscin JM. A case-control study on adverse effects: H2 blocker or proton pump inhibitor use and risk of vitamin B12 deficiency in older adults. J Clin Epidemiol. 2004 Apr;57(4):422-8. PMID: 15135846

949 Maggio M, Lauretani F, Ceda GP, et al. Use of proton pump inhibitors is associated with lower trabecular bone density in older individuals. Bone. 2013 Dec;57(2):437-42. Epub 2013 Sep 26. PMID: 24076021

950 Arj A, Razavi Zade M, Yavari M, et al. Proton pump inhibitors use and change in bone mineral density. Int J Rheum Dis. 2016 Sep;19(9):864-8. Epub 2016 May 31. PMID: 27242025

951 Freedberg DE, Haynes K, Denburg MR, et al. Use of proton pump inhibitors is associated with fractures in young adults: a population-based study. Osteoporos Int. 2015 Oct;26(10):2501-7. Epub 2015 May 19. PMID: 25986385

952 Chapman LE, Darling AL, Brown JE. Association between metformin and vitamin B12 deficiency in patients with type 2 diabetes: A systematic review and meta-analysis. Diabetes Metab. 2016 Nov;42(5):316-327. Epub 2016 Apr 26. PMID: 27130885

953 Mintzer S, Skidmore CT, Sperling MR. B-vitamin deficiency in patients treated with antiepileptic drugs. Epilepsy Behav. 2012 Jul;24(3):341-4. Epub 2012 May 31. PMID: 22658435

954 Palmery M, Saraceno A, Vaiarelli A, Carlomagno G. Oral contraceptives and changes in nutritional require- ments. Eur Rev Med Pharmacol Sci. 2013 Jul;17(13):1804-13. PMID: 23852908 https://www.ncbi.nlm.nih.gov/ pubmed/?term=23852908

955 Porter K, Hoey L, Hughes CF, et al. Causes, Consequences and Public Health Implications of Low B-Vitamin Status in Ageing. Nutrients. 2016 Nov 16;8(11). pii: E725. PMID: 27854316

956 Abrahamsen B, Madsen JS, Tofteng CL, et al. A common methylenetetrahydrofolate reductase (C677T) polymorphism is associated with low bone mineral density and increased fracture incidence after menopause: longitudinal data from the Danish osteoporosis prevention study. J Bone Miner Res. 2003 Apr;18(4):723-9. PMID: 12674333

957   Bai R, Liu W, Zhao A, et al. Quantitative assessment of the associations between MTHFR C677T and A1298C polymorphisms and risk of fractures: a meta-analysis. Mol Biol Rep. 2013 Mar;40(3):2419-30. PMID: 23229495

958   Wang H, Liu C. Association of MTHFR C667T polymorphism with bone mineral density and fracture risk: an updated meta-analysis. Osteoporos Int. 2012 Nov;23(11):2625-34. Epub 2011 Dec 21. PMID: 22187009

959   Castro R, Barroso M, Rocha M, et al. The TCN2 776CNG polymorphism correlates with vitamin B(12) cellular delivery in healthy adult populations. Clin Biochem. 2010 May;43(7-8):645-9. Epub 2010 Feb 6. PMID: 20144600

960   Gaby A, Chapter 20, "B12" in Nutritional Medicine, 2nd edition, pgs. 94-101

961   Gaby A. "Vitamin B6," Chapters 14, 15, 16, 18 & 61 Nutritional Medicine, 2nd edition, 2017.

962   Kennedy DO. B Vitamins and the Brain: Mechanisms, Dose and Efficacy--A Review. Nutrients. 2016 Jan 27;8(2):68. PMID: 26828517

963   Gaby A. Chapter 16, Folic acid (Folate) in Nutritional Medicine, 2nd edition, Fritz Perlberg Publishing: Concord, NH, pp. 75-81

964   Mudryj AN, de Groh M, Aukema HM, et al. Folate intakes from diet and supplements may place certain Canadians at risk for folic acid toxicity. Br J Nutr. 2016 Oct;116(7):1236-1245. Epub 2016 Sep 9. PMID: 27609220

965   Mason JB . Folate, cancer risk, and the Greek god, Proteus: a tale of two chameleons. Nutr Rev. 2009 Apr;67(4):206-12. Review. PMID: 19335714

966   https://www.nationalgeographic.com/science/article/scurvy-disease-discovery-jonathan-lamb

967   Sekhar RV, Patel SG, Guthikonda AP, et al. Deficient synthesis of glutathione underlies oxidative stress in aging and can be corrected by dietary cysteine and glycine supplementation. Am J Clin Nutr. 2011 Sep;94(3):847-53. Epub 2011 Jul 27. PMID: 21795440

968   Calder PC, Albers R, Antoine JM, et al. Inflammatory disease processes and interactions with nutrition. Br J Nutr. 2009 May;101 Suppl 1:S1-45. PMID: 19586558

969   Bellanti F, Matteo M, Rollo T, et al. Sex hormones modulate circulating antioxidant enzymes: impact of estrogen therapy. Redox Biol. 2013 Jun 19;1:340-6. eCollection 2013. PMID: 24024169 PMCID: PMC3757703

970   Priyanka HP, Sharma U, Gopinath S, et al. Menstrual cycle and reproductive aging alters immune reactivity, NGF expression, antioxidant enzyme activities, and intracellular signaling pathways in the peripheral blood mononuclear cells of healthy women. Brain Behav Immun. 2013 Aug;32:131-43. Epub 2013 Mar 27. PMID: 23542336

971   Lean JM, Davies JT, Fuller K, et al. A crucial role for thiol antioxidants in estrogen-deficiency bone loss. J Clin Invest. 2003 Sep;112(6):915-23. PMID: 12975476 PMCID: PMC193670

972   De Tullio MC. Beyond the antioxidant: the double life of vitamin C. Subcell Biochem. 2012;56:49-65. PMID: 22116694

973   Aghajanian P, Hall S, Wongworawat MD, et al. The Roles and Mechanisms of Actions of Vitamin C in Bone: New Developments. J Bone Miner Res. 2015 Nov;30(11):1945-55. Epub 2015 Oct 7. PMID: 26358868

974   Shen Y, Liu HX, Ying XZ, et al. Dose-dependent effects of nicotine on proliferation and differentiation of human bone marrow stromal cells and the antagonistic action of vitamin C. J Cell Biochem. 2013 Aug;114(8):1720-8. PMID: 23386463

975   Sahni S, Hannan MT, Gagnon D, Blumberg J, et al. High vitamin C intake is associated with lower 4-year bone loss in elderly men. J Nutr. 2008 Oct;138(10):1931-8. PMID: 18806103

976   Tucker KL, Chen H, Hannan MT, et al. Bone mineral density and dietary patterns in older adults: the Framingham Osteoporosis Study. Am J Clin Nutr. 2002 Jul;76(1):245-52. PMID: 12081842

977   Kim YA, Kim KM, Lim S, et al. Favorable effect of dietary vitamin C on bone mineral density in postmenopausal women (KNHANES IV, 2009): discrepancies regarding skeletal sites, age, and vitamin D status. Osteoporos Int. 2015 Sep;26(9):2329-37. Epub 2015 Apr 24. PMID: 25906241

978   Sahni S, Marian T, Blumberg J, et al. Protective effect of total and supplemental vitamin C intake on the risk of hip fracture - A 17-year follow-up from the Framingham Osteoporosis Study. Osteoporos Int. 2009 Nov;20(11):1853-61. Epub 2009 Apr 4. PMID: 19347239 PMCID: PMC2766028

979   National Institutes of Health, Office of Dietary Supplements, Vitamin C https://ods.od.nih.gov/factsheets/VitaminC-HealthProfessional/#h2

980   Nieves JW. Skeletal effects of nutrients and nutraceuticals, beyond calcium and vitamin D. Osteoporos Int. 2013 Mar;24(3):771-86. Epub 2012 Nov 14. PMID: 23152094

981   Calder PC, Albers R, Antoine JM, et al. Inflammatory disease processes and interactions with nutrition. Br J Nutr. 2009 May;101 Suppl 1:S1-45. PMID: 19586558

982   Hart A, Cota A, Makhdom A, et al. The Role of Vitamin C in Orthopedic Trauma and Bone Health. Am J Orthop (Belle Mead NJ). 2015 Jul;44(7):306-11. PMID: 26161758

983   Gaby A. Vitamin C, in Nutritional Medicine, 2nd edition, 2017: Fritz Perlberg Publishing, Concord, NH, p. 105.

984   Hathcock JN, Azzi A, Blumberg J, et al. Vitamins E and C are safe across a broad range of intakes. Am J Clin Nutr. 2005 Apr;81(4):736-45. PMID: 15817846

985   Ipsen DH, Tveden-Nyborg P, Lykkesfeldt J. Does vitamin C deficiency promote fatty liver disease development?

Nutrients. 2014 Dec 16(12):5473-99. PMID: 25533004

986 Michels AJ, Joisher N, Hagen TM. Age-related decline of sodium-dependent ascorbic acid transport in isolated rat hepatocytes. Arch Biochem Biophys. 003 Feb 1;410(1):112-20. PMID: 12559983

987 Lykkesfeldt J, Moos T. Age-dependent change in Vitamin C status: a phenomenon of maturation rather than of ageing. Mech Ageing Dev. 2005 Aug;126(8):892-8. Epub 2005 Apr 25. PMID: 15992612

988 Palmery M, Saraceno A, Vaiarelli A, Carlomagno G. Oral contraceptives and changes in nutritional requirements. Eur Rev Med Pharmacol Sci. 2013 Jul;17(13):1804-13. PMID: 23852908

989 Zal F, Mostafavi-Pour Z, Amini F, Heidari A. Effect of vitamin E and C supplements on lipid peroxidation and GSH-dependent antioxidant enzyme status in the blood of women consuming oral contraceptives. Contraception. 2012 Jul;86(1):62-6. Epub 2012 Apr 9. PMID: 22494786

990 Lee S, Choi Y, Jeong HS, Lee J, Sung J. Effect of different cooking methods on the content of vitamins and true retention in selected vegetables. Food Sci Biotechnol. 2017 Dec 12;27(2):333-342. PMID: 30263756; PMCID

991 Levine M, Conry-Cantilena C, Wang Y, et al. Vitamin C pharmacokinetics in healthy volunteers: evidence for a recommended dietary allowance. Proc Natl Acad Sci U S A. 1996 Apr 16;93(8):3704-9. PMID: 8623000 PMCID: PMC39676

992 Gaby A. Vitamin C, in Nutritional Medicine, 2nd edition, 2017: Fritz Perlberg Publishing, Concord, NH, p. 105.; "Vitamin C," Linus Pauling Institute: http://lpi.oregonstate.edu/mic/vitamins/vitamin-C, accessed 5-29-17

993 Georgetown University Center for Hypertension, Kidney & Vascular Research, https://hypertension.gumc. georgetown.edu/patientcare/dietarysaltrestriction

994 Johnston CS, Luo B. Comparison of the absorption and excretion of three commercially available sources of vitamin C. J Am Diet Assoc. 1994;94(7):779-781. PMID: 8021423

995 Carr AC, Vissers MC. Synthetic or food-derived vitamin C--are they equally bioavailable? Nutrients. 2013 Oct 28;5(11):4284-304. PMID: 24169506

996 Hathcock JN, Azzi A, Blumberg J, et al. Vitamins E and C are safe across a broad range of intakes. Am J Clin Nutr. 2005 Apr;81(4):736-45. PMID: 15817846

997 http://lpi.oregonstate.edu/mic/vitamins/vitamin-C#reference133

998 Dahl C, Søgaard AJ, Tell GS, et al, plus Norwegian Epidemiologic Osteoporosis Study (NOREPOS) Core Research Group. Do cadmium, lead, and aluminum in drinking water increase the risk of hip fractures? A NOREPOS study. Biol Trace Elem Res. 2014 Jan;157(1):14-23. Epub 2013 Nov 29. PMID: 24287706

999 Gaby A, "Vitamin C" in Nutritional Medicine, 2nd edition, p. 109.

1000 Chang CY, Ke DS, Chen JY. Essential fatty acids and human brain. Acta Neurol Taiwan. 2009 Dec;18(4):231-41. PMID: 20329590

1001 Pekmezci D. Vitamin E and immunity. Vitam Horm. 2011;86:179-215. PMID: 21419272

1002 Mandal A. Lipid biological functions, November 6, 2016, http://www.news-medical.net/life-sciences/Lipid-Biological-Functions.aspx

1003 Chang CY, Ke DS, Chen JY. Essential fatty acids and human brain. Acta Neurol Taiwan. 2009 Dec;18(4):231-41. PMID: 20329590

1004 Reiter E, Jiang Q, Christen S. Anti-inflammatory properties of a- and γ-tocopherol. Mol Aspects Med. 2007 Oct-Dec;28(5-6):668-91. Epub 2007 Jan 11. PMID: 17316780

1005 Jiang Q. Natural forms of vitamin E: metabolism, antioxidant, and anti-inflammatory activities and their role in disease prevention and therapy. .Free Radic Biol Med. 2014 Jul;72:76-90. Epub 2014 Apr 3. PMID: 24704972

1006 Hyman M, Pizzorno J, Weil A. A rational approach to antioxidant therapy and vitamin E. Altern Ther Health Med. 2005 Jan-Feb;11(1):14-7. PMID: 15712759

1007 Schwab S, Zierer A, Schneider A, et al. Vitamin E supplementation is associated with lower levels of C-reactive protein only in higher dosages and combined with other antioxidants: The Cooperative Health Research in the Region of Augsburg (KORA) F4 study. Br J Nutr. 2015 Jun 14;113(11):1782-91. Epub 2015 Apr 21. PMID: 25895432

1008 Ochi H, Takeda S. The Two Sides of Vitamin E Supplementation. Gerontology. 2015;61(4):319-26. Epub 2014 Nov 22. PMID: 25428288

1009 Hamidi MS, Corey PN, Cheung AM. Effects of vitamin E on bone turnover markers among US postmenopausal women. J Bone Miner Res. 2012 Jun;27(6):1368-80. PMID: 22308007

1010 Bender, DA. Vitamin E: Tocopherols and tocotrienols. In "Nutritional Biochemistry of the Vitamins," (D. A. Bender, Ed.), pp. 109–130. Cambridge University Press: New York, 2003.

1011 Traber MG. Vitamin E and K interactions--a 50-year-old problem. Nutr Rev. 2008 Nov;66(11):624-9. PMID: 19019024

1012 Shearer MJ, Newman P. Recent trends in the metabolism and cell biology of vitamin K with special reference to vitamin K cycling and MK-4 biosynthesis.J Lipid Res. 2014 Mar;55(3):345-62. Epub 2014 Jan 31. PMID: 24489112

1013 Shi WQ, Liu J, Cao Y, et al. Association of dietary and serum vitamin E with bone mineral density in middle-aged and elderly Chinese adults: a cross-sectional study. Br J Nutr. 2016 Jan 14;115(1):113-20. Epub 2015

Oct 28. PMID: 26507315

1014 Michaëlsson K, Wolk A, Byberg L, et al. Intake and serum concentrations of α-tocopherol in relation to fractures in elderly women and men: 2cohort studies. Am J Clin Nutr. 2014 Jan;99(1):107-14. PMID: 24225359

1015 Guralp O. Effects of vitamin E on bone remodeling in perimnopausal women: mini review. Maturitas. 2014 Dec;79(4):476-80. Epub 2014 Sep 6. PMID: 25248856

1016 Mata-Granados JM, Cuenca-Acebedo R, Luque de Castro MD, et al. Lower vitamin E serum levels are associated with osteoporosis in early postmenopausal women: a cross-sectional study. J Bone Miner Metab. 2013 Jul;31(4):455-60. Epub 2013 Mar 28. PMID: 23536191

1017 Food and Nutrition Board, and Institute of Medicine (2000). Vitamin E. In "Dietary Reference Intakes for Vitamin C, Vitamin E, Selenium, and Carotenoids," pp. 186–283. National Academy Press, Washington

1018 Pekmezci D. Vitamin E and immunity. Vitam Horm. 2011;86:179-215. PMID: 21419272

1019 Serafini M. Dietary vitamin E and T cell-mediated function in the elderly: effectiveness and mechanism of action. Int J Dev Neurosci. 2000 Jul-Aug;18(4-5):401-10. Review. PMID: 10817923

1020 Calder PC, Albers R, Antoine JM, et al. Inflammatory disease processes and interactions with nutrition. Br J Nutr. 2009 May;101 Suppl 1:S1-45. PMID: 19586558

1021 Weber P, Bendich A, Machlin LJ. Vitamin E and human health: rationale for determining recommended intake levels. Nutrition. 1997 May;13(5):450-60. PMID: 9225339

1022 Meydani SN, Meydani M, Blumberg JB, et al. Assessment of the safety of supplementation with different amounts of vitamin E in healthy older adults. Am J Clin Nutr. 1998 Aug;68(2):311-8. PMID: 9701188

1023 Food and Nutrition Board, and Institute of Medicine (2000). Vitamin E. In "Dietary Reference Intakes for Vitamin C, Vitamin E, Selenium, and Carotenoids," pp. 186–283. National Academy Press, Washington.

1024 Hathcock JN, Azzi A, Blumberg J, et al. Vitamins E and C are safe across a broad range of intakes. Am J Clin Nutr. 2005 Apr;81(4):736-45. PMID: 15817846

1025 Pekmezci D. Vitamin E and immunity. Vitam Horm. 2011;86:179-215. PMID: 21419272

1026 Kalyan S, Huebbe P, Esatbeyoglu T, et al. Nitrogen-bisphosphonate therapy is linked to compromised coenzyme Q10 and vitamin E status in postmenopausal women. PMID: 24423355

1027 Sylvester PW. Vitamin E and apoptosis. Vitam Horm. 2007;76:329-56

1028 Hathcock JN, Azzi A, Blumberg J, et al. Vitamins E and C are safe across a broad range of intakes. Am J Clin Nutr. 2005 Apr;81(4):736-45. PMID: 15817846

1029 Schaffler M, Cheung W, Majeska R, et al. Osteocytes: master orchestrators of bone. Review Calcif Tissue Int. 2014 Jan;94(1):5-24. Epub 2013 Sep 17. PMID: 24042263

1030 Lu Y, Rosner B, Chang G, et al. Twelve-Minute Daily Yoga Regimen Reverses Osteoporotic Bone Loss, Topics in Geriatric Rehabilitation: April/June 2016 - Volume 32 - Issue 2 - p 81-87 doi: 10.1097/TGR.0000000000000085

1031 Azuma K, Adachi Y, Hayashi H, et al. Chronic Psychological Stress as a Risk Factor of Osteoporosis. J UOEH. 2015 Dec 1;37(4):245-53. PMID: 26667192

1032 Fishman, Loren M. MD, BPhil(Oxon) Yoga for Osteoporosis, Topics in Geriatric Rehabilitation: July 2009 - Volume 25 - Issue 3 - p 244-250 doi: 10.1097/TGR.0b013e3181b02dd6

1033 Lu YH, Rosner B, Chang G, Fishman LM. Twelve-Minute Daily Yoga Regimen Reverses Osteoporotic Bone Loss. Top Geriatr Rehabil. 2016;32(2):81-87 PMID: 27226695

1034 Morris HA, Eastell R, Jorgensen NR, et al; IFCC-IOF Working Group for Standardisation of Bone Marker Assays (WG-BMA). Clinical usefulness of bone turnover marker concentrations in osteoporosis. Clin Chim Acta. 2017 Apr;467:34-41. Epub 2016 Jun 30. PMID: 27374301

1035 Szulc P, Naylor K, Pickering ME, et al. Use of CTX-I and PINP as bone turnover markers: National Bone Health Alliance recommendations to standardize sample handling and patient preparation to reduce pre-analytical variability. Ann Biol Clin (Paris). 2018 Aug 1;76(4):373-391. English. PMID: 30078776

1036 Shearer MJ, Fu X, Booth SL. Vitamin K nutrition, metabolism, and requirements: current concepts and future research. Adv Nutr. 2012 Mar 1;3(2):182-95. PMID: 22516726

1037 Porter K, Hoey L, Hughes CF, Ward M, McNulty H. Causes, Consequences and Public Health Implications of Low B-Vitamin Status in Ageing. Nutrients. 2016 Nov 16;8(11):725. PMID: 27854316; PMCID: PMC5133110

1038 Pizzorno J. Homocysteine: Friend or Foe? Integr Med (Encinitas). 2014 Aug;13(4):8-14. PMID: 26770102; PMCID: PMC4566450

1039 https://www.kidney.org/atoz/content/gfr

1040 Lipski L. Digestive Wellness, 5th edition, McGraw Hill: NY, 2020, p. 170

1041 Wang L, Li T, Liu J. et al. Association between glycosylated hemoglobin A1c and bone biochemical markers in type 2 diabetic postmenopausal women: a cross-sectional study. BMC Endocr Disord 19, 31 (2019). PMID: 30866902

1042 Yamamoto M, Yamaguchi T, Yamauchi M, et al. Serum Pentosidine Levels Are Positively Associated with the Presence of Vertebral Fractures in Postmenopausal Women with Type 2 Diabetes, The Journal of Clinical Endocrinology & Metabolism, Volume 93, Issue 3, 1 March 2008, Pages 1013–1019, PMID: 18160470

1043 Kida, Y., Saito, M., Shinohara, A. et al. Non-invasive skin autofluorescence, blood and urine assays of the advanced glycation end product (AGE) pentosidine as an indirect indicator of AGE content in human bone. BMC Musculoskelet Disord 20, 627 (2019). PMID: 31881872

1044 Campillo-Sánchez F, Usategui-Martín R, Ruiz-de Temiño Á, et al. Relationship between Insulin Resistance (HOMA-IR), Trabecular Bone Score (TBS), and Three-Dimensional Dual-Energy X-ray Absorptiometry (3D-DXA) in Non-Diabetic Postmenopausal Women. J Clin Med. 2020;9(6):1732. Published 2020 Jun 3. PMID: 32503328

1045 Lee DH, Ha MH, Kim JH, Christiani DC, Gross MD, Steffes M, Blomhoff R, Jacobs DR Jr. Gamma-glutamyltransferase and diabetes--a 4 year follow-up study. Diabetologia. 2003 Mar;46(3):359-64. PMID: 12687334

1046 Mun H, Liu B, Pham THA, et al. C-reactive protein and fracture risk: an updated systematic review and meta-analysis of cohort studies through the use of both frequentist and Bayesian approaches. Osteoporos Int. 2021 Mar;32(3):425-435. Epub 2020 Sep 15. PMID: 32935169.

1047 Pizzorno J. Homocysteine: Friend or Foe? Integr Med (Encinitas). 2014 Aug;13(4):8-14. PMID: 26770102; PMCID: PMC4566450

1048 Yang J, Hu X, Zhang Q, et al. Homocysteine level and risk of fracture: A meta-analysis and systematic review. Bone. 2012 Sep;51(3):376-82. Epub 2012 Jun 26. PMID: 22749888

About the Authors

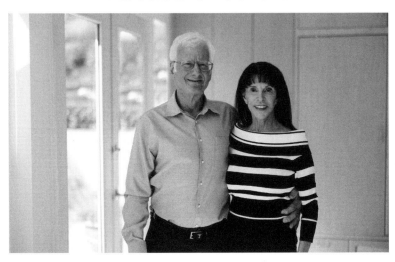

Lara Pizzorno, MDiv, MA, LMT, is the best-selling author of *Your Bones: How YOU Can Prevent Osteoporosis & Have Strong Bones for Life—Naturally.* A 25-year member of the American Medical Writers Association, editor of *Longevity Medicine Review,* and senior medical editor for Integrative Medicine Advisors, LLC, Lara publishes review articles in *Integrative Medicine: A Clinician's Journal* covering the latest bone research, which she also shares in online articles, video presentations, and lectures at medical conferences worldwide. A member of the American College of Nutrition, she is a contributing author to several textbooks, including the *Textbook of Natural Medicine* and the *Textbook of Functional Medicine,* and co-author of *The Encyclopedia of Healing Foods.* Lara is currently completing her M.S., Clinical Nutrition, at MUIH (Maryland University Integrative Health).

Dr. Joe Pizzorno, N.D., is one of the world's leading authorities on science-based natural/integrative medicine. He co-founded and served 22 years as president of Bastyr University, the country's first and largest fully accredited university of natural medicine. He is the author or co-author of more than a dozen books, including the *Textbook of Natural Medicine, Clinical Environmental Medicine, The Encyclopedia of Natural Medicine,* and *The Toxin Solution.* He is a founder and Board Chair of the Institute for Functional Medicine and editor in chief of *Integrative Medicine, A Clinician's Journal*, the field's leading peer-reviewed journal. He was appointed by Presidents Clinton and Bush to two prestigious government commissions to advise the President and Congress on the integration of natural medicine into the healthcare system. Joe travels worldwide, consulting, lecturing, and teaching physicians about science-based natural medicine.

Lara and Joe live in Seattle, Washington, where they love to provide entertainment for their cats, work in their garden, and eat the abundantly healthful food it provides. They delight in spending time with their daughter Raven, son-in-law Eugene and amazing grandchild Hiro, and (when he can get away from his work as an Emergency Medicine doctor and come home to visit) son Galen and his increasingly significant other, Emma.